Transbronchial cryobiopsy in diffuse parenchymal lung disease

Venerino Poletti
Editor

Transbronchial cryobiopsy in diffuse parenchymal lung disease

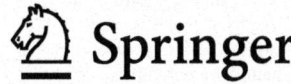 Springer

Editor
Venerino Poletti
Department of Diseases of the Thorax
Ospedale Morgagni-Pierantoni
Forlì
Italy

ISBN 978-3-030-14890-4   ISBN 978-3-030-14891-1   (eBook)
https://doi.org/10.1007/978-3-030-14891-1

This Springer imprint is published by the registered company Springer Nature Switzerland AG.
The registered company address is: Gewerbestrasse 11, 6330 Cham, Switzerland

Preface

This book originates from postgraduate meetings on transbronchial lung cryo-biopsy annually held in Ravenna (Italy) since 2014 (endorsed by the Italian Association of Hospital Pulmonologists (Associazione Italiana Pneumologi Ospedalieri, AIPO)), during which collaborations with experts around the world on this specific topic were started or consolidated. It is also the fruit of the experience acquired in the GB Morgagni Hospital in Forlì (Italy) in which transbronchial cryobiopsy was introduced in clinical activities since 2010. In this center, more than 1000 transbronchial lung biopsy procedures were carried out so far. Finally during this period, I had the opportunity to be invited in different centers around the world to present and discuss data on this new technique and also to be appointed as Full Professor of Pulmonary Medicine in the Aarhus University Hospital, Aarhus (Denmark). In this period, this procedure was introduced in the clinical practice also in that institute. Therefore, suggestions provided by people I met during these meetings and the experience accumulated in Denmark contributed to build up the Forlì approach to transbronchial cryobiopsy and are condensed in this book.

The objective of this book—after a concise clinical and radiologic overview of diffuse parenchymal lung diseases—is to provide technical information on this new technique, illustrate the modalities by which lung samples may be obtained using the machinery, and discuss the advantages and limits of transbronchial cryobiopsy compared to surgical lung biopsy (performed in intubated patients or in the "awaked" modality). The last part of the book is dedicated to specific disorders approached also using information obtained using this new bioptic method.

The book is meant to be practical, clinically oriented, and up-to-date. Also, despite being it a multiauthored work, it was my intention to have a uniform style, and at the end, it wasn't a great effort to reach it since a large part of the authors have been collaborating, sharing ideas and projects for a long time, and the younger are or have been students of the older ones.

I hope that the positive feedbacks will far outweigh any negative ones. However, if the objectives were not reached, the responsibility is only mine.

The book is dedicated to the memory of my parents Elisabetta and Francesco, as well as to all students and pupils who gave and are giving me enthusiasm and always new ideas.

Forlì, Italy   Venerino Poletti
23 January 2019

Contents

Part III   Clinical Role of Transbronchial Cryobiopsy

Part I

Introduction to Diffuse Parenchymal Lung Disease

Diffuse Parenchymal Lung Disease: A Clinical Overview

Venerino Poletti

1.1 Introduction

Diffuse parenchymal lung disease (DPLD) is a generic term for a large group of disorders. A definition based on precise criteria to identify these disorders is not yet universally accepted. A "morphologic definition" includes in this group all the disorders that are characterized by a pathologic accumulation/infiltration of extracellular substances, fluids, or cells in the structures of the secondary pulmonary lobule [1]. Secondary pulmonary lobule is an anatomic and functional unit supplied by a cluster of three to five terminal bronchioles, and it is usually separated from other secondary pulmonary lobules by connective tissue septa. It is irregularly polyhedral in shape and approximately 1–2.5 on each side [2]. This accumulation/infiltration is, by definition, not limited to one single lobe. This definition is quite inclusive because almost all lung disorders may present with this morphologic background. However in this huge group are included systemic disorders in which the lung is one of the main organs involved, idiopathic diseases limited to the lungs, and diffuse parenchymal disorders of known cause or well-known pathogenesis (Table 1.1).

The clinical profiles with which these diseases manifest are variegated from very acute onset with respiratory failure needing invasive respiratory supports to mild chronic symptoms lasting for more than 6 months (dry cough, dyspnea on effort) (Table 1.2). Diagnosis is a complex process beset with pitfalls—often representing the balancing of different uncertainties—that starts having in mind a model based on pathophysiologic elements and other scientific knowledges. Thereafter it requires acquisition of data deriving from a comprehensive clinical history, a careful physical examination, as well as clues provided by laboratory and pulmonary function tests. Imaging, mainly high-resolution CT has a pivotal role in the detection of these disorders and in the diagnostic workup providing information robust enough to draw up a differential diagnosis list and sometimes identifying pathognomonic features. More invasive procedures are deemed necessary only when these steps are inconclusive or do not allow a confident clinical-radiological hypothesis.

1.2 Pathophysiology of DPLD

Due to the variety of entities included under the DPLD umbrella term, it is virtually impossible to have a common pathogenetic scheme. The structures injured are heterogeneous including bronchioles (terminal and respiratory), alveolar septa,

V. Poletti (✉)
Department of Diseases of the Thorax,
Ospedale Morgagni-Pierantoni, Forlì, Italy

Department of Respiratory Diseases and Allergy,
Aarhus University Hospital, Aarhus, Denmark

© Springer Nature Switzerland AG 2019
V. Poletti (ed.), *Transbronchial cryobiopsy in diffuse parenchymal lung disease*,
https://doi.org/10.1007/978-3-030-14891-1_1

Table 1.1 Classification of diffuse parenchymal lung disorders

Systemic disorders	Unknown cause	Known cause/pathogenesis
Sarcoidosis	IPF	Drugs/radiation
		Infections
CVDs	NSIP	Organic exposure (*hypersensitivity pneumonitis*)
Neoplastic (*metastases, lymphoproliferative disorders, LAM, LCH, myeloid disorders*)	COP	Inorganic exposure (*silicosis, asbestosis*)
Immunodeficiencies	AIP	Smoking related (*RB-ILD, DIP, SRIF*)
Telomeropathies (*Dyskeratosis congenita, ...*)	LIP	Pulmonary alveolar proteinosis
Inborn errors of metabolism (*Niemann-Pick, Gaucher, Hermansky-Pudlak, Fabry, Mucopolysaccharidoses*)	PPFE	Pulmonary alveolar microlithiasis
Neurofibromatosis	Chronic eosinophilic pneumonia	Mutations in genes coding for surfactant proteins or in ABCA3 transporter gene
Tuberous sclerosis		
Hypereosinophilic syndrome	Acute eosinophilic pneumonia	
IgG4-related disease		
Infections		

CVD collagen vascular disease, *LAM* lymphangioleiomyomatosis, *LCH* Langerhans cell histiocytosis, *IPF* idiopathic pulmonary fibrosis, *NSIP* nonspecific interstitial pneumonia, *COP* cryptogenic organizing pneumonia, *AIP* acute interstitial pneumonia, *LIP* lymphocytic interstitial pneumonia, *PPFE* pleuroparenchymal fibroelastosis, *RB* respiratory bronchiolitis, *DIP* desquamative interstitial pneumonia, *SRIF* smoking-related interstitial fibrosis, *ABCA3* ATP-binding cassette subfamily A member 3

Table 1.2 Time course of disease onset

Acute (in days to few weeks)	Subacute (<3 months)	Chronic (>3 months)
AIP	HP	IPF
		Smoking-related ILDs
		HP
AEP	COP	LCH
DAH/capillaritis	NSIP	LAM
Drug-induced ILDs	Drug-induced ILDs	Drug-induced ILDs
Antisynthetase syndrome	Sarcoidosis	Sarcoidosis
AFOP		Chronic eosinophilic pneumonia
Infections	Infections	Infections
Acute exacerbation of IPF		

AIP acute interstitial pneumonia, *AEP* acute eosinophilic pneumonia, *DAH* diffuse alveolar hemorrhage, *AFOP* acute fibrinous organizing pneumonia, *IPF* idiopathic pulmonary fibrosis, *HP* hypersensitivity pneumonitis, *COP* cryptogenic organizing pneumonia, *NSIP* nonspecific interstitial pneumonia, *LCH* Langerhans cell histiocytosis, *LAM* lymphangioleiomyomatosis

interlobular septa, small pulmonary and bronchiolar arteries, capillaries and veins, and lymphatics. These structures have also a different embryogenic origin and different regenerative machineries. The pathogenetic events in DPLD may be divided into five patterns. The neoplastic and infectious processes have pathogenetic events that are in common with all the other organs or systems. However in the lungs some events taking place in the alveolar spaces (production of degradating enzymes in lymphangioleiomyomatosis) may lead to characteristic cystic changes. Recently lymphangioleiomyomatosis has been reclassified as a low-grade sarcoma (belonging to the so-called PEComas) and Langerhans cell histiocytosis and Erdheim-Chester disease as inflammatory myeloid neoplasms with specific drug-targetable mutations along the RAS-RAF mitogen-activated protein kinase (MEK) and extracellular signal-regulated kinase (ERK) signaling cascade [3–5].

The other three pathophysiologic patterns left are granulomatous inflammation/fibrosis, inflammation/fibrosis, and, finally, alveolar stem cell senescence-bronchiolar dysplastic proliferation/ fibrosis. Genetic predispositions have been clearly documented in some disorders and are suspected to have a role in the large majority of the others.

Granulomatous inflammation/fibrosis is usually the morphologic background of sarcoidosis, hypersensitivity pneumonitis, and berylliosis. The inflammatory process is, at least in the florid phases, driven by Th1 cells (with release of interferon-gamma, IL-2, and IL-12) and macrophages. Granuloma formation is the key marker of these disorders [6]. When the disorders evolve to fibrosis, a switch to a Th2-like response seems to represent an important pathogenetic step. B-cell dysregulation and B-T cell interconnections may also have a role in granulomatous disorders as suggested by the association between granulomatous-lymphocytic interstitial lung disease (GLILD) and common variable immunodeficiency or 22q11.2 deletion syndrome [7].

In nongranulomatous inflammatory/fibrotic DPLDs, the exact composition of inflammation and the distribution of inflammatory cells in the secondary pulmonary lobule vary depending on the individual disorders. Neutrophils are predominant in vasculitis, lymphocytes in nonspecific interstitial pneumonia (NSIP), eosinophils in chronic eosinophilic pneumonia, and macrophages in smoking-related diseases. Typical giant cells are a hallmark of hard metal lung disease. Necrosis (ischemic or apoptotic) is usually observed when the inflammatory cells are predominantly neutrophils. In the majority of these disorders, autoimmunity has a significant role. Accumulation of type I collagen and fibroblasts/ myofibroblasts represents a progression toward the irreversible stage. These complex events are driven by activation of a variety of pathways that are very similar regardless the cause or the clinical settings in which these disorders appear [8].

The prototype of alveolar stem cell senescence-bronchiolar dysplastic proliferation/fibrosis is idiopathic pulmonary fibrosis (IPF). The pathogenetic mechanisms leading to lung parenchymal derangement typically observed in this disorder are only partly elucidated. The cross talk between different cell components is provided by an extremely complex exchange of molecular signals, depending on a discrete number of pathways, signaling molecules, receptors, and transcription factors, including among others TGF-beta, Wnt, Notch, BMP, SOX2, and Hedgehog signaling pathways that are also involved in lung development and cancer. Their aberrant expression has been proposed as relevant in the pathogenesis of IPF [9, 10]. In this pathogenic scheme, alveolar stem cell failure is the crucial event. When precursor cell exhaustion is reached for the concurrent action of intrinsic defects (genetic predisposition such as TERT/TERC mutations, mutations of genes coding for surfactant proteins, etc.) and extrinsic agents (smoke, air pollution), the damage caused to alveolar epithelial cells by endoplasmic reticulum and oxidative stress at sites of maximal mechanical stress in lower lobes cannot be properly repaired. Frustrated attempts of epithelial regeneration trigger an exaggerated activation of proliferative and/or antiapoptotic signals. Senescent aspects and oncogene-induced senescence features have been identified in this context. In IPF senescent alveolar stem cells behave as robust secretors that interfere ["senescence-associated secretory phenotype" (SASP) or "senescence-messaging secretome" (SMS)] with the correct tissue renewal. When this wave of damage reach the bronchiolar epithelial basal cells, these cells start to proliferate, and bronchiolar proliferative lesions (these lesions are unproperly called "honeycomb changes") represent the irreversible phase in IPF remodeling as also suggested by the recent demonstration of abnormal production of mucins in bronchiolar cysts. There are evidences that a common polymorphism in the promoter of MUC5B gene is a predisposing factor for IPF development [11–13].

1.3 Clinical History

Patients should be divided in different subsets mainly considering two elements: how the disease manifests (Table 1.2) and if accompanying signs/symptoms are limited to the respiratory system or are also systemic and/or extrathoracic. Patients with acute lung injury (having usually as histological background diffuse alveolar damage without or with eosinophils, capillaritis, and alveolar hemorrhage or organizing pneumonia with accumulation of fibrin) tend to seek medical attention for rapidly progressive dyspnea. In this group the more characteristic disorders are acute eosinophilic pneumonia (AEP), rapidly progressive cryptogenic organizing pneumonia (COP), acute interstitial pneumonia, subacute hypersensitivity pneumonitis (HP) and a not yet clear entity or group of entities called acute fibrinous and organizing pneumonia (AFOP), and collagen vascular disorders (mainly anti-synthetase syndrome and systemic lupus erythematosus) or ANCA-associated vasculitis. Rarely idiopathic pulmonary fibrosis may manifest with acute respiratory failure being acute exacerbation the first clinical overt event. The prototype of chronic DPLD is IPF, manifesting with long-lasting dry cough and exertional dyspnea. Fever, asthenia, and weight loss are frequently present when a diffuse parenchymal lung disease has an acute/subacute presentation or when it has a manifestation of a systemic disorder. Extrathoracic manifestations may draw attention addressing toward a diagnosis of a systemic disorder: skin and/or articular lesions or alterations in other organs in collagen vascular diseases; vasculitis, oculocutaneous albinism, and colitis in Hermansky-Pudlak disease; dyskeratosis, early hair graying, in telomeropathies; and fibrofolliculomas in Birt-Hogg-Dubè syndrome. Some forms present with short and episodic events (mainly dyspnea or dry cough with or without fever). In this group HP and COP are most frequently represented. The age is an important diagnostic clue. Sarcoidosis, lymphangioleiomyomatosis (LAM), and hereditary forms such as Hermansky-Pudlak syndrome, telomeropathies, and Langerhans cell histiocytosis (LCH) present usually in the first 40–50 years of age. IPF is a disorder of elderly (mean age at diagnosis 64). Some disorders are strictly related to gender. LAM is almost always limited to women. Also lung injury associated to collagen vascular diseases is, except rheumatoid arthritis, more frequently observed in females. Pneumoconioses is, because of professional exposure, more frequently observed in males. Familial history is fundamental to identify subjects affected by neurofibromatosis and tuberous sclerosis. Early gray hair, the presence of cryptogenic liver cirrhosis, or myelodysplastic syndrome in the family suggest a diagnosis of telomeropathy. Hermansky-Pudlak, Gaucher and Niemann-Pick diseases have an autosomal recessive pattern of inheritance. Finally smoking habit (IPF is mainly observed in smokers or former smokers, and other disorders—LGH, pulmonary alveolar proteinosis, lung hemorrhage due to Goodpasture syndrome and the so-called smoking-related DPLDs—are almost always detected in current or former smokers), professional exposure, assumption of licit and illicit drugs [cocaine is the cause of a variety of lung injuries; a long list of drugs have been associated to a variety of diffuse lung injury patterns (www.pneumotox.com)], and the immunologic status [common variable immunodeficiency, HIV infection) should be elicited from all patients with known or suspected DPLD.

1.4 Physical Examination

Teleinspiratory, bibasilar, and dry crackles are typically auscultated in patients with IPF or fibrosing interstitial pneumonias and very rarely in granulomatous disorders. Scattered late inspiratory high-pitched rhonchi, called squeaks, are heard in patients with bronchiolitis. Hemoptysis may be observed in patients with vasculitis but also in sarcoidosis (mainly when it is associated to lung aspergillomas). Digital clubbing is a marker of fibrotic DPLD and may precede the appearance of the lung disease for years. Extrathoracic signs are present in patients with collagen vascular disease, and some of them are quite specific [Gottron nodules, mechanic's hands and heliotrope rash in dermatomyositis, cutaneous and oral ulcerations, panniculitis and alopecia in anti-melanoma differentiation-associated gene 5 (MDA5) dermatomyositis]. Tattoo or scar granulomatous reaction is a specific sign of sarcoidosis. Pneumothorax may be a manifestation of LAM or LCG.

1.5   Laboratory Testing

Some laboratory tests are quite specific enabling a definite diagnosis. Identification of obligatory pathogens on body fluids (*Mycobacterium tuberculosis*), autoantibodies against GM-CSF in autoimmune alveolar proteinosis, D-VEGF in lymphangioleiomyomatosis, and blood or bronchoalveolar lavage (BAL) beryllium lymphocyte proliferation test (BeLPT) is used to confirm the beryllium as cause of DPLD. Other tests may strongly support the diagnosis already hypothesized on the basis of clinical and radiological features: autoantibodies seen in association with antisynthetase syndrome (anti-Jo-1, anti-PL-7, anti-PL-12, anti-EJ, anti-OJ, etc.), anti-MDA5 antibodies, ANCA autoantibodies, serum monoclonal heavy chains, or Bence Jones proteins in urine. However the presence of autoantibodies does not automatically address to a diagnosis of an "autoimmune" disorder as autoantibodies may merely be considered an epiphenomenon of senescence. Finally some laboratory findings may simply represent a clue to hypothesize specific disorders. Precipitins indicate specific exposures; a huge increase of LDH is typically present when intravascular lymphoma is the cause of the interstitial infiltrates. Eosinophils in peripheral blood are significantly increased in chronic eosinophilic pneumonia or in hypereosinophilic syndrome. Lymphopenia is a marker of advanced HIV infection, but it may be observed also in cases of lymphomatoid granulomatosis. Decreased levels of immunoglobulins suggest a diagnosis of common variable immunodeficiency. Hemophagocytic syndrome (fever, hepatosplenomegaly, blood cytopenia, increased liver enzymes, hypofibrinogenemia, high triglyceride levels, and hemophagocytic features in the bone marrow) may be associated to NK nasal type lymphoma appearing first in the lungs.

In well-known genetic disorders manifesting with lung infiltrates, specific mutations are already clearly identified (i.e., Birt-Hogg-Dubè syndrome, Hermansky-Pudlak syndrome, neurofibromatosis, tuberous sclerosis, etc.). Furthermore genetic tests are increasingly becoming an important piece of information for identification of some forms of familial or sporadic DPLD. Telomere-related mutations account for up to 10% of sporadic IPF, 25% of familial IPF, and 10% of connective tissue disease-associated interstitial lung disease. Furthermore, single-nucleotide polymorphisms (SNPs) in TERT, TERC, OBFC1, and RTEL1, as well as short telomere length, have been associated with several DPLDs. Additionally, it was found that also SNPs in telomere-related genes are risk factors for the development of pulmonary disease. Mutations in gene coding for surfactant proteins A1, A2, and C and for ABCA3 are associated to peculiar forms of interstitial lung disease. The MUC5B promoter variant rs35705950 accounts for a substantial risk of developing IPF.

1.6   Pulmonary Function Tests

Most forms of diffuse parenchymal lung disease produce a restrictive defect with reduced total lung capacity, functional residual capacity, and residual volume. A minority of disorders are associated to an obstructive defect (lymphangioleiomyomatosis, bronchiolitis, rarely in sarcoidosis, and hypersensitivity pneumonitis). Pulmonary function studies have been proved to have prognostic value in patients with IPF. The resting arterial blood gases may be normal, but hypoxemia is detected in the majority of cases even during the first visit. Usually hypocapnia precedes the appearance of hypoxemia at rest. A 6-min walking test or, more precisely, a cardiopulmonary test may reveal the disease in the early stage.

1.7   Chest Imaging

The radiograph in patients with suspected DPLD has substantial limitations due to the intrinsic defects of the technique. However a correct diagnostic hypothesis (based on the distribution of the shadows and the prevalence of nodules, lines, or honeycombing) may be done in around 30% of cases. High-resolution CT scan is superior to the plain chest X-ray for higher definition of the images (elementary lesions) and the capacity to identify the distribution of the lesions in the structures of the secondary pulmonary lobules. The combination of these elements defines different reproducible patterns [14, 15]:

1. Septal pattern (linear pattern with preserved architecture)
2. Fibrotic pattern (linear pattern with distorted architecture)
3. Nodular pattern
4. Alveolar pattern
5. Tree in bud pattern
6. Cystic pattern
7. Dark lung pattern

A *septal* pattern is present when a network of white lines representing thickened perilobular septa is appreciable. Thickening of the sleeves wrapping the bronchovascular bundles may be identifiable as well. The white lines or the thickened sleeves around bronchovascular bundles may be regular, smooth, or irregular, and beaded, but the intralobular architecture is preserved. Hilar and mediastinal lymph node enlargement is frequently observed as an ancillary finding. An important diagnostic clue is represented by the preferential distribution of the lesions. This pattern may be observed in a variety of disorders: pulmonary edema due to heart failure, venoocclusive disease, carcinomatous lymphangitis, sarcoidosis, lymphoproliferative disorders, Erdheim-Chester disease, and amyloidosis.

Fibrotic pattern is defined by the loss of volume, presence of irregular linear opacities in the intralobular zones, traction bronchiectasis and bronchiolectasis, and honeycomb changes. At the pulmonary interface, a pleural line with shaggy margins and connections with parenchymal irregular lines (the so-called interface sign) may be evident. When the honeycomb changes are predominant in the subpleural zones and mainly in the lower lobes, the descriptive term usual interstitial pneumonia (UIP) pattern is used. This pattern is observed mainly in IPF, collagen vascular disorders with lung involvement, idiopathic fibrosing nonspecific interstitial pneumonia (NSIP), chronic hypersensitivity pneumonitis, asbestosis, and chronic drug-induced lung disease. A subset of fibrotic pattern (called also "tug-of-war" pattern) is defined by the presence of irregular linear opacities stretching between the mediastinum and the thoracic boundaries, bridging over variably involved bronchi, fissures, and more generally anatomic structures and even pathologic elements found on their way. This pattern may be found in chronic sarcoidosis, berylliosis, and pleuroparenchymal fibroelastosis.

The *nodular* pattern is defined by the presence of multiple roundish opacities ranging from 2 to 10 mm. These nodules may be solid or may have a ground-glass density; they may be distributed along the lymphatic routes, in a random way, or may be centrilobular. Disorders that may have this pattern are subacute hypersensitivity pneumonitis, respiratory bronchiolitis, follicular bronchiolitis, Langerhans cell histiocytosis, sarcoidosis, silicosis, miliary tuberculosis, viral or fungal infections, and hematogenous metastases. Mainly infections, Langerhans cell histiocytosis and metastases may present cavitation (so-called "cheerios in the lung" pattern).

The *alveolar* pattern is characterized by an increase in pulmonary attenuation that obscures the vessels and the airway walls (alveolar consolidation). The bronchial lumen may remain visible inside the consolidation (air bronchogram). When the increase of lung attenuation does not cancel the vascular margins, the term ground-glass attenuation is used. Subsets included in this group are the so-called "crazy paving pattern" (a smooth, regular network of white lines superimposed on a background of ground-glass attenuation), the halo sign (a central area of consolidation surrounded by a halo of ground-glass attenuation), the reverse halo sign (a ring or crescent of dense consolidation that surrounds a core of ground-glass attenuation), and the perilobular pattern (poorly defined band-like opacities with an arcade-like or polygonal appearance with a pleural base). In this group are included all the disorders characterized by filling of distal airways by cells, exudates, or proteins or, more rarely, diseases with a significant thickening of alveolar septa. The list is quite long: infectious pneumonia, organizing pneumonia (cryptogenic or secondary), alveolar proteinosis, lymphomas, mucinous adenocarcinoma, alveolar hemorrhage, pneumocystosis, acute and chronic eosinophilic pneumonia, acute interstitial pneumonia, acute respiratory distress syndrome, desquamative interstitial pneumonia, lipoid pneumonia, and nonspecific interstitial pneumonia.

The *tree in bud* pattern is characterized by centrilobular dense branching linear structures originating from a single stalk and often ending in a nodular form (thus resembling a budding tree). This pattern is typical of cellular bronchiolitis (the most frequent being infectious bronchiolitis). Rarely a similar pattern may be due to thrombotic neoplastic microangiopathy.

Cystic pattern is present when multiple roundish, well-defined air-containing spaces are variably scattered throughout the lung parenchyma. Distribution of the cysts, their shape, association with nodules, or content (usually it is air but in infections mainly they may contain fluid) are useful information for discriminating between different disorders. Disorders that typically have this pattern are Langerhans cell histiocytosis, lymphangioleiomyomatosis, Birt-Hogg-Dubè syndrome, cystic metastases, lymphocytic interstitial pneumonia (LIP), and pneumocystosis. Rarely hypersensitivity pneumonitis and bronchiolitis (constrictive or proliferative) may appear with cysts in the lung.

When variable portions of lung parenchyma present a reduced attenuation to the X-rays, the descriptive term *dark lung* is used. When patchy the aspect is called mosaic perfusion. This aspect is due to lower perfusion, and lower perfusion recognizes two causes: vascular obstruction or bronchiolar obstruction. In patients with "dark lung" secondary to bronchiolar disease, hyperlucent areas of lobule size are common, usually with well-defined margins. When the disorder is characterized by vascular obstruction, the areas of low attenuation are often larger and poorly defined. The differentiation between vascular versus bronchiolar origin of

the decreased attenuation may be done also using the dynamic CT (CT expiratory scan compared to inspiratory CT scan). In the dark lung of vascular origin, a homogenous increase in density occurs everywhere. On the other hand, when the dark lung is due to constrictive bronchiolitis, the contrast increases (expiratory air trapping). The list of diseases presenting with dark lung includes chronic thromboembolism, primary pulmonary hypertension, constrictive bronchiolitis, and diffuse idiopathic pulmonary neuroendocrine cell hyperplasia. In the last disorder small, well-defined, randomly distributed nodules may also be identified. These nodules represent histologically tumorlets or even small carcinoids.

A significant number of diseases may manifest with combined patterns, or they may present different patterns during the course. The so-called *headcheese* pattern is characterized by areas of mosaic oligemia along with ground-glass attenuation or alveolar consolidation. It may be mainly observed in subacute hypersensitivity pneumonitis or *mycoplasma pneumoniae* pneumonia. Acute exacerbation of IPF presents with areas of ground-glass attenuation or even alveolar consolidation superimposed on a fibrotic pattern. Langerhans cell histiocytosis has a nodular pattern in the active phase and appears cystic or even with features of "dark" lung in the fibrotic stage.

1.8 The Invasive Diagnostic Procedures

Bronchoalveolar lavage (BAL) is a safe procedure that may even been carried out in ventilated patients [16]. The fluid recovered by the maneuver may be subjected to a variety of investigations: microbiological tests, cytological analysis and cell count, flow cytometry analysis, and assessment of various biochemical mediators. In the daily clinical practice, microbiological tests, cytological analysis, cell count, and flow cytometry are routinely done. BAL may be diagnostic in a minority of cases when specific "signatures" may be recognized: alveolar proteinosis, Langerhans cell histiocytosis (when >3.5% of macrophages express CD1a protein or Langerhin), epithelial neoplasms, low-grade B-cell lymphomas, infections (pneumocystosis, etc.), atypical type II pneumocytes in diffuse alveolar damage, hemosiderin laden macrophages in alveolar hemorrhage, macro-vacuolated, oil red positive histiocytes in lipoid pneumonia, and asbestos bodies in exposed subjects. Cytological and immunophenotypical profiles may represent a clue for the final diagnosis: lymphocytosis in granulomatous disorders, in drug-induced lung disorders, or in viral infections, mixed pattern (increase of lymphocytes and, in a lesser degree, of eosinophils and neutrophils associated to scattered mast cells) in organizing pneumonia, eosinophilia in chronic and acute eosinophilic pneumonia or in desquamative interstitial pneumonitis, neutrophilia (+/− scattered eosinophils) in fibrosing processes or in bacterial infections, foamy macrophages in amiodarone lung-induced injury or in Niemann-Pick disease, and "wrinkled paper" macrophages in Gaucher disease.

Bronchial biopsy may be diagnostic in carcinomatous lymphangitis, sarcoidosis, and even in low-grade B-cell lymphomas.

Transbronchial lung biopsy with flexible forceps is also a safe procedure (the more frequent complication being pneumothorax, observed in around 5% of cases; the most life-threatening complication being bleeding observed in less than 1% of cases). With this approach the sampling is mainly in the centrilobular parenchyma. However samples so obtained are tiny and usually with crush artifacts. Therefore it is diagnostic mainly in sarcoidosis, carcinomatous lymphangitis, organizing pneumonia, chronic eosinophilic pneumonia, diffuse alveolar damage, subacute hypersensitivity pneumonitis, low-grade B-cell lymphomas. Very rarely the morphological pattern UIP (with patchy fibrosis and fibroblastic foci with or without honeycomb changes) may be identified in these smaller samples. However recently it has been suggested that with the use of a genomic-based machine trained to identify a specific molecular signature identified from RNA sequencing on tiny transbronchial lung biopsy samples, the sensitivity of the procedure increases significantly. In this study the classifier identified UIP pattern in TBLB with an 88% specificity and 70% sensitivity. Considering all the DPLDs as a group, transbronchial lung biopsy appears to have a diagnostic yield varying from 30 to 70%, being it higher in disorders with simple morphology and in those located mainly in the centrilobular zones.

Surgical lung biopsy and nowadays video-assisted thoracoscopy was and is considered the gold standard for obtaining decent lung tissue samples to reach a specific morphological diagnosis. This approach is suggested when a morphological diagnosis of interstitial pneumonia (UIIP, NSIP, DIP, etc.) need to be validated, or when HRCT scan documents scattered nodules in the subpleural zones. However complications related to this approach are no longer negligible. Mortality is around 2% in 1 month, and it increases significantly when there is a clinical suspicion of IPF or collagen vascular disease, in elderly (patients >67 years) or with a reduced lung function (DLCO <45% of the predicted value). Mortality rate is significantly higher (around 16%) for not elective admissions, i.e., when the procedure is carried out in patients with rapidly decline of lung function. Morbidities are represented by subcutaneous emphysema, prolonged air leakage, empyema, chronic thoracic pain, and wound paraesthesia. These complications seem to be significantly reduced when a uniportal tubeless video-assisted thoracoscopy is applied. The limitation of this approach is, however, that areas easy to sample are mainly located on the lingula, the middle lobe, or on the anterior basal segment of the lower lobes.

Transbronchial cryobiopsy is a recently developed technique to obtain larger portions of lung tissue in an attempt to improve the yield of diagnostic tissue in lieu of an open surgical lung biopsy [17–19]. The main histologic benefits of cryobiopsy compared to transbronchial lung biopsy are the capacity to obtain larger and well-preserved samples. Complex morphological patterns such as usual interstitial pneumonia (UIP) may be recognizable.

References

1. Colby TV, Carrington CB. Interstitial lung disease. In: Thurlbeck WM, Churg AM, editors. Pathology of the lung. New York: Thieme; 1995. p. 589–737.
2. Nagaishi C. Functional anatomy and histology of the lung. Baltimore: University Park Press; 1972. p. 26–41.
3. Martignoni G, Pea M, Righellin D, et al. Molecular pathology of lymphangioleiomyomatosis and other perivascular epithelioid cell tumors. Arch Pathol Lab Med. 2010;134:33–40.
4. Durham BH. Molecular characterization of the histiocytosis: neoplasia of dendritic and macrophages. Semin Cell Dev Biol. 2019;86:62–76.
5. Milne P, Bigley V, Bacon CM, et al. Hematopoietic origin of Langerhans cell histiocytosis and Erdheim Chester disease in adults. Blood. 2017;130:167–75.
6. Korsten P, Tampa B, Konig MF, Nikiphorou E. Sarcoidosis and autoimmune diseases: differences, similarities and overlaps. Curr Opin Pulm Med. 2018;24:504–12.
7. Sood AK, Funkhouser W, Handly B, Weston B, Wu EY. Granulomatous-lymphocytic interstitial lung disease in 22q11.2 deletion syndrome: case report and literature review. Curr Allergy Asthma Rep. 2018;18:14.
8. Atzeni F, Gerardi MC, Barillaro G, Masala IF, Benucci M, Sarzi-Puttini P. Interstitial lung disease in systemic autoimmune rheumatic diseases: a comprehensive review. Expert Rev Clin Immunol. 2018;14:69–82.
9. Chilosi M, Caliò A, Rossi A, et al. Epithelial to mesenchymal transition-related proteins ZEB1, beta-catenin, and beta-tubulin III in idiopathic pulmonary fibrosis. Mod Pathol. 2017;30:26–36.
10. Chilosi M, Carloni A, Rossi A, Poletti V. Premature lung aging and cellular senescence in the pathogenesis of idiopathic pulmonary fibrosis and COPD/emphysema. Transl Res. 2013;162:156–73.
11. Kaur A, Mathai SK, Schwartz DA. Genetics in idiopathic pulmonary fibrosis. Pathogenesis, prognosis and treatment. Front Med. 2017;4:154.
12. Hoffman TW, van Moorsel CHM, Borie R, Crestani B. Pulmonary phenotypes associated with genetic variation in telomere-related genes. Curr Opin Pulm Med. 2018;24:269–80.
13. Allen RJ, Porte J, Braybrooke R, et al. Genetic variants associated with susceptibility to idiopathic pulmonary fibrosis in people of European ancestry: a genome-wide association study. Lancet Respir Med. 2017;5:869–80.
14. Dal Piaz G. Computed tomography of diffuse lung diseases and solitary pulmonary nodules. In: Leslie KO, Wick MR, editors. Practical pulmonary pathology: a diagnostic approach. 3rd ed. Amsterdam: Elsevier; 2018. p. 35–98.
15. Cagle PT, Kerr KM. Pulmonary pathology. Berlin: Springer; 2018.
16. Costabel U, du Bois RM, Egan JJ, Herth F, Bolliger CT. Diffuse parenchymal lung disease. Basel: Karger; 2007.
17. Hetzel J, Maldonado F, Ravaglia C, et al. Transbronchial cryobiopsies for the diagnosis of diffuse parenchymal lung diseases. Expert statement from the cryobiopsy working group on safety and utility and a call for standardization of the procedure. Respiration. 2018;95:188–200.
18. Poletti V, Casoni GL, Gurioli C, Ryu JH, Tomassetti S. Lung cryobiopsies: a paradigm shift in diagnostic bronchoscopy? Respirology. 2014;19:645–54.
19. Ravaglia C, Wells AU, Tomassetti S, Gurioli C, Gurioli C, Dubini A, Cavazza A, Colby TV, Piciucchi S, Puglisi S, Bosi M, Poletti V. Diagnostic yield and risk/benefit analysis of trans-bronchial lung cryobiopsy in diffuse parenchymal lung diseases: a large cohort of 699 patients. BMC Pulm Med. 2019;19(1):16.

Radiologic-Pathologic Correlations in Diffuse Parenchymal Lung Diseases

2

Sara Piciucchi

2.1 Introduction

The diagnosis of interstitial lung diseases is mostly the result of integration of clinical, radiologic, and pathologic data.

In the recent years, several updates and classifications have been published trying to focus the different features of idiopathic forms compared with secondary entities.

The 2013 ATS/ERS statement subdivided the idiopathic interstitial pneumonias into major and rare [1].

The major IIPs were again subgrouped into three groups.

The first group was represented by the chronic fibrosing IIPs: idiopathic pulmonary fibrosis (IPF) and nonspecific interstitial pneumonia (NSIP).

The second group was represented by smoking-related IIPs: respiratory bronchiolitis/interstitial lung disease (RB ILD) and desquamative interstitial pneumonia (DIP).

The third one included acute/subacute IIP including cryptogenic organizing pneumonia (COP) and acute interstitial pneumonia (AIP) (Table 2.1).

The rare IIPs included the idiopathic lymphocytic pneumonia (LIP) and the idiopathic pleuroparenchymal fibroelastosis (IPPFE).

S. Piciucchi (✉)
U.O. Radiologia, Ospedale G.B. Morgagni, Azienda USL Romagna-Sede di Forlì, Forlì, Italy

Table 2.1 Major idiopathic interstitial pneumonias

Major idiopathic interstitial pneumonias	Clinical-radiologic-pathologic entities
Chronic fibrosing IPs	IPF and i-NSIP
Smoking-related IPs	RB-ILD and DIP
Acute/subacute IPs	COP and AIP

Adapted from Travis WD, Costabel U, Hansell DM, et al. An Official American Thoracic Society/European Respiratory Society Statement: Update of the International Multidisciplinary Classification of the Idiopathic Interstitial Pneumonias. Am J Respir Crit Care Med Vol 2013; 188: 733–748

Finally, a subgroup of unclassifiable IIPs was recognized.

Beside the idiopathic forms, some interstitial pneumonia can be in association with known etiologies such as hypersensitivity pneumonitis (HP) and collagen vascular diseases (CVDs) [2].

2.2 UIP Pattern in Idiopathic Pulmonary Fibrosis

In the diagnostic workup, a valid approach to interstitial lung diseases is analyzing whether CT findings are suggestive of a UIP in IPF with high confidence or not [3].

Idiopathic pulmonary fibrosis (IPF) is a specific form of chronic, progressive fibrosing interstitial pneumonia occurring primarily in adults and allegedly limited to the lungs.

© Springer Nature Switzerland AG 2019
V. Poletti (ed.), *Transbronchial cryobiopsy in diffuse parenchymal lung disease*,
https://doi.org/10.1007/978-3-030-14891-1_2

Table 2.2 Summary of the features of new nomenclature of UIP pattern

	Sagittal distribution	Axial distribution	Honeycombing	Reticulation	Traction bronchiectasis
Typical UIP	Basal	Subpleural and heterogeneous	Yes	Yes	Yes
Probable	Basal	Subpleural and heterogeneous	No	Yes	Yes
Indeterminate	Variable or diffuse	Variable or diffuse	Not highly evocative for a non-UIP pattern	Not highly evocative for a non-UIP pattern	Not highly evocative for a non-UIP pattern

Adapted from Lynch DA, Sverzellati N, Travis WD, Brown KK, Colby TV, Galvin JR, Goldin JG, Hansell DM, Inove Y, Johkoh T, Nicholson AG, Knight SL, Raoof S, Richeldi L, Ryerson CJ, Ryu JH, Wells A. Diagnostic criteria for idiopathic pulmonary fibrosis a Fleischner Society White Paper. Lancer Respir Med 2017

It is characterized by progressive worsening of dyspnea and lung function and is associated with a poor prognosis [4].

Pulmonary function test results may be normal in patients with mild disease, but usually they show some degree of restriction at diagnosis. Diffusion capacity is also commonly decreased.

Usual interstitial pneumonia represents the pattern at the basis of radiologic and histologic diagnosis of IPF.

Guidelines published in 2011 [4] have defined the role of CT in the diagnosis of IPF, listing the main CT features of UIP that account a reticular pattern with honeycombing, often associated with traction bronchiectasis; ground-glass opacity may be depicted, but it should be less extensive than the reticular abnormalities. These abnormalities show a peripheral and basal predominance.

Honeycombing, defined as clustered cystic spaces, measuring between 3 and 5 mm, has been recognized as a key feature of the UIP pattern. Traction bronchiectasis and bronchiolectasis are the hallmark of lung fibrosis on chest imaging and have been described as important prognostic marker [5]. More recently Lynch et al. [6] have published a white paper that clarified and updated the approach to diagnosis of IPF. The authors emphasized the role of CT features in diagnostic process. The typical CT findings of a UIP pattern still include honeycombing and traction bronchiectasis with a basal and peripheral predominance. However, the authors assert that the absence of honeycombing should not exclude the diagnosis of UIP pattern if the remaining fea-

tures are already present. So, CT findings previously considered as "possible" now can define a "probable UIP pattern." Cases without a typical or probable UIP pattern previously described as "inconsistent" should be named as "indeterminate" (Table 2.2). Furthermore, the histology of UIP in IPF is characterized by a regionally and temporally variegated pattern of peripheral accentuated fibrosis, typically with numerous sub epithelial foci of ongoing fibroblastic proliferation [7] (Fig. 2.1).

2.3 Early IPF: UIP Pattern and Ancillary Findings

In the recent years, cryobiopsy has allowed significant advance in knowledge in the tissue characterization of the early forms of IPF.

On the other hand, another revolutionary tool in the identification of subtle changes is represented by micro-CT [8]. These two important applications of interventional pulmonology and imaging have widened the spectrum of findings traditionally described in the UIP-IPF.

2.3.1 Ground Glass

Interpretation of ground-glass attenuation is still challenging in UIP pattern.

In the advanced stage of IPF, Rabeyrin et al. [9] identified that GG correlated with focal exacerbation and with focal areas of coexisting NSIP (Fig. 2.2).

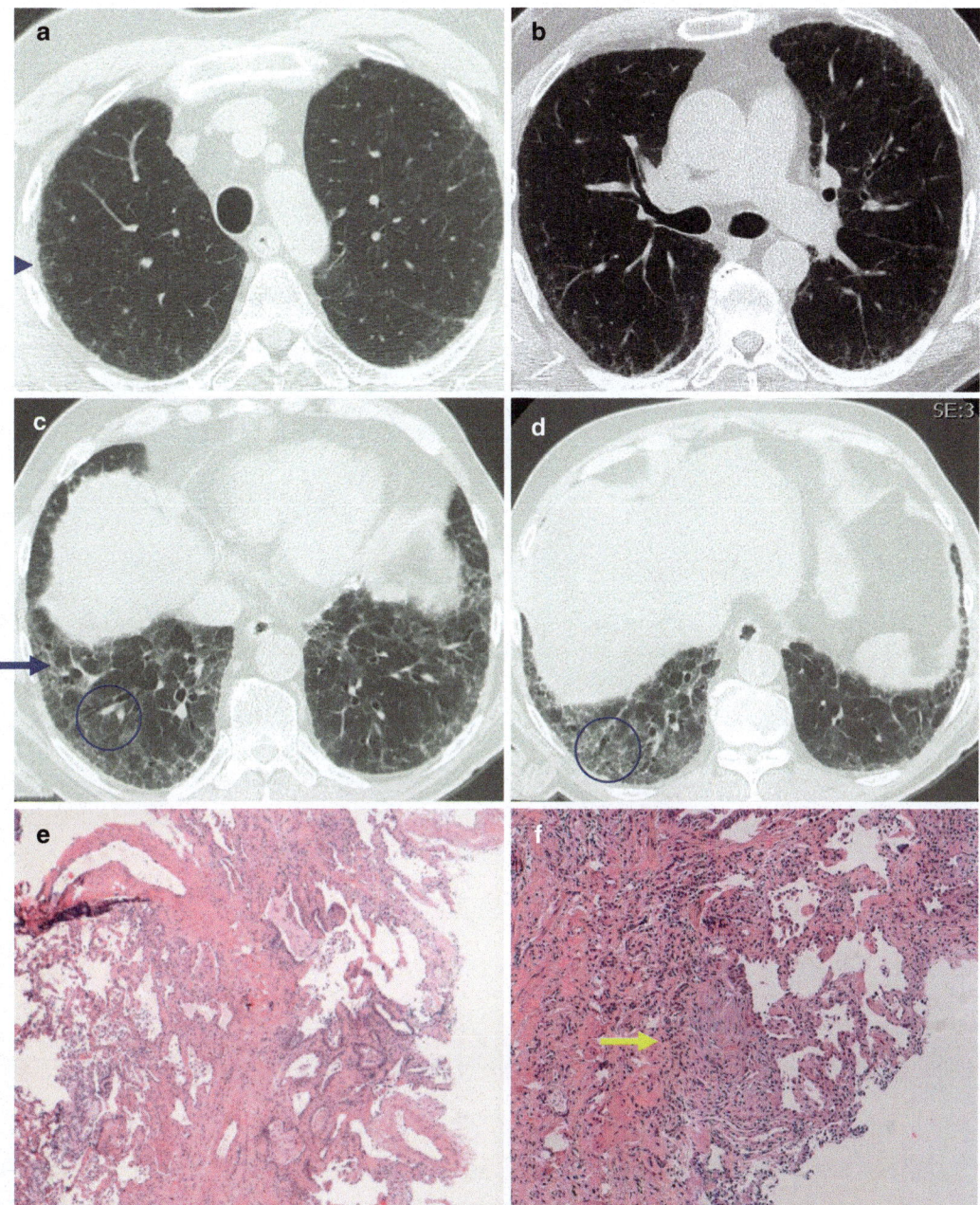

Fig. 2.1 CT scan of a 65-year-old, male, never smoked, with history of GERD. CT findings are suggestive of a probable UIP pattern (**a–d**): bilateral, peripheral reticulation with basal predominance (blue arrow); traction bronchiectasis in both lower lobes, mainly on the right side (blue circle). Cryobiopsy (**e**, **f**) shows patchy fibrosis (**e**) and some fibroblastic foci (**f**, yellow arrow). Histology meets the criteria for UIP pattern. The final diagnosis is UIP-IPF

However, ground glass can be seen also in the early stages of IPF. Micro-CT studies [8] have identified that it may correspond to some micro areas of hypoventilation in the dependent zones and minimal fibrotic changes. Moreover, these minimal changes have been identified in cases studied with cryobiopsy and actually can be related to areas of "young fibrosis" associated with fibrin remnant and with subclinical exacerbation (Fig. 2.3).

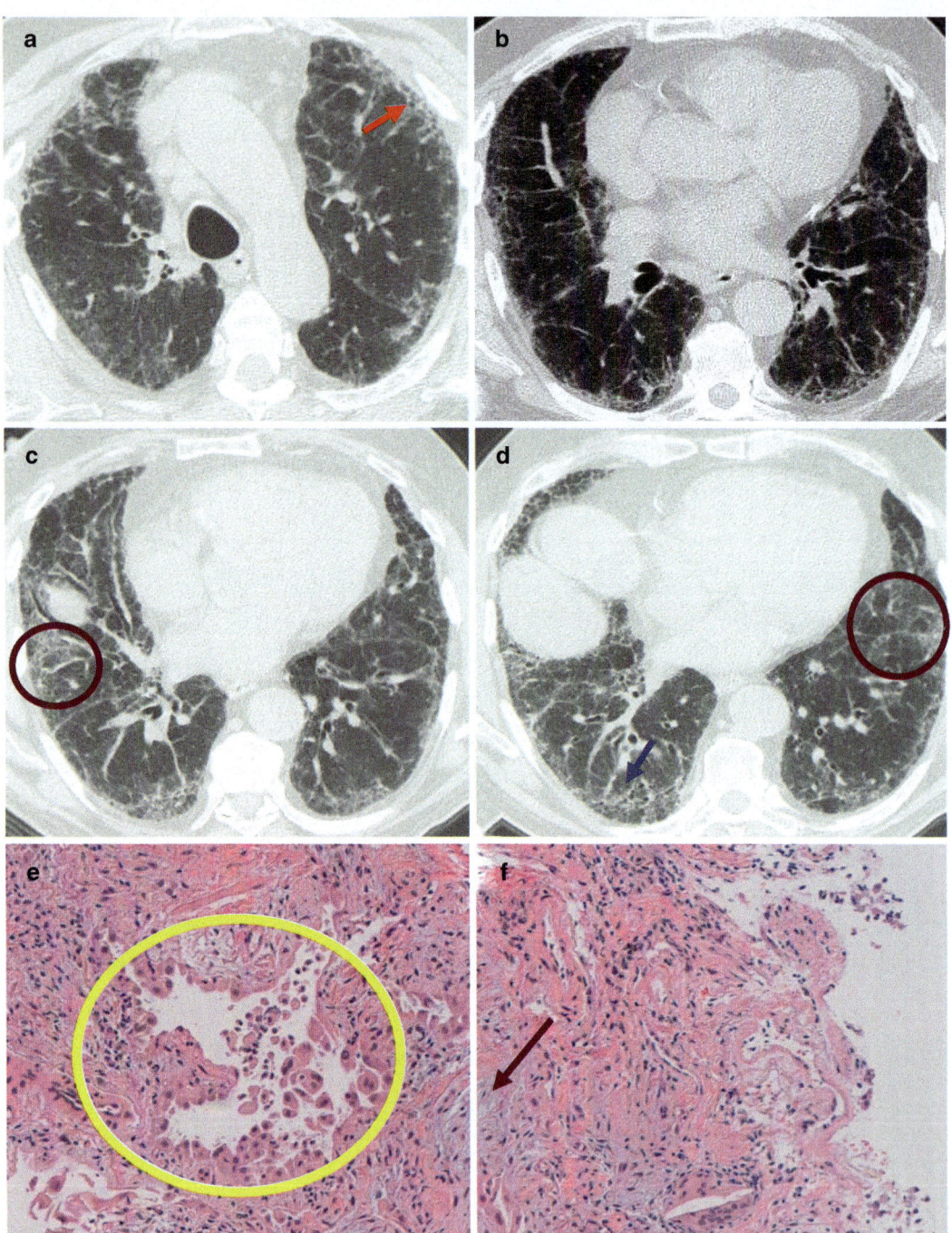

Fig. 2.2 CT scan of a 73-year-old male, former smoker, with 3 years history of chronic cough and dyspnea on exertion. Peripheral reticulation (**a**; red arrow) and lobular distortion are present in both hemithoraces (**a–d**), associated with traction bronchiectasis mainly in lower lobes (**d**; blue arrow). Some areas of patchy ground-glass attenuation are present bilaterally (**c**, **d**; circles). No honeycomb-ing is visible. Cryobiopsy shows a context of alveolar stem cells proliferation associated with foci of young fibrosis and fibrin remnants. CT findings are suggestive of probable UIP likely associated with areas of acute damage. Histology confirms the acute/subacute damage, and radiologic-pathologic integration defines IPF with subclinical exacerbation

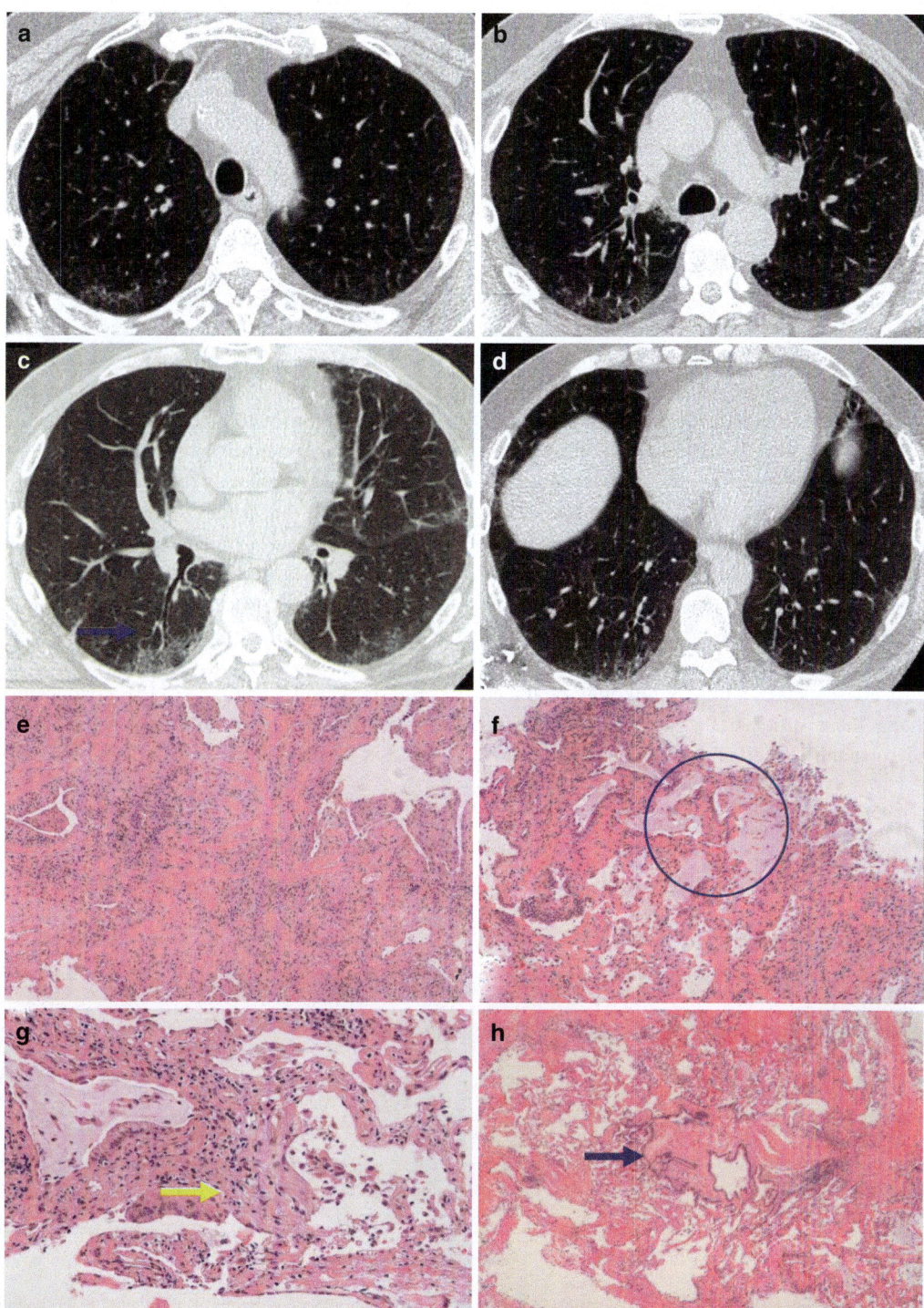

Fig. 2.3 CT scan shows mild ground-glass attenuation in mid to lower zones of both the lungs, mainly in the right side (**a**–**d**). The distribution is peripheral. Rare traction bronchiectasis are present, mainly in the periphery (**c**, blue arrow). Cryobiopsy showed a dense scarring (**e**), alveolar septal fibrosis (**f**) with mucus stasis (blue circle), some fibroblastic foci (**g**, yellow arrow), and areas of peribronchiolar metaplasia (**h**, blue arrow). Histology is consistent with UIP pattern. Axial and sagittal distributions of CT findings correlate with a probable UIP. Ground-glass attenuation in this case is likely an expression of young and active fibrotic process

2.3.2 Minimal Reticular Changes and ILA

Mai et al. [8] have correlated the presence of minimal changes, resembling interstitial lung abnormalities (ILA), with native collagen adjacent to the interlobular septum and in the alveolar walls, seen on the histology.

ILA have already been described by Jin and coworkers [10] as collateral findings present in the CT scans of the lung cancer screening program. In a cohort of 884 patients, 9.7% showed ILA ($n = 86$). Among these patients, 5.9% had a non-fibrotic pattern; 2.1% had a fibrotic pattern, and finally, 1.7% had a mixed pattern. Interestingly, 37% of the fibrotic ILA showed progression.

Furthermore, Putman RK et al. [11] recently have pointed the attention on the association between ILA and occurring of distress respiratory syndromes, concluding that the cohorts of patients with sepsis and respiratory distress may have some undiagnosed cases of ILA [11].

As consequence, a unique link may be traced among these articles: the possibility of acute and subacute exacerbations in subclinical early

IPF [12, 13]. Screening for ILA might eventually provide a mean for the early identification of IPF, and a further crucial step is differentiating ILAs representing early UIP-IPF from smoking-related changes (that sometimes can overlap with the first) and others, like foci of organizing pneumonia (Fig. 2.4).

2.3.3 Bony Metaplasia

Bony metaplasia in the lung is represented by a localized or diffuse ossification [14]. Localized form is common in injured lung tissue such as abscess, old TB, and tumors -(Fig. 2.5).

The diffuse form can be nodular (usually associated with the various causes of pulmonary venous hypertension) or dendriform (also called racemose or branching).

The dendriform ossification is usually associated with chronic fibrosing lung disease, especially IPF.

Egashira and coworkers [15] conducted a retrospective analysis on 892 patients (452 with diagnosis of IPF, 244 with NSIP, and 192 with

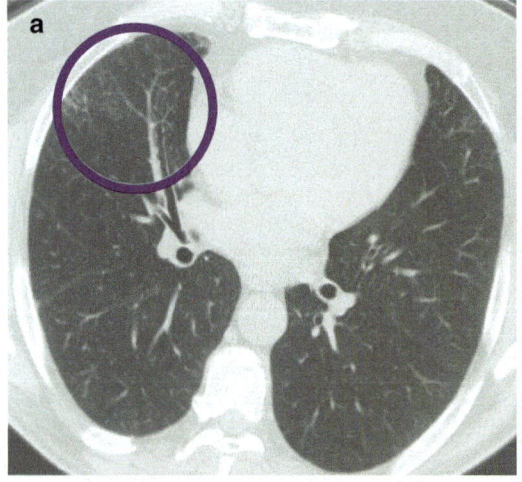
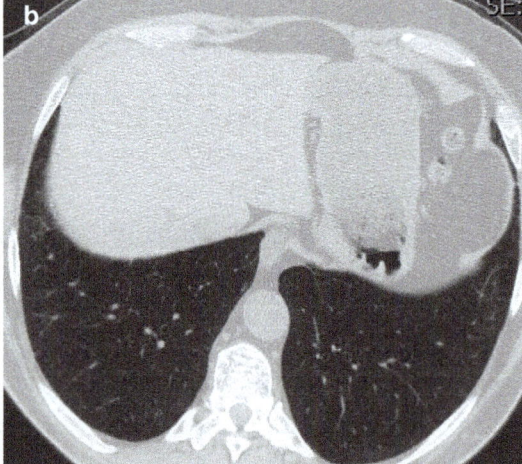
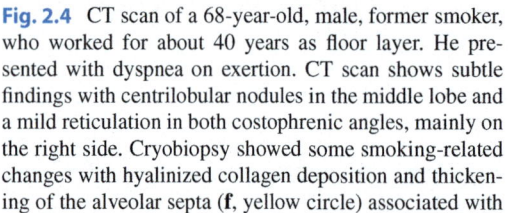

Fig. 2.4 CT scan of a 68-year-old, male, former smoker, who worked for about 40 years as floor layer. He presented with dyspnea on exertion. CT scan shows subtle findings with centrilobular nodules in the middle lobe and a mild reticulation in both costophrenic angles, mainly on the right side. Cryobiopsy showed some smoking-related changes with hyalinized collagen deposition and thickening of the alveolar septa (**f**, yellow circle) associated with a peribronchial accumulation of pigmented macrophages (**g**, yellow arrow). However, in the sample of lower lobe, some fibroblastic foci and patchy fibrosis are present (**h**, blue circle). Even though CT findings are in a context of the indeterminate pattern, histologic findings are consistent with smoking-related ILD associated with UIP pattern. Integration of these data delineates a context of early IPF

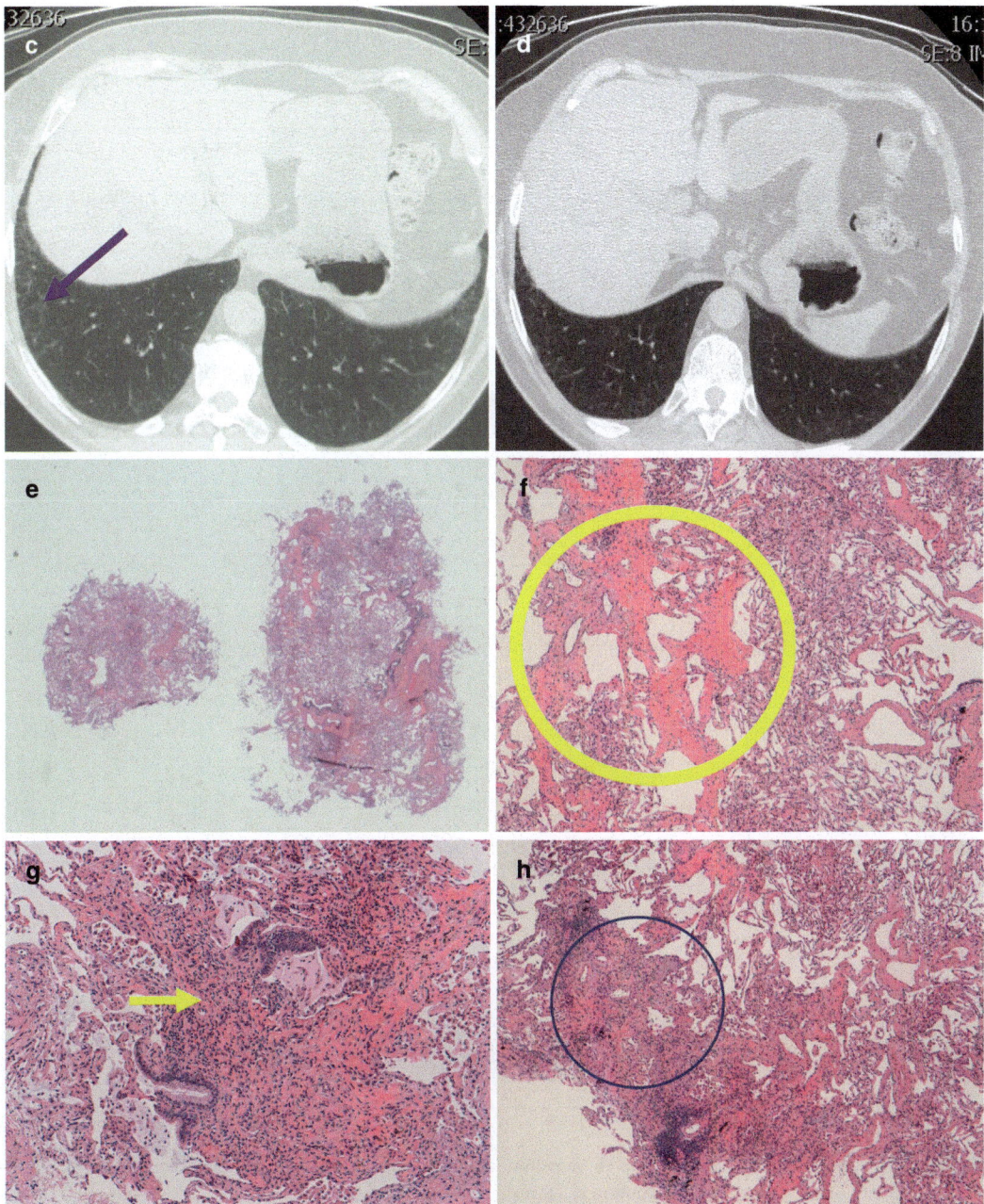

Fig. 2.4 (continued)

HP), classifying pulmonary ossification into two definitions.

The ossification definition 1 consisted in ten or more, bilateral, was significantly higher in the group of IPF patients with a prevalence of 28.5%. Moreover, the multivariate analysis showed that definition 1 was an independent predictor of IPF diagnosis ($P < 0.011$) and for male sex ($P = 0.003$).

Coarseness of fibrosing ILD ($P = 0.011$) and IPF diagnosis ($P = 0.016$) was independently associated to pulmonary ossification. In IPF

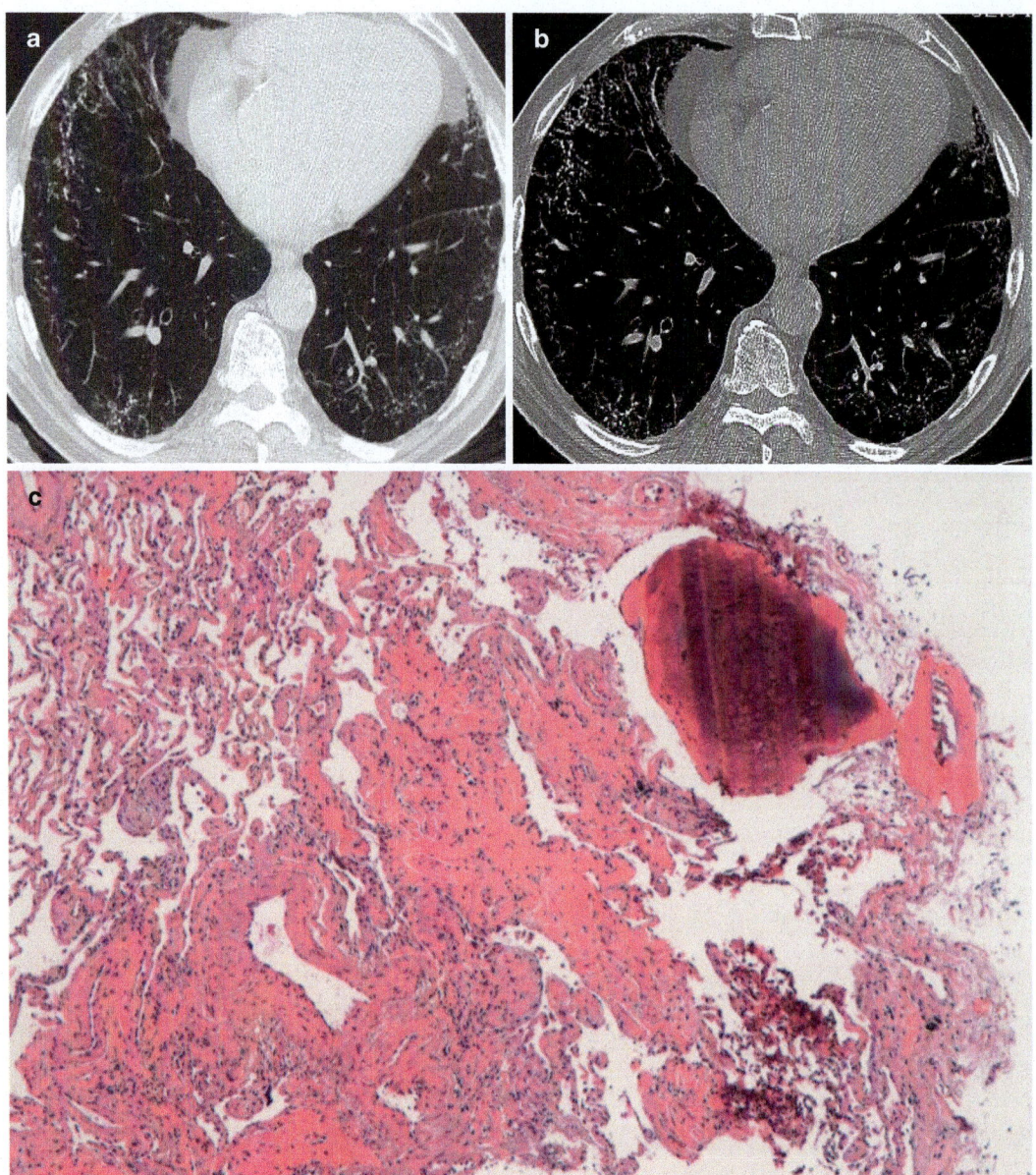

Fig. 2.5 CT scan with lung (**a**) and bone (**b**) window shows dendriform ossification that are confirmed by the corresponding sample (**c**), in which dense fibrosis, spatial, and temporal heterogeneity are associated with a focal bony metaplasia

patients, bony metaplasia could be interpreted as consequence of the aberrant activation of the Wnt pathway [16].

Tsai APY et al. [17] described a case of relapsing pneumothoraces in a patient with DPO. The etiology of pneumothorax was postulated as consequence of bony spicules that induce punctures on the pleura (Fig. 2.6).

2.3.4 Fatty Metaplasia

The significance of fatty metaplasia is still to determine. In 2000, Travis et al. [18] evaluated the main pathologic features, on lung biopsies, from patients with idiopathic pneumonias.

These features included changes related to the different structures of the chest (alveolar and

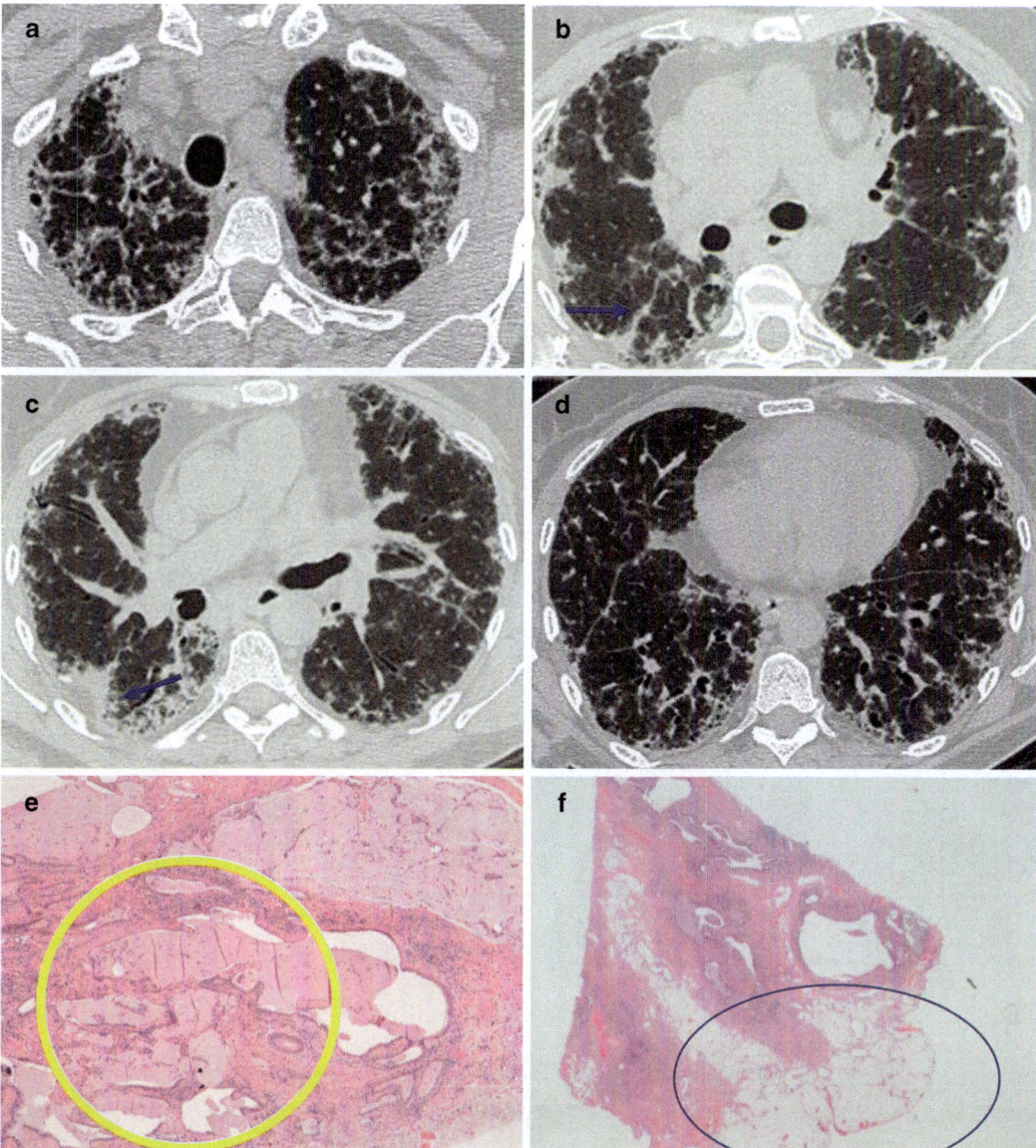

Fig. 2.6 CT scan shows a diffuse, severe interstitial thickening associated with lobular distortion (**a–d**). No peripheral and basal predominance is present. The patient underwent surgical biopsy that showed an UIP pattern characterized by dense fibrosis and honeycombing with mucus stasis (**e**; yellow circle). On the edge of the sample, in low power, a fatty metaplasia of the pleura is visible (**f**), likely related to the focal thickening on the CT scan (**b**, **c**, blue arrow)

interstitial cellularity, findings related to fibrosis like fibroblastic foci, stromal changes, airways changes, vascular changes), including pleural changes, investigating presence of pleuritis, presence of pleural plaques, blebs, and finally fat. In the analysis of IPF (*n* cases, 54), the subpleural fat was the only feature to have a prognostic significance in the multivariate analysis.

2.3.5 PPFE and UIP Pattern

Pleuroparenchymal fibroelastosis (PPFE) is a rare entity first described in 2004 [19] characterized by pleural and subpleural fibrosis mainly in the apical regions (Fig. 2.7).

In the recent years, PPFE has been described in association with UIP (Fig. 2.8) by Oda et al.

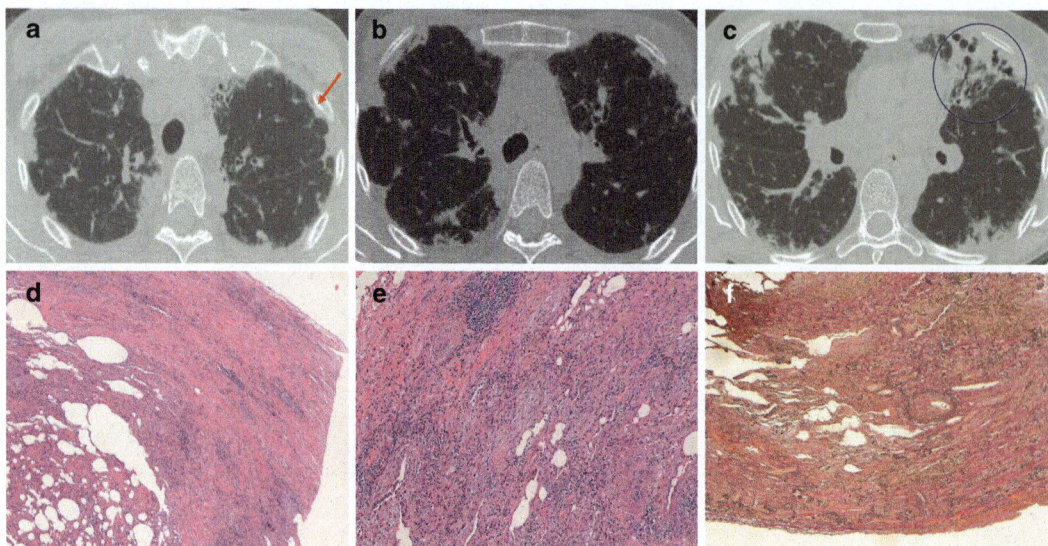

Fig. 2.7 CT (**a–c**) and histology (**d–f**) suggestive of pleuroparenchymal fibroelastosis CT scan shows a severe thickening of the pleura (**a**, red arrow) associated with sub-pleural consolidation and traction bronchiectasis (**c**, blue circle). Histology confirms the dense pleural and subpleural fibrosis and the presence of elastic fibers (**f**)

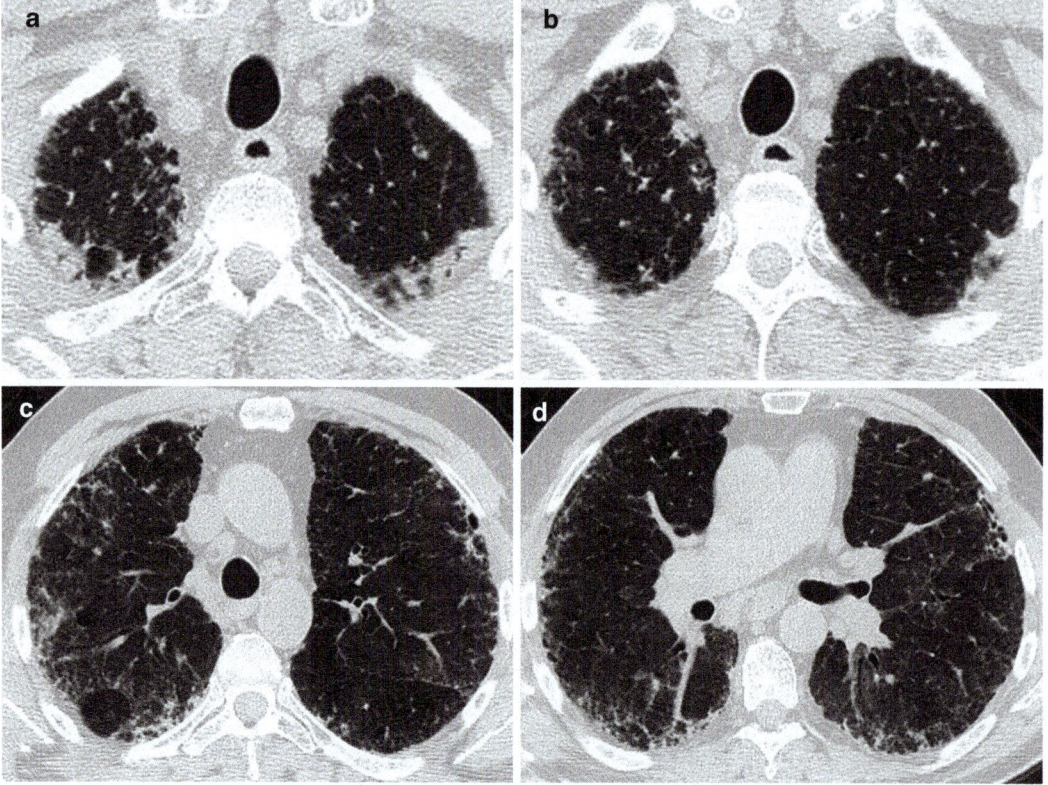

Fig. 2.8 CT findings suggestive of a combination of UIP pattern in the lower lobes and PPFE in the upper lobes. Dense subpleural and pleural fibrosis in both upper lobes suggestive of pleuroparenchymal fibroelastosis (**a**, **b**) associated with reticulation in the lower lobes and peripheral traction bronchiectasis (**c**, **d**)

[20]. The authors retrospectively reviewed 291 consecutive patients with IPF who underwent surgical lung biopsy and identified 9 cases that met criteria both radiologically and pathologically of PPFE in upper lobes and UIP pattern in lower lobes. The PPFE with UIP showed a significantly higher $PaCO_2$ (44.6 mmHg vs 41.7 mmHg, $P = 0.04$) and higher complication rate of pneumothorax and pneumomediastinum compared with the group of UIP-IPF. Moreover, survival time tended to be shorter in patients with PPFE and UIP.

2.4   Non-idiopathic UIP Patterns

2.4.1   UIP and Connective Tissue Diseases

Pulmonary fibrosis is a well-recognized complication of systemic CTD, most commonly in rheumatoid arthritis, progressive systemic sclerosis, systemic lupus erythematosus, polymyositis/dermatomyositis, and Sjogren syndrome [21]. Due to the exaggerated immune response to autoantigens, the response can progressively destroy the parenchyma. UIP pattern on CT scan can overlap the UIP in IPF, with criteria of a definite UIP: basal and peripheral predominance, reticular abnormalities, honeycombing, and absence of all the features listed as inconsistent. Recently Chung et al. [21] described features that could be helpful in differential diagnosis of CTD-UIP vs UIP in IPF, particularly, anterior upper lobe, exuberant honeycombing, and straightedge signs. Histopathology shows distinctive features. First, at low magnification, RA-associated ILD often shows a mixed pattern of fibrosis NSIP and UIP. Second, the boundary between fibrotic areas and preserved parenchyma in RA-associated ILDs tends to be indistinct compared with UIP in IPF where the boundary between fibrosis and normal parenchyma is sharp and well-defined. Finally, a prominent lymphoid hyperplasia is more common in CTD-ILD. Lymphoid aggregates are more prominent around the airways, in the areas of fibrosis, and adjacent to the pleura (Fig. 2.9).

2.4.2   Chronic Hypersensitivity Pneumonitis with UIP-Like Pattern

Chronic hypersensitivity pneumonitis (CHP) represents a fibrotic interstitial pneumonia secondary to environmental exposure. Separating UIP-IPF from CHP with an UIP-like pattern is by far the most challenging issue in diagnosis of CHP. CT findings that CHP and UIP in IPF have in common include fibrosis with reticulation, architectural distortion, and traction bronchiectasis. Honeycombing, even if a requirement for UIP in IPF, has been reported in 16–69% of CHP [22–24]. The most typical features of CHP, compared with UIP-IPF, are that fibrosis tends to be predominantly mid and upper zonal with basal sparing, subpleural fibrosis is less marked, the subacute HP findings may superimpose, and lobular areas of decreased attenuation and vascularity are present in approximately 80% of patients (Fig. 2.10). Poorly defined centrilobular nodules are also present in 50% of cases. In contrast, in UIP-IPF, reticulation is mainly in the lower zones, and honeycombing has a basal and peripheral predominance. Organizing pneumonia can be an ancillary sign of CHP [25]. Moreover, Yousem et al. [26] reported ten cases under the name bronchiolocentric interstitial pneumonia. All the cases showed a bronchiolar scarring with interstitial fibrosis following the alveolar walls and covered by metaplastic bronchiolar epithelium radiating away from the bronchioles. This fibrosis sometimes reached the pleura. Again Churg et al. [27] described 12 cases with a process termed airway-centered interstitial fibrosis that was like the cohort described by Yousem: fine interstitial fibrosis covered by metaplastic bronchiolar epithelium.

2.5   Nonspecific Interstitial Pneumonia

2.5.1   Idiopathic NSIP

In 2013 the ATS/ERS classification accepted NSIP as a distinct clinicopathologic entity that

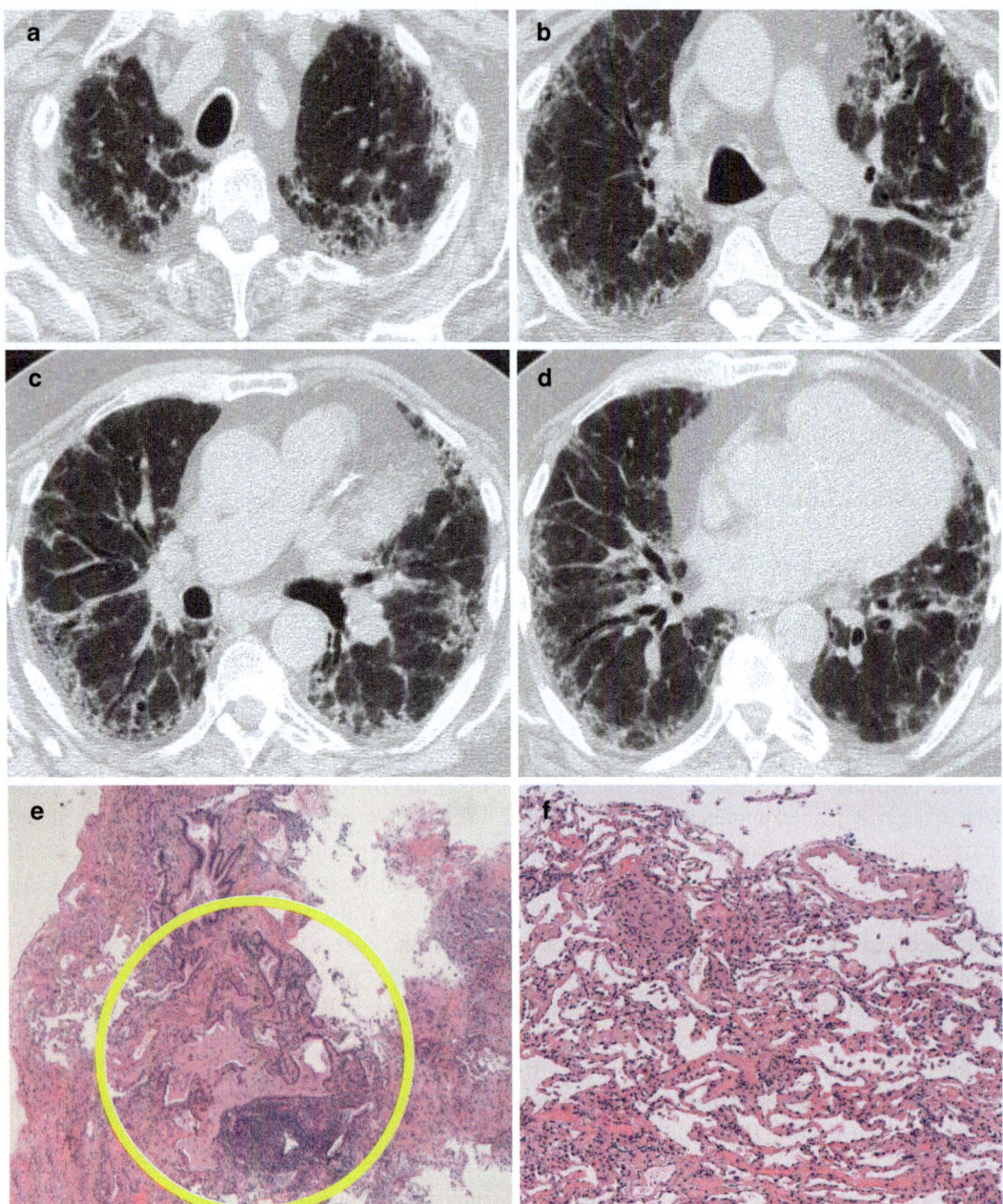

Fig. 2.9 Radiologic-pathologic findings suggestive of a UIP pattern secondary to Rheumathoid Arthritis. CT scan (**a–d**) of a 70-year-old, male, non-smoker, with recent history of xerostomia and positive serology for rheumatoid arthritis. Fibrotic findings characterized by reticulation and traction bronchiectasis are associated with ground glass. Cryobiopsy samples show a UIP pattern with a honeycomb chanes (e; yellow circle), lymphoid follicle (**e**) and a nonspecific interstitial pattern (**f**) diffuse inflammatory infiltrate (yellow circle)

was no more provisional. Moreover, it was subdivided into cellular and fibrotic. CT scan of NSIP typically shows ground-glass density associated with reticulation and traction bronchiectasis. The histopathology of idiopathic NSIP is characterized by varying degrees of interstitial inflammation and fibrosis, with uniform appearance. The fibrosis develops in the original alveolar walls and does not cause significant distortion. Two distinct histologic patterns are recognized: cellular

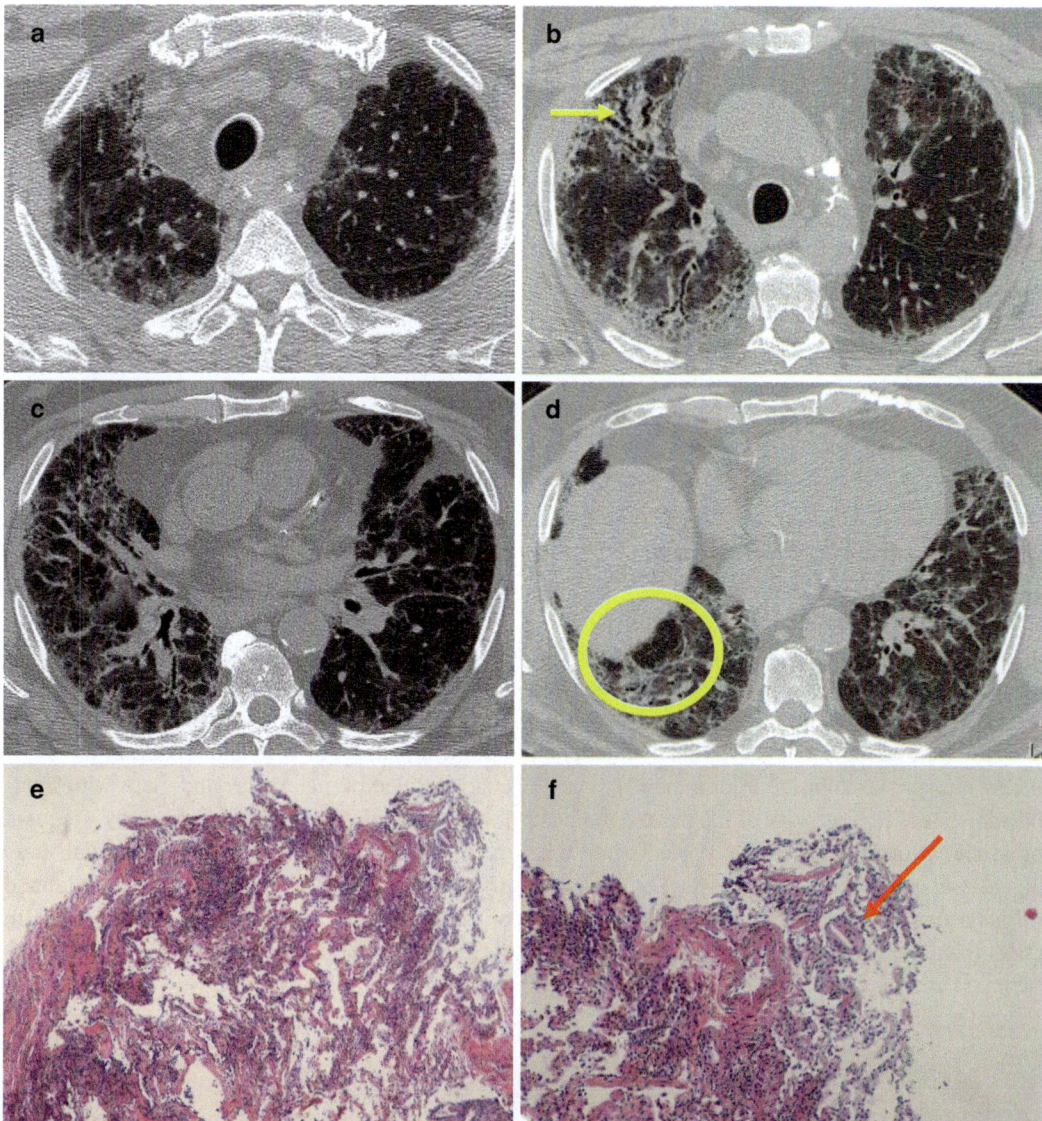

Fig. 2.10 CT scan of a 69-year-old, male, non-smoker, with progressive shortness of breath. CT findings are characterized by extensive fibrotic distortion of the secondary lobule (**a–d**), associated with traction bronchiectasis (**b**, yellow arrow) and ground glass. The distribution is mainly in mid to upper lobes. In both costophrenic angles, some areas of lobular air trapping are present (**d**; yellow circle). Pattern is indeterminate for UIP. Cryobiopsy shows some important ancillary findings: lymphoid aggregates (**e**) and giant cells (**f**, red arrow)

and fibrotic. Cellular NSIP shows a predominant mononuclear interstitial inflammation. Fibrous NSIP has a predominately uniform interstitial fibrosis. Although the extent of changes can vary along a spectrum ranging from cellular to fibrous, the pulmonary architecture is overall preserved.

The most challenging distinction between UIP and NSIP is represented by the most advanced fibrosis. However, in these cases the distinction can be based on the diffusely abnormal alveolar septa, UIP pattern.

2.5.2 NSIP in Connective Tissue Diseases

NSIP represents the most common histologic pattern in interstitial pneumonia associated with CDV [28]. It has been estimated that up to 15–20% of patients with chronic IP have occult CVD [29]. Kono M et al. [30] and Romagnoli et al. [31] demonstrated the association between NSIP and subsequent onset of CVD. Kono also observed that no significant difference was present in clinical characteristics and survival among patients with NSIP preceding CVD with those with NSIP-CVD [29].

2.6 Organizing Pneumonia

Organizing pneumonia (OP) is a common pattern of lung injury of a variable etiology. It can be a common manifestation of drug reaction, connective tissue diseases, transplant rejection, GVHD, and radiation therapy. It begins as an alveolar epithelial injury consisting of predominantly type 1 pneumocytes. The integrity of the basal lamina is breached, allowing coagulative proteins into the alveolar airspaces. Fibrin is deposited in the alveoli as result of coagulative cascade. On histology, OP is characterized by fibrous plugs composed of fibroblasts and myofibroblasts within airspaces admixed with inflammatory cells. AFOP can be a component of or be the predominant pattern in diffuse alveolar disease, represented by patchy intra-alveolar fibrin balls. Radiologically, OP can be characterized by focal or multiple consolidations, nodular pattern, and reversed halo sign.

OP can present with a single focus of consolidation or multifocal migratory consolidations with or without air bronchograms [32]. The typical distribution is in the peripheral and lower lungs. Peripheral consolidations also occur in chronic eosinophilic pneumonia, pulmonary hemorrhage, and vasculitis. The bronchocentric form of OP can occur in up to one-third of patients and is associated with peribronchovascular consolidation. This pattern is frequently seen in association with polymyositis and dermatomyositis. Unusual patterns include an upper zone involvement, crazy paving, nodular pattern, perilobular thickening, and reverse halo. The upper lobe predominance that can mimic CEP have mixed histological features of CEP and OP. Crazy paving is characterized by patchy ground glass with interlobular septal thickening, particularly frequent as nitrofurantoin drug-related interstitial lung disease. Smaller nodules can have well-defined or poorly defined margins, measuring from 3 to 10 mm. When nodules are associated with centri-

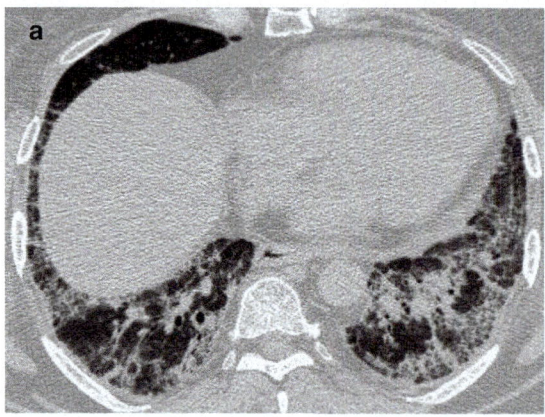
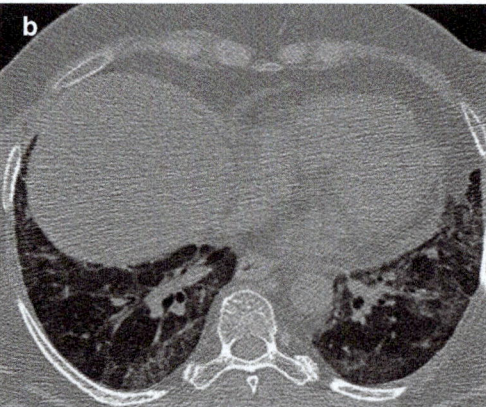
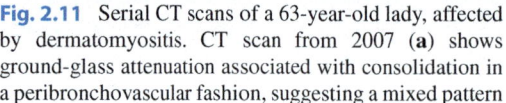

Fig. 2.11 Serial CT scans of a 63-year-old lady, affected by dermatomyositis. CT scan from 2007 (**a**) shows ground-glass attenuation associated with consolidation in a peribronchovascular fashion, suggesting a mixed pattern NSIP-OP. CT scan 2 years later (**b**), 3 years later (**c, d**) show a wax and wane behavior of the ground-glass attenuation expression of the partial relapse of OP component

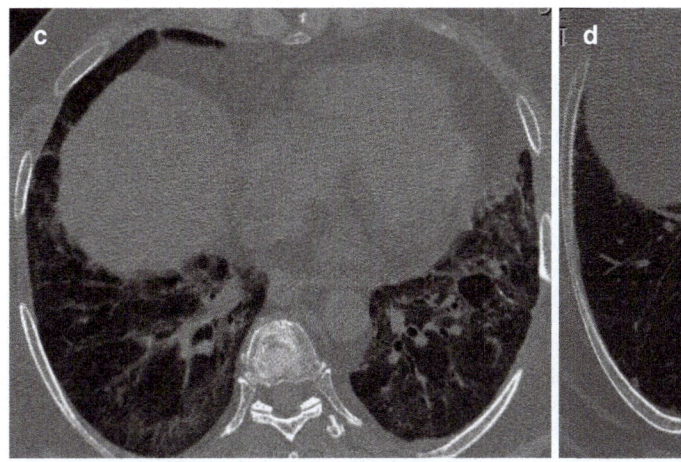
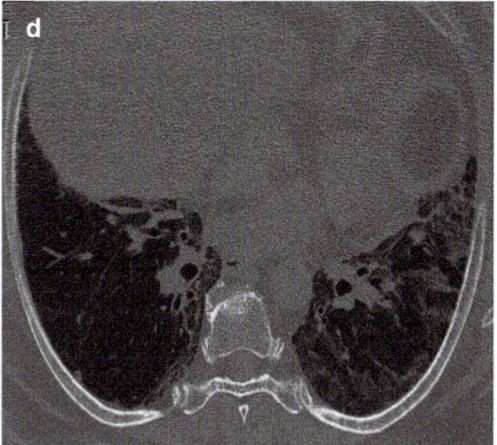

Fig. 2.11 (continued)

lobular nodules with tree-in-bud, they are expression of OP coexisting with infection. Perilobular thickening has an arcade-like opacity correlated with accumulation of organizing exudate in the peripheral lobules. Finally, the reverse halo, or atoll sign, has been described as possible expression of OP. It is characterized by a focal area of ground glass surrounded by a crescent or ring of consolidation [32]. Differential diagnosis of reversed halo includes lymphomatous granulomatosis, granulomatosis with polyangiitis, lipoid pneumonia, and sarcoid (Fig. 2.11).

2.7 Smoking-Related Interstitial Lung Diseases

Respiratory bronchiolitis is an asymptomatic lesion of small airways of cigarette smokers. When RB becomes more extensive, typically in heavy smokers, RB-ILD may develop. CT scan depicts ill-defined centrilobular nodules. Emphysema and bronchial wall thickening can be ancillary signs. In a small percentage reticular pattern can coexist. Histologically, two are the key features: accumulation of smoker macrophages inside the respiratory bronchiole lumen. Inflammation around the terminal airways is minimal. Recently Katzenstein [33] described

features of smoking-related interstitial fibrosis (SRIF) as a distinct type of hyalinized interstitial fibrosis associated with emphysema and RB [34]. In SRIF, the affected alveolar septa are thickened by deposition of dense eosinophilic ropey-appearing collagen often with admixed hyperplastic smooth muscle bundles. Occasional foci of mild chronic inflammation are admixed with the interstitial collagen, but inflammation is never prominent. Differential diagnosis between SRIF and UIP is based on enlarged airspaces, lined by bronchiolar epithelium of honeycombing. Distinction between SRIF and fibrosing NSIP is based on the deeply eosinophilic and hyalinized collagen of SRIF compared with the loose collagen fibrosis typical of NSIP. Scars in Langerhans cell histiocytosis (LCH) can be also differentiated due to the presence of their peribronchiolar and stellate-shaped scars.

2.8 Summary

Cryobiopsy has opened a new frontier in the radiologic diagnosis of ILD. In fact the correlation of imaging and pathology, particularly in cases of subtle CT findings, offers the opportunity of the identification of signs for the early stages of disease [35].

References

1. Travis WD, Costabel U, Hansell DM, et al. An official American Thoracic Society/European Respiratory Society statement: update of the international multidisciplinary classification of the idiopathic interstitial pneumonias. Am J Respir Crit Care Med. 2013;188:733–48.
2. Batra K, Butt Y, Gokaslan T, Burguete D, Glazer C, Torrealba JR. Pathology and radiology correlation of idiopathic interstitial pneumonias. Hum Pathol. 2018;72:1–17.
3. Sverzellati N, Lynch DA, Hansell DM, Jonkoh T, King TE, Travis WD. American Thoracic Society-European Respiratory Society Classification of the idiopathic interstitial pneumonias: advances in knowledge since 2002. Radiographics. 2015;35:1849–72.
4. Raghu G, Collard HR, Egan JJ, et al. An official ATS/ERS/JRS/ALAT statement: idiopathic pulmonary fibrosis: evidence-based guidelines for diagnosis and management. Am J Respir Crit Care Med. 2011;183:788–824.
5. Walsh S, Wells AU, Sverzellati N, Devaraj A, Von der Thusen J, Yousem SA, Colby TV, Nicholson A, Hansell DM. Relationship between fibroblastic foci profusion and high resolution CT morphology in fibrotic lung disease. BMC Med. 2015;13:241.
6. Lynch DA, Sverzellati N, Travis WD, Brown KK, Colby TV, Galvin JR, Goldin JG, Hansell DM, Inove Y, Johkoh T, Nicholson AG, Knight SL, Raoof S, Richeldi L, Ryerson CJ, Ryu JH, Wells A. Diagnostic criteria for idiopathic pulmonary fibrosis a Fleischner Society White Paper. Lancet Respir Med. 2018;6:138–53.
7. Larsen BT, Smith ML, Elicker BM, Fernandez JM, Arbo Oze de Morvil G, Pereira CA, Leslie KO. Diagnostic approach to advanced fibroblastic interstitial lung disease. Arch Pathol Lab Med. 2017;141:901–15.
8. Mai C, Verleden SE, McDonough JE, Willems S, et al. Thin-section CT features of idiopathic pulmonary fibrosis correlated with micro-CT and histologic analysis. Radiology. 2017;283:252–63.
9. Rabeyrin M, Thivolet F, Ferretti GR, et al. Usual interstitial pneumonia end-stage features from explants with radiologic pathologic correlations. Ann Diagn Pathol. 2015;19:269–76.
10. Jin GY, et al. Interstitial lung abnormalities in a CT lung cancer screening population: prevalence and progression rate. Radiology. 2013;268:563–71.
11. Putman RK. Interstitial lung abnormalities are associated with acute respiratory distress syndrome. Am J Respir Crit Care Med. 2017;195:138–41.
12. Araki T, Putman RK, Hatabu H, Gao W, Dupuis J, Latourelle JC, Nishino M, Zazueta OE, Kurugol S, Ross JC, et al. Development and progression of interstitial lung abnormalities in the Framingham heart study. Am J Respir Crit Care Med. 2016;195:1514–22.
13. Wells AU. Subclinical interstitial lung abnormalities: toward the early detection of idiopathic pulmonary fibrosis? Am J Respir Crit Care Med. 2016;194:1445–6.
14. Bisceglia M, Chiaromonte A, Panniello G, et al. Selected case from the Arkadi M. Rywlin international pathology slide series: diffuse dendriform pulmonary ossification report of 2 cases with review of the literature. Adv Anat Pathol. 2015;22:59–68.
15. Egashira R, Jacob J, Kokosi MA, Brun AL, Rice A, Nicholson AG, Wells AU, Hansell DM. Diffuse pulmonary ossification in fibrosing interstitial lung diseases: prevalence and associations. Radiology. 2017;284:255–63.
16. Chilosi M, Carloni A, Rossi A, et al. Premature lung aging and cellular senescence in the pathogenesis of idiopathic pulmonary fibrosis and COPD/emphysema. Transl Res. 2013;162:156–73.
17. Tsai AP, English JC, Murphy D, Sin DD. Recurrent pneumothorax related to diffuse dendriform pulmonary ossification in genetically predisposed individual. Respirol Case Rep. 2016;5:e00211.
18. Travis WD, Matsui K, Moss J, Ferans VJ. Idiopathic nonspecific interstitial pneumonia: prognostic significance of cellular and fibrosing patterns. Am J Surg Pathol. 2000;24:19–33.
19. Frankel SK, Cool CD, Lynch DA, Brown KK. Idiopathic pleuroparenchymal fibroelastosis: description of a novel clinicopathologic entity. Chest. 2004;126:2007–13.
20. Oda T, Ogura T, Kitamyra H, et al. Distinct characteristics of pleuroparenchymal fibroelastosis with usual interstitial pneumonia compared with idiopathic pulmonary fibrosis. Chest. 2014;146:1248–55.
21. Chung JH, Cox CW, Montner SM, et al. CT features of the usual interstitial pneumonia pattern: differentiating connective tissue disease–associated interstitial lung disease from idiopathic pulmonary fibrosis. AJR. 2018;210:307–13.
22. Leslie KO, Trahan S, Gruden J. Pulmonary pathology of the rheumatic diseases. Semin Respir Crit Care Med. 2007;28:369–78.
23. Spagnolo P, Rossi G, Cavazza A, et al. Hypersensitivity pneumonitis: a comprehensive review. J Investig Allergol Clin Immunol. 2015;25:288–97.
24. Akashi T, Takemura T, Ando N, et al. Histopathologic analysis of sixteen autopsy cases of chronic hypersensitivity pneumonitis and comparison with idiopathic pulmonary fibrosis/usual interstitial pneumonia. Am J Clin Pathol. 2009;131:405–15.
25. Selman M, Pardo A, Barrera L, et al. Gene expression profiles distinguish idiopathic pulmonary fibrosis from hypersensitivity pneumonitis. Am J Respir Crit Care Med. 2006;173:188–98.
26. Yousem SA, Dacis S. Idiopathic bronchiolocentric interstitial pneumonia. Mod Pathol. 2002;15:1148–53.
27. Churg A, Myers J, Suarez T, et al. Airway-centered interstitial fibrosis: a distinct form of aggressive diffuse lung disease. Am J Surg Pathol. 2004;28:62–8.

28. Bouros D, Wells AU, Nicholson AG, et al. Histopathologic subsets of fibrosing alveolitis in patients with systemic sclerosis and their relationship to outcome. Am J Respir Crit Care Med. 2002;165:1581–6.
29. Strange C, Highland KB. Interstitial lung disease in the patient who has connective tissue disease. Clin Chest Med. 2004;25:549–59.
30. Kono M, Nakamura Y, Yoshimura K, et al. Nonspecific interstitial pneumonia preceding diagnosis of collagen vascular disease. Respir Med. 2016;117:40–7.
31. Romagnoli M, Nannini C, Piciucchi S, et al. Idiopathic nonspecific interstitial pneumonia: an interstitial lung disease associated with autoimmune disorder? Eur Respir J. 2011;38:384–91.
32. Torrealba JR, Fisher S, Kanne JP, Butt YM, Glazer C, Kershaw C, Burguete D, Gokaslan T, Batra K. Pathology-radiology correlation of common and uncommon computed tomographic patterns of organizing pneumonia. Hum Pathol. 2018;71:30–40.
33. Katzeinstein A. Smoking-related interstitial fibrosis-SRIF: pathologic findings and distinction from other chronic fibrosing lung diseases. J Clin Pathol. 2013;66:882–7.
34. Katzeinstein A-LA, Mukhopadhyay S, Zanardi S. Clinically occult interstitial fibrosis in smokers: classification and significance of a surprisingly common finding in lobectomy specimens. Hum Pathol. 2010;41:316–25.
35. Ravaglia C, Wells AU, Tomassetti S, Gurioli C, Gurioli C, Dubini A, Cavazza A, Colby TV, Piciucchi S, Puglisi S, Bosi M, Poletti V. Diagnostic yield and risk/benefit analysis of trans-bronchial lung cryobiopsy in diffuse parenchymal lung diseases: a large cohort of 699 patients. BMC Pulm Med. 2019;19(1):16.

Multidisciplinary Discussion in Diffuse Parenchymal Lung Disease

Silvia Puglisi, Jay H. Ryu, Sara Tomassetti, and Venerino Poletti

3.1 Introduction

Interstitial lung disease (ILD) is a heterogeneous group of disorders with varying clinical-radiological presentation and evolution. The most common idiopathic ILD is IPF which has an unpredictable clinical course, including cases with slowly progressive decline and cases with rapid deterioration. Prognosis is poor, with a median survival of 3–5 years. In the last decade, many advances have been made in the understanding of IPF pathogenesis, and two antifibrotic drugs, pirfenidone [1] and nintedanib [2], have become available for IPF treatment. In this context, an accurate IPF diagnosis is of particular importance to optimize the care of patients with ILDs, discriminating those who may benefit from steroid and immunosuppressive treatments from IPF patients for whom the immunosuppressive therapy may be detrimental. The ATS/ERS/ JRS/ALAT guidelines emphasize the importance of the multidisciplinary team (MDT) diagnosis to correctly identify IPF patients [3]. The MDT should be composed of specialists of relevant disciplines, to integrate all available clinical, radiological, and pathological data.

3.2 The Past: The Role of Histology and Radiology

Before the recognition of the multidisciplinary diagnosis as the gold standard for ILD diagnosis, pathology was considered the reference standard for many years. The preeminent role of pathology was based on two historical developments. Firstly, Averill Liebow, the founding father of modern lung pathology, was the first to classify the interstitial lung diseases in 1965, and the current classification of ILDs still takes its root from this classification scheme [4]. Secondly, several studies proved that pathology carries important prognostic information, particularly distinguishing usual interstitial pneumonia (UIP) form other patterns [5].

However pathology in the diagnosis of ILDs has several limitations and alone is patently insufficient. It has been shown that the interobserver agreement between pathologists in ILD diagnosis is poor, with an overall kappa value of only 0.38 for the first-choice diagnosis, and a high confidence diagnosis could be achieved by expert pathologists in only 39% of cases [6].

S. Puglisi · S. Tomassetti
Department of Diseases of the Thorax,
Ospedale Morgagni-Pierantoni, Forlì, Italy

J. H. Ryu
Pulmonary and Critical Care Medicine, Mayo Clinic,
Rochester, MN, USA

V. Poletti (✉)
Department of Diseases of the Thorax,
Ospedale Morgagni-Pierantoni, Forlì, Italy

Department of Respiratory Diseases and Allergy,
Aarhus University Hospital, Aarhus, Denmark

© Springer Nature Switzerland AG 2019
V. Poletti (ed.), *Transbronchial cryobiopsy in diffuse parenchymal lung disease*,
https://doi.org/10.1007/978-3-030-14891-1_3

Other limitation of histopathology is related to the observation that two or more biopsies taken from the same patient can manifest divergent histopathological patterns as described by Flaherty et al. [7]. With regard to the histological distinction between UIP and nonspecific interstitial pneumonia (NSIP), 26% of patients presented different histopathological patterns in different lobes, proving that the UIP diagnosis based on a single lung specimen from one lobe can be misleading.

As for radiology, the level of interobserver agreement among practising thoracic radiologists in the diagnosis of idiopathic interstitial pneumonias (IIPs) has been estimated by Aziz et al. as moderate or very good on the basis of HRCT features, especially for IPF [8]. Several other studies have reported on the interobserver agreement for a CT diagnosis of IPF/UIP with conflicting results. All of these studies involved thoracic radiologists with high expertise in the interpretation of diffuse parenchymal lung diseases on CT [9].

Walsh et al. showed that interobserver agreement for the ATS/ERS/JRS/ALAT CT criteria for UIP among an international group of thoracic radiologists of varying levels of experience is at best moderate and is not significantly increased among thoracic radiologists with greater levels of experience. The most frequent diagnostic difficulty in the interpretation of CT scan was the separation of patients with IPF/UIP, fibrotic NSIP, and CHP which can only be achieved based on CT appearances alone in approximately 50% of cases [10].

Several studies have shown that radiology alone is patently insufficient to discriminate IPF form other fibrotic ILDs, when IPF doesn't have the typical UIP pattern appearance. Sverzellati et al. showed that three expert radiologists, blinded to any clinical information, when asked to make an IPF diagnosis on the basis of CT scan, missed it in 62% of cases. Among 123 patients with various chronic ILDs, including a core group of 55 biopsy-proved cases of IPF, 34 (62%) of 55 biopsy-proved IPF cases were regarded as alternative diagnoses, and the first-choice diagnoses, expressed with high probability, were NSIP (53%), chronic hypersensitivity

pneumonitis (HP, 12%), sarcoidosis (9%), and organizing pneumonia (3%). This study clearly demonstrates that CT scan findings when nondiagnostic for UIP may overlap with other ILDs [11]. Similarly Flaherty et al. showed that 26 (35%) of 73 patients with UIP at biopsy had a thin-section CT appearance more akin to that of NSIP [12].

The recognition of the limitations in using pathology, clinical evaluation, and radiology data in isolation led to the creation and implementation of multidisciplinary discussion of ILD cases. Several other studies have reported on the interobserver agreement for a CT diagnosis of IPF/UIP with conflicting results. All of these studies involved thoracic radiologists with high expertise in the interpretation of diffuse lung diseases on CT [9].

3.3   The MDT

The multidisciplinary diagnosis is a dynamic process that requires the integration of clinical, radiologic, and pathologic data. The benefits of integrating radiological, histopathological, and clinical data in IIPs diagnosis have been reported in several studies. Flaherty et al. demonstrated that a consensus diagnosis, reached after exchange of clinical, radiological, and histopathologic information, often differs from the initial diagnosis reached by the individual clinician, radiologist, or pathologist working in isolation, leading to the idea of a multidisciplinary approach to the IIP diagnosis might be more accurate. Radiologists, pathologists, and chest physicians took part in this study and were allowed to change their initial diagnosis as more information were added. Physicians changed more often their initial diagnosis when patients had a clinical and radiographic scenario suggestive of non-IPF IIP, while in patients with a presentation considered typical for IPF, the diagnosis was accurate in more than 95% of cases emphasizing the central role for HRCT in the cases presenting with the UIP radiologic pattern.

When clinical and radiological information were added, pathologists changed their diagnosis in 19% of cases. This result empathizes the importance of combining histological, radiological, and clinical data and that neither radiology nor histology alone can provide a secure diagnosis of ILD. The level of agreement was particularly high between radiologists, even if they changed more frequently their diagnosis compared to clinicians after revision of histological data. The level of agreement between all participants improved with discussion and with the addition of subsequent clinical, radiological and particularly pathological information, thus confirming the importance of integrating those information in the dynamic scenario of multidisciplinary team discussion [13].

Similarly Thomeer et al. showed that although the level of agreement between radiologists for IPF diagnosis was only moderate (κw = 0.40) and the level of agreement between pathologists was fair (κw = 0.30), the overall accuracy of the multidisciplinary team diagnosis of IPF was good (87.2%). The IPF diagnosis proposed by chest physician was rejected in 12.8% of cases after the revision of CT scan and pathological data by groups of radiologist expert committee, underlining the importance of MDT in the correct diagnosis [14].

The 2002 ATS/ERS classification of IIPs [15], the 2013 update, and the 2011 guidelines [3] for the diagnosis of IPF strongly recommend the interaction and information exchange between radiologists, pathologists, and clinicians to reach the final diagnosis. Thus, the MDT is proposed as the gold standard for ILD diagnosis. Despite ERS/ATS recommendations, no guideline statement regulating MDT has been published, and there are some unresolved issues regarding the composition of the MDT, its governance, its validation, the selection of cases to be discussed, its purpose, and the optimal frequency of the MDT meetings (MDTM).

The first study evaluating the level of agreement between international multidisciplinary teams (MDTs) of experts in IIPs since the 2013 ATS/ERS update was conducted by Walsh et al. [16]. In this study each MDT, consisting of at least 1 clinician, radiologist, and pathologist, from 7 countries (Denmark, France, Italy, Japan, the Netherlands, Portugal, and the UK), evaluated

70 cases of interstitial lung disease in a two-stage process: (1) the radiologist, pathologist, and clinician independently evaluated each case and selected up to five differential diagnoses from a group of ILDs. Clinicians had only access to clinical information and high-resolution CT scan without report or pathology results. Radiologists and pathologists just knew age, sex, and smoking status for the patient with high-resolution CT (for radiologist) and digitalized surgical lung biopsy slides (pathologist). (2) These specialists participated in MDT reviewing all data and selecting up to five differential diagnoses. The inter-MDT agreement on diagnostic likelihoods was good for IPF (weighted kappa coefficient (κw) of 0.71, interquartile range (IQR) 0.64–0.77) and connective tissue disease (CTD)-related ILD (κw = 0.73, IQR 0.68–0.78), moderate for NSIP (κw = 0.42, IQR 0.37–0.49), and fair for HP (κw = 0.29, IQR 0.24–0.40). High-confidence diagnoses of IPF were given in 77% of cases by MDT, in 65% of cases by clinicians, and in 66% of cases by radiologists showing that inter-MDT agreement for the diagnosis of IPF is good, with clinicians having only marginally lower levels of agreement than MDTs for this diagnosis. Compared to clinicians or radiologists, MDT made diagnosis of IPF with high confidence more frequently. In patients without surgical lung biopsy, inter-MDT agreement and interobserver agreement between clinicians for the diagnosis of IPF were similar (κw = 0.71 [IQR 0.64–0.77]), thus implying that in cases in which the clinical-radiological scenario of IPF is sound and clear, the MD discussion of cases has a marginal role and probably can be neglected.

By contrast, MDT agreement for the diagnosis of HP and NSIP was low (κ value, respectively, κw = 0.29 [0.24–0.40], NSIP κw = 0.42 [0.37–0.49]) (in both cases with or without lung biopsy), reflecting the urgent need for clarity and standardized diagnostic international criteria.

Diagnostic agreement between MDTs was higher compared to agreement between clinicians, radiologists, and pathologists in the setting of ILDs, especially assessing IPF diagnosis. Moreover, the good diagnostic accuracy of MDT diagnosis was validated by the nonsignificant greater prognostic separation of an IPF diagnosis made by MDTs than by individual specialists; in particular a significant prognostic separation was observed in seven of seven MDTs (HR 2.61–5.30 $p < 0.05$), in five of seven clinician teams, and in four of seven radiologist teams. The same analysis for pathologist team was not significant probably due to the small number of cases.

3.4 Composition of MDT

Despite the clear utility and importance of ILD-MDTs, the constitution and governance of these meetings have not been explicitly addressed. Based on the original studies by Flaherty et al. [13], it might be suggested that MDT should at a minimum be composed by a clinician, a radiologist, and a pathologist. In recent times, more expansive models including rheumatologists, thoracic surgeons, and ILD nurses have been suggested. The role of the rheumatologists in the MDTs has been investigated in a recent study showing that among seven international expert multidisciplinary groups evaluating ILD cases, new diagnoses of CTD-ILD were constructed in approximately 10% of patients [16]. The authors of this study suggest that rheumatologists should take part in MDT because some patients present with subtle clinical features or serological abnormalities that imply an autoimmune process without meeting established criteria for a specific CTD. Recently, an ERS/ATS task force was formed in order to establish consensus on how to classify these patients, and specific diagnostic criteria were established to define cases of interstitial pneumonia with autoimmune features (IPAF) lacking the criteria for a specific rheumatologic disease [17].

Determining whether a patient has a diagnosis of CTD-ILD rather than IIP may impact treatment decisions and influence prognosis, especially in cases presenting with UIP pattern on CT scan that may be difficult to differentiate from IPF. Despite the fact that IPF antifibrotic drugs have been recently tested in clinical trials for CTD-ILD treatment, the treatment of IPF and CTD-ILD remains strikingly divergent, and the use of antifibrotic is still not approved in CTD-ILDs. Currently CTD-ILDs are treated with immunosuppression [18] in contrast to IPF, in which immunosuppression is ineffective or potentially harmful [19]. CTD-ILDs occur most commonly in the context of an established CTD, but can be the first and/or only manifestation of an occult CTD or occur in patients who have features suggestive of an autoimmune process, but not meeting diagnostic criteria for a defined CTD (IPAF) [17]. The identification of IPAF or of some complex CTD-ILDs cases requires the combination of specific clinical, serologic, and morphologic features. The identification of IPAF patients and the difficulties related to clinical diagnosis of some CTD cases may require the rheumatologist evaluation; this implies that rheumatologist should participate in MDT discussions only after a careful clinical evaluation of the patient.

3.5 MDT Diagnosis Is Influenced by Components

Although MDTM diagnoses are more confident and they reach higher levels of agreement compared to individual participants, the performance of the MDT is dependent on the experience of its components, as demonstrated by Flaherty et al. who evaluated the diagnostic agreement between academic and community-based physicians in ILD diagnosis in an interactive approach involving radiologists, clinicians, and pathologists and found a significant disagreement between academic-based clinicians and community-based physicians. The most evident discordance was for the evaluation of cases of HP, NSIP, and IPF. Final diagnostic agreement was higher between academic physicians (κ 0.55–0.71) and community physicians (κ 0.11–0.56). Interestingly, community pathologists were more influenced in their final diagnosis by interaction with clinicians and radiologists compared to academic pathologists. This study also showed that academic physicians in a multidisciplinary setting display better diagnostic agreement and consider a greater range of diagnoses, compared to community physicians [20].

Walsh et al. have recently conducted an international study aimed to evaluate the importance of expertise in the MDT diagnosis of IPF made by nonacademic clinicians, university-affiliated clinicians, and an international panel of IPF experts using three surrogates of diagnostic accuracy: diagnostic confidence, diagnostic agreement, and prognostic accuracy. No randomized trials have ever been conducted to demonstrate MDT diagnosis results in improved patient survival. In the absence of a reference standard, separations in mortality between patients diagnosed with IPF and those diagnosed with other ILDs have been used to evaluate the diagnostic skills of clinicians. A total of 1141 respiratory physicians and 34 IPF experts participated to the study, evaluating 60 cases of ILDs without interdisciplinary consultation.

Accuracy of IPF diagnosis made by university hospital-based practitioners with greater than 20 years of experience was equivalent to that of international IPF experts, proving that academic status and experience level of physicians are independently associated with greater prognostic discrimination between diagnoses of IPF and other ILDs. Participating in weekly MDT meetings by nonacademic physicians increased prognostic accuracy of IPF diagnosis to that achieved by IPF experts [21].

MDT diagnosis is defined as a "consensus" among participants and may be influenced by individual personalities in the dynamics of MDT so that the final diagnosis may ultimately be more reflective of the strongest voice in the room. Jo et al. conducted a study among 12 expert centres based on an internet questionnaire regarding the constitution and governance of their MDT. Interestingly, chest physicians adopted a dominant role in MDT diagnosis in 90% of meetings, and for 70% of cases, the referring physician was also responsible for documenting the diagnosis. Just in 30% of cases, the final diagnosis was left to the clinician following multidisciplinary discussion [22].

3.6 Final Scope of MTD

A great debate is ongoing regarding the role of MDT meetings in the evaluation of patients with ILDs. In oncology, multidisciplinary boards are widely applied and have demonstrated a sig-

nificant impact on treatment decisions through collaboration between specialists, including palliative care. In contrast, the role of MDT in ILDs is limited to the diagnostic evaluation even though there is an increasing range of therapeutic choices for ILDs, including antifibrotic therapy for IPF, antigen avoidance for chronic hypersensitivity pneumonitis, immune suppression for inflammatory and connective tissue disease-related ILD, and lung transplantation and palliative care in case of end-stage lung disease [23].

Therapeutic choices available, including the availability of active clinical trials, patient's own wishes, and clinical context including frailty, have a great impact on the MDTM decision. In addition to evaluating new cases, revising diagnoses based upon disease behaviour and response to therapy is an important role of MDTM discussion especially for patients whose disease behaviour is unexpected and could not have been predicted on initial assessment. Revisiting existing diagnoses on the basis of clinical behaviour and evolution may lead to change the initial diagnosis and to change therapeutic approach.

3.6.1 Comparison Between Cryobiopsy and Surgical Biopsy in MDT Discussion

Surgical lung biopsy (SLB) is still considered an important diagnostic step in the diagnosis of ILDs when the clinical-radiological features are not specific even though SLB has never been validated as a gold standard test. However surgical lung biopsy is associated with significant mortality (2–4%) and adverse effects such as chronic chest pain observed in more than 50% of the cases lasting for months, prolonged air leakage, infections, and prolonged hospitalization [24]. In addition, many patients with suspected ILD may be unable to undergo SLB because of their comorbidities, even if histopathological confirmation may be helpful to reach the correct diagnosis. For all those reasons, SLB is obtained in <15% of ILD cases, and the indication to biopsy has to be carefully considered by the MDT. Regarding the interobserver agreement in SLBs, some studies have shown that it is higher ($\kappa = 0.42$) when UIP pattern is identified; but is low when NSIP pattern ($\kappa = 0.29$) or chronic HP patterns ($\kappa = 0.36$) are evaluated [6].

Transbronchial cryobiopsy is a new diagnostic approach recently introduced into clinical practice as a promising and less invasive alternative to SLB to diagnose ILDs. Cryobiopsy allows attainment of larger, higher quality lung tissue samples without the crush artefacts seen with conventional transbronchial lung biopsy using flexible forceps [25]. It has been shown that the specimen size is directly related to the diagnostic yield and the sampling of different segments of the same lobe appears to increase the diagnostic confidence or at least to reduce the number of samples needed to identify the UIP pattern [26].

A recent study by Casoni et al. has also demonstrated that pathologists can detect UIP pattern with high confidence in about half of the cases with a very good overall interobserver agreement [27]. Our group reported a sensitivity for UIP detected by transbronchial forceps biopsy of only 30% for expert pathologists, and these data have recently been confirmed in a study that found transbronchial forceps biopsy useful to reach a confident and accurate multidisciplinary diagnosis in only 20–30% of patients with ILDs, with the majority of cases requiring SLB to reach a definite diagnosis. In suspected cases of non-IPF, particularly HP and NSIP, the diagnosis is much more difficult, and in this setting, transbronchial forceps biopsy has little role, with a negative predictive value for a UIP diagnosis ranging between 46 and 55% [28].

In a recent study, we evaluated the impact of the addition of transbronchial cryobiopsy/SLB information to the multidisciplinary diagnosis of ILDs. Transbronchial cryobiopsy increased diagnostic confidence in the multidisciplinary diagnosis of IPF and also increased self-reported confidence levels, to a similar extent compared to SLB. Specifically, the proportion of IPF cases diagnosed with a high degree of confidence increased from 16 to 63% after adding cryobiopsy [29]. Moreover, cryobiopsy changed the initial clinical-radiological impression in 26% of cases, reclassifying 73% of those as IPF. In line with previously published studies, these data

show that in cases in which the initial clinical-radiological scenario is inconclusive, pathology adds the most important piece of information, regardless if it is obtained by surgery or transbronchial cryobiopsy.

3.7 Conclusion

According to the current ATS/ERS/JRS/ALAT guidelines, the MDT consensus has replaced histopathology alone as the gold standard for the diagnosis of ILDs. MDT discussion of cases improves diagnostic confidence and agreement compared to individual observers. However, no guidelines exist in literature to describe in detail how the MDTs should be conducted and many of the specifics remain unclear. There are no published guidelines concerning the composition, frequency of MDTs, or the kind of ILD cases that really need to be discussed. There is a need for evidence-based clinical guidelines regarding the constitution and governance to reach the best clinical outcomes [30, 31].

References

1. Noble PW, Albera C, Bradford WZ, et al. Pirfenidone in patients with idiopathic pulmonary fibrosis (CAPACITY): two randomized trials. Lancet. 2011;377:1760–9.
2. Richeldi L, Costabel U, Selman M, et al. Efficacy of a tyrosine kinase inhibitor in idiopathic pulmonary fibrosis. N Engl J Med. 2011;365:1079–87.
3. Raghu G, Collard HR, Egan JJ, et al. An official ATS/ERS/JRS/ALAT statement: idiopathic pulmonary fibrosis: evidence-based guidelines for diagnosis and management. Am J Respir Crit Care Med. 2011;183:788–824.
4. Smith GJ. Averill Abraham Liebow: contributions to pulmonary pathology. Yale J Biol Med. 1981;54(2):139–46.
5. Katzenstein AL, Myers JL. Idiopathic pulmonary fibrosis: clinical relevance of pathologic classification. Am J Respir Crit Care Med. 1998;157:1301–15.
6. Nicholson AG, Addis BJ, Bharucha H, et al. Interobserver variation between pathologists in diffuse parenchymal lung disease. Thorax. 2004;59:500–5.
7. Flaherty KR, Travis WD, Colby TV, et al. Histopathologic variability in usual and nonspecific interstitial pneumonias. Am J Respir Crit Care Med. 2001;164:1722–7.

8. Aziz ZA, Wells AU, Hansell DM, et al. HRCT diagnosis of diffuse parenchymal lung disease: interobserver variation. Thorax. 2004;59:506–11.
9. Lynch DA, Godwin JD, Safrin S, et al. High-resolution computed tomography in idiopathic pulmonary fibrosis: diagnosis and prognosis. Am J Respir Crit Care Med. 2005;172:488–93.
10. Walsh SL, Calandriello L, Sverzellati N, Wells AU, Hansell DM, UIP Observer Consort. Interobserver agreement for the ATS/ERS/JRS/ALAT criteria for a UIP pattern on CT. Thorax. 2016;71:45–51.
11. Sverzellati N, Wells AU, Tomassetti S, et al. Biopsy-proved idiopathic pulmonary fibrosis: spectrum of nondiagnostic thin-section CT diagnoses. Radiology. 2010;254(3):957–64.
12. Flaherty KR, Thwaite EL, Kazerooni EA, et al. Radiological versus histological diagnosis in UIP and NSIP: survival implications. Thorax. 2003;58(2):143–8.
13. Flaherty KR, King TE Jr, Raghu G, et al. Idiopathic interstitial pneumonia: what is the effect of a multidisciplinary approach to diagnosis? Am J Respir Crit Care Med. 2004;170:904–10.
14. Thomeer M, Demedts M, Behr J, et al. Multidisciplinary interobserver agreement in the diagnosis of idiopathic pulmonary fibrosis. Eur Respir J. 2008;31:585–91.
15. American Thoracic Society, European Respiratory Society. American Thoracic Society/European Respiratory Society international multidisciplinary consensus classification of the idiopathic interstitial pneumonias. Am J Respir Crit Care Med. 2002;165:277–304.
16. Walsh SL, Wells AU, Desai SR, et al. Multicentre evaluation of multidisciplinary team meeting agreement on diagnosis in diffuse parenchymal lung disease: a case–cohort study. Lancet Respir Med. 2016;4:557–65.
17. Fischer A, Antoniou KM, Brown KK, et al. An official European Respiratory Society/American Thoracic Society research statement: interstitial pneumonia with autoimmune features. Eur Respir J. 2015;46:976–87.
18. Fischer A, Krishnamoorthy M, Olson AL, Solomon JJ, Fernandez-Perez ER, Huie TJ, et al. Mycophenolate mofetil (MMF) in various interstitial lung diseases (abstract). Am J Respir Crit Care Med. 2012;185:A3638.
19. PANTHER National Heart Lung and Blood Institute. Commonly used three-drug regimen for idiopathic pulmonary fibrosis found harmful. www.nih.gov/news/health/oct2011/nhlbi-21.htm. Accessed 2 Nov 2011.
20. Flaherty KR, Andrei AC, King TE Jr, Raghu G, Colby TV, Wells A, et al. Idiopathic interstitial pneumonia: do community and academic physicians agree on diagnosis? Am J Respir Crit Care Med. 2007;175(10):1054–60.
21. Walsh LFS, Maher TM, Kolb M, et al. Diagnostic accuracy if a clinical diagnosis of idiopathic pulmonary fibrosis: an international case cohort study. Eur Respir J. 2017;50:1700936.
22. Jo HE, Corte TJ, Moodley Y, et al. Evaluating the interstitial lung disease multidisciplinary meeting: a survey of expert centres. BMC Pulm Med. 2016;16:22.
23. Caminati A, Cassandro R, Torre O, Harari S. Severe idiopathic pulmonary fibrosis: what can be done? Eur Respir Rev. 2017;26(145).
24. Hutchinson JP, Fogarty AW, McKeever TM, et al. In-hospital mortality after surgical lung biopsy for interstitial lung disease in the United States. 2000 to 2011. Am J Respir Crit Care Med. 2016;193:1161–7.
25. Poletti V, Ravaglia C, Gurioli C, et al. Invasive diagnostic techniques in idiopathic interstitial pneumonias. Respirology. 2016;21:44–50.
26. Ravaglia C, Wells AU, Tomassetti S, et al. Transbronchial lung cryobiopsy in diffuse parenchymal lung disease: comparison between biopsy from 1 segment and biopsy from 2 segments—diagnostic yield complications. Respiration. 2017;93(4):285–92.
27. Casoni GL, Tomassetti S, Cavazza A, Colby TV, Dubini A, Ryu JH, Carretta E, Tantalocco P, Piciucchi S, Ravaglia C, et al. Transbronchial lung cryobiopsy in the diagnosis of fibrotic interstitial lung diseases. PLoS One. 2014;9:e86716.
28. Tomassetti S, Cavazza A, Colby TV, et al. Transbronchial biopsy is useful in predicting UIP pattern. Respir Res. 2012;13:96.
29. Tomassetti S, Wells AU, Costabel U, et al. Bronchoscopic lung cryobiopsy increases diagnostic confidence in the multidisciplinary diagnosis of idiopathic pulmonary fibrosis. Am J Respir Crit Care Med. 2016;193:745–52.
30. Cottin V, Castillo D, Poletti V, Kreuter M, Corte TJ, Spagnolo P. Should patients with interstitial lung disease be seen by experts? Chest. 2018;154:713–4.
31. Richeldi L, Launders N, Marrtinez F, Walsh SLF, Myers J, Wang B, et al. The characterisation of interstitial lung disease multidisciplinary team meetings: a pilot study. EJR Open Res. In press.

Part II

Transbronchial Cryobiopsy

Cryobiopsy: Physics

4

Sara Colella

4.1 Introduction: Cold Temperatures in Lung Diseases

Cold temperatures have been used in medicine for several decades, mainly for therapeutic purposes in several fields [1]; in the airway, cold temperatures were initially used to restore airway patency from endobronchial tumours [2] and further on were used in other diseases such as benign central airway obstructions or for the treatment of low-grade endobronchial malignancy [3]. Compared to other debulking techniques, cryotherapy does not show an immediate result since it needs a second procedure to remove the treated tissue. Cryoextraction, that is, the use of cold temperature to remove tissues, was subsequently developed to remove an endobronchial lesion immediately, without the need of a clean-up bronchoscopy: this procedure is useful for therapeutic purposes in endoluminal obstructions and also in foreign body removal. It has become a diagnostic tool in the place of conventional endobronchial biopsy with forceps since samples obtained with cryoextraction were found in selected cases more suitable for histological and molecular analyses [4]. Thus, the use of cold temperatures led to observe larger and better-quality specimens with no

or few morphologic crush artefacts, and this opened the way to transbronchial lung cryobiopsy (TBLC) in the diagnostic algorithm of diffuse parenchymal lung diseases [5].

4.2 Physic Principle of TBLC

The operating principle of TBLC differs from other endoscopic lung biopsy techniques such as transbronchial biopsy (TBB) with conventional forceps or with jumbo forceps: cryoprobes use very low temperatures, below the freezing point, to obtain lung specimens.

The underlining physic principle is the "Joule-Thomson" effect: it is a phenomenon in which the temperature of a real gas increases or decreases following, respectively, its compression or its expansion—as a result from a pressure difference—that is carried out without extracting a work.

4.3 "Joule-Thomson" Effect in TBLC

The "Joule-Thomson" effect works through a cryoequipment consisting of a tank that contains the cooling agents—liquefied gas, a footswitch that allows the release of the gas, and a cryoprobe where the gas is finally released, with a consequent freeze of the lung tissue around the probe.

S. Colella (✉)
Pulmonary Unit, Ascoli Piceno, Italy

© Springer Nature Switzerland AG 2019
V. Poletti (ed.), *Transbronchial cryobiopsy in diffuse parenchymal lung disease*,
https://doi.org/10.1007/978-3-030-14891-1_4

In comparison to TBB with forceps, the obtained specimens are significantly larger and contain more alveolated tissue and with fewer morphological artefacts, and this entails a better interpretation of the biopsy [6].

The physics of the biopsy process is influenced by several factors such as the type of the cryogenic gas used, the tissue cryosentitivity, which probe is used and its activation time, and the thawing phase.

4.3.1 Cryogenic Gases

The cooling agents used in TBLC are the carbon dioxide (CO_2) or the nitric oxide (N_2O): both are liquefied under high pressure in a tank, and no differences in the working mechanism of the two gases are found, but there are differences in terms of temperatures reached, costs, and occupational exposure.

The cryogenic effect of CO_2 is less pronounced than the one of N_2O, since a drop of temperature to minus 75 °C is reached with CO_2 and to minus 89 °C with the N_2O [7].

A list of the cooling gases used in some studies with the corresponding freezing times is shown in Table 4.1.

CO_2 is less costly than N_2O [14] and its use appears to be safer for the operators. Indeed, the use of N_2O could raise some concerns regarding the occupational exposure because an exhausting system is needed, and thus CO_2 has been proposed as a valid alternative [15].

Moreover, another property of CO_2 is that when it cools, a mixture of its gaseous and solid form is created, the so-called CO_2 snow [16].

Table 4.1 Cryogenic gases and temperatures reached

Author	Cooling gas	Temperature (°C)
Almeida, 2017 [8]	N_2O	−85
Echevarria-Uraga, 2016 [9]	N_2O	−89
Ravaglia, 2016 [10]	CO_2	−75
Gershman, 2015 [11]	N_2O	−89
Griff, 2014 [12]	CO_2	−77
Casoni, 2014 [13]	CO_2	−75

4.3.2 Tissue Cryosensitivity

Different tissues have different sensitivities to cold temperatures: this characteristic, also called cryosensitivity, depends mainly on the tissue water content and the microcirculation—tissues composed of a higher water content are more prone to be frozen [5]. For example, because of their higher water content and vascularization, the skin, granulation tissue, or tumour tissue is more cryosensitive than fat, cartilage, or collagen.

About the lung, structures located in the central airways have a different composition from peripheral lung parenchyma because the latter has lower connective tissue content, and therefore it is easier to freeze whilst the bronchial wall is less susceptible to cold due to the higher rate of connective tissue. This different tissue composition may also explain the bleeding that is a common complication of TBLC: because of the lack of complete cartilaginous structures in the middle third part of the lung, taking a biopsy from those zones may result in a higher bleeding risk since the vasculature could be damaged [17].

4.3.3 Probes

Cryoprobes are available in two diameters, 1.9 and 2.4 mm: obviously, because the 2.4 mm probe is larger, it provides larger samples than the 1.9 mm, and in order for the sample dimension to be equal with different probes, a longer freezing time is needed with the smaller one (1.9 mm) [5].

Moreover, since the cold has a concentric expansion, the optimal position of the probe is perpendicular to the biopsy site; however this is not always possible to ensure.

Lastly, the biopsy size may be increased when the probe was pressed on the tissue during cooling [18].

4.3.4 Activation of the Probe

Once the probe is activated, the cooling gas goes from the tank to the tip of the probe where it is released at atmospheric pressure and is propagated

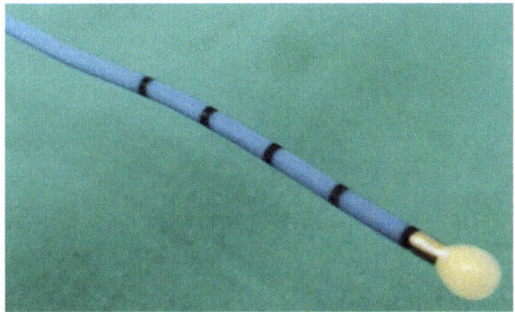

Fig. 4.1 The "iceball" with a 2.4 mm probe, activation time: 10 s

within the surrounding lung tissue, with a concentric propagation of the frozen zone that radiates from the probe. The lung tissue is then quickly frozen, within few seconds, and this frozen lung tissue is called "iceball" (Fig. 4.1).

The longer activation time, the larger the specimen will be: indeed, there is a positive correlation between freezing time and cross-sectional biopsy area [4], since a prolonged activation time will result in an increased weight and diameter of the cryobiopsies; thus, by increasing freezing times, a larger surface area and subsequently larger biopsies can be generated [19].

4.3.5 Thawing Phase

Once the probe is taken away from the airway, the "iceball" could be removed from the tip of the probe: now starts the thawing phase that occurs relatively slowly in a hand-warmed water bath with a gentle removal of the tissue from the probe—with the aid of a needle, for example—in order to minimize damages.

4.4 The "Joule-Thomson" Effect on Living Tissues: Mechanism of Tissue Damage

Despite the mechanism of cell damage of cryotherapy is well known, the tissue damages created in TBLC were poorly investigated.

Cell destruction during cryotherapy occurs with two different mechanisms: an immediate and a delayed injury. The immediate damages are due to the formation of extra- and intracellular ice crystals that damage the organelles and the cell membrane with consequent transcellular fluid shift (mechanical damage). The delayed injury is due to a local vasoconstriction and thrombosis with consequent ischaemia (vascular damage): when the circulation is restored in the thawing phase, a hyperaemic response with consequent oedema, increasing capillary permeability, platelet aggregation, and micro-thrombi formation are observed, and those lead to the apoptosis, promoted by DNA fragmentation, cytokine release, inflammation, and ischemic injury (immunological mechanism) [1].

As already said, the cell survivability depends also on the thawing phase: a greater number of cells is observed to survive when higher thawing temperatures are employed because there is a lower probability of recrystallization, and if the freezing takes place again, like in cryotherapy, the size of crystals is smaller [20]. Finally, the more freezing-thawing cycles are performed, the more destructive effects on living tissue will be.

However, the above-mentioned mechanisms lead to irreversible tissue damage, useful to treat endobronchial lesions, whilst the aim of TBLC is not to destroy tissue but to collect and preserve it. The optimal temperature and time in the freezing process that has to be correlated to the biological damage rather than to the tissue preservation is not known [20].

Evidences to explain cell survivability could be extrapolated from studies conducted in cryosurgery, but some differences have to be underlined in comparison to TBLC: in TBLC higher temperatures—but below zero in both cases—are employed, only one freeze-thaw cycle is performed, and the thawing phase is passive and slow.

Some studies have investigated the relation between cooling rate and direct cell damage [21]. The extracellular and intracellular ice formation occurs, respectively, during slow and rapid freezing rate: so, a characteristic shape of survival curve has been hypothesized (Fig. 4.2), in

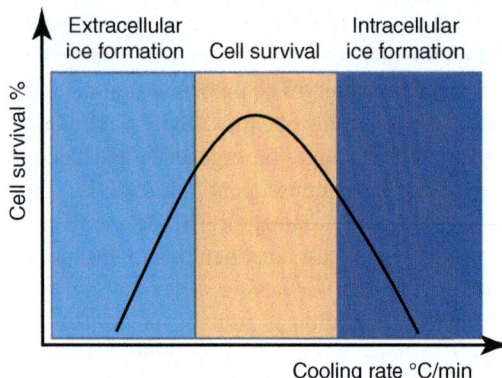

Fig. 4.2 The survival curve of cells depending on the cooling rate

which there are two domains of tissue damage at the extreme part of the curve and an intermediate domain in which the range of cooling rates for cells survival is optimal. Which is the exact rate of cooling that creates the extracellular ice formation rather than the intracellular ice or the cell survival is unknown.

Moreover, the cells closer to the probe are more susceptible to cold temperatures, whilst further away near the edge of the ice front, cooling rates are lower and fewer cells are killed because little ice crystallization takes place [20].

To sum up, the exact mechanism of tissue damage in TBLC is not known: some hypotheses could be done starting from studies about cryotherapy, but further research is needed to better elucidate this point.

References

1. Colella S, Ravaglia C, Tomassett S, Gurioli CH, Gurioli C, Poletti V. Cryotherapy: application in the airways. In: Diaz-Jimenez JP, Rodriguez AN, editors. Interventions in pulmonary medicine. Cham: Springer; 2018.
2. Maiwand MO. Cryotherapy for advanced carcinoma of the trachea and bronchi. Br Med J (Clin Res Ed). 1986;293(6540):181–2.
3. DiBardino DM, Lanfranco AR, Haas AR. Bronchoscopic cryotherapy. Clinical applications of the cryoprobe, cryospray, and cryoadhesion. Ann Am Thorac Soc. 2016;13(8):1405–15.
4. Hetzel J, Eberhardt R, Herth FJ, Petermann C, Reichle G, Freitag L, Dobbertin I, Franke KJ, Stanzel F, Beyer T, Möller P, Fritz P, Ott G, Schnabel PA, Kastendieck H, Lang W, Morresi-Hauf AT, Szyrach MN, Muche R, Shah PL, Babiak A, Hetzel M. Cryobiopsy increases the diagnostic yield of endobronchial biopsy: a multicentre trial. Eur Respir J. 2012;39(3): 685–90.
5. Poletti V, Casoni GL, Gurioli C, Ryu JH, Tomassetti S. Lung cryobiopsies: a paradigm shift in diagnostic bronchoscopy? Respirology. 2014;19(5):645–54.
6. Griff S, Ammenwerth W, Schönfeld N, Bauer TT, Mairinger T, Blum TG, Kollmeier J, Grüning W. Morphometrical analysis of transbronchial cryobiopsies. Diagn Pathol. 2011;6:53.
7. Poletti V, Hetzel J. Transbronchial cryobiopsy in diffuse parenchymal lung disease: need for procedural standardization. Respiration. 2015;90(4):275–8.
8. Almeida LM, Lima B, Mota PC, Melo N, Magalhães A, Pereira JM, Moura CS, Guimarães S, Morais A. Learning curve for transbronchial lung cryobiopsy in diffuse lung disease. Rev Port Pneumol (2006). 2017. pii: S2173-5115(17)30148-3. https://doi.org/10.1016/j.rppnen.2017.09.005.
9. Echevarria-Uraga JJ, Pérez-Izquierdo J, García-Garai N, Gómez-Jiménez E, Aramburu-Ojembarrena A, Tena-Tudanca L, Miguélez-Vidales JL, Capelastegui-Saiz A. Usefulness of an angioplasty balloon as selective bronchial blockade device after transbronchial cryobiopsy. Respirology. 2016;21(6):1094–9.
10. Ravaglia C, Bonifazi M, Wells AU, Tomassetti S, Gurioli C, Piciucchi S, Dubini A, Tantalocco P, Sanna S, Negri E, Tramacere I, Ventura VA, Cavazza A, Rossi A, Chilosi M, La Vecchia C, Gasparini S, Poletti V. Safety and diagnostic yield of transbronchial lung cryobiopsy in diffuse parenchymal lung diseases: a comparative study versus video-assisted thoracoscopic lung biopsy and a systematic review of the literature. Respiration. 2016;91(3):215–27.
11. Gershman E, Fruchter O, Benjamin F, Nader AR, Rosengarten D, Rusanov V, Fridel L, Kramer MR. Safety of cryo-transbronchial biopsy in diffuse lung diseases: analysis of three hundred cases. Respiration. 2015;90(1):40–6.
12. Griff S, Schönfeld N, Ammenwerth W, Blum TG, Grah C, Bauer TT, Grüning W, Mairinger T, Wurps H. Diagnostic yield of transbronchial cryobiopsy in non-neoplastic lung disease: a retrospective case series. BMC Pulm Med. 2014;14:171.
13. Casoni GL, Tomassetti S, Cavazza A, Colby TV, Dubini A, Ryu JH, Carretta E, Tantalocco P, Piciucchi S, Ravaglia C, Gurioli C, Romagnoli M, Gurioli C, Chilosi M, Poletti V. Transbronchial lung cryobiopsy in the diagnosis of fibrotic interstitial lung diseases. PLoS One. 2014;9(2):e86716.
14. Seamans Y, et al. Effect of cough technique and cryogen gas on temperatures achieved during simulated cryotherapy. BMC Womens Health. 2007;7:16.
15. Maiti H, Cheyne MF, Hobbs G, Jeraj HA. Cryotherapy gas—to use nitrous oxide or carbon dioxide? Int J STD AIDS. 1999;10(2):118–20.
16. Mariategui J, Santos C, Taxa L, Jeronimo J, Castle PE. Comparison of depth of necrosis achieved by

CO$_2$- and N$_2$O-cryotherapy. Int J Gynaecol Obstet. 2008;100(1):24–6.

17. Hetzel J, Maldonado F, Ravaglia C, Wells AU, Colby TV, Tomassetti S, Ryu JH, Fruchter O, Piciucchi S, Dubini A, Cavazza A, Chilosi M, Sverzellati N, Valeyre D, Leduc D, Walsh SLF, Gasparini S, Hetzel M, Hagmeyer L, Haentschel M, Eberhardt R, Darwiche K, Yarmus LB, Torrego A, Krishna G, Shah PL, Annema JT, Herth FJF, Poletti V. Transbronchial cryobiopsies for the diagnosis of diffuse parenchymal lung diseases: expert statement from the cryobiopsy working group on safety and utility and a call for standardization of the procedure. Respiration. 2018;95(3):188–200.

18. Franke KJ, Szyrach M, Nilius G, Hetzel J, Hetzel M, Ruehle KH, Enderle MD. Experimental study on biopsy sampling using new flexible cryoprobes: influence of activation time, probe size, tissue consistency, and contact pressure of the probe on the size of the biopsy specimen. Lung. 2009;187(4):253–9.

19. Ing M, Oliver RA, Oliver BG, Walsh WR, Williamson JP. Evaluation of transbronchial lung cryobiopsy size and freezing time: a prognostic animal study. Respiration. 2016;92(1):34–9.

20. Chua KJ, Chou SK, Ho JC. An analytical study on the thermal effects of cryosurgery on selective cell destruction. J Biomech. 2007;40(1):100–16.

21. Mazur P, Leibo SP, Farrant J, Chu EHY, Hanna MG Jr, Smith LH. Interactions of cooling rate, warming rate and protective additive on the survival of frozen mammalian cells. In: Wolstenholme GEW, O'Connor M, editors. Ciba foundation symposium on the frozen cell. London: J&A Churchill Publication; 1970. p. 69–88.

Technique and Equipment in Transbronchial Cryobiopsy

5

Sara Colella

5.1 Introduction

There is a large amount of evidence that underlines the importance of technical aspects in transbronchial lung cryobiopsy (TBLC) since, as in many other medical procedures, optimizing the technique means consequently optimizing its safety and its utility (diagnostic yield).

In the published studies, a variability in the technique and in the equipment used is found; therefore a call for standardization was proposed in a recent document by Hetzel et al. [1], in which technical recommendations to enhance safety and optimize the diagnostic yield were proposed.

In the following chapter, the potential variability of the technical aspects of TBLC will be analysed, pointing out advantages and disadvantages in the various techniques and equipment proposed.

5.2 A Summary of What TBLC Needs to Be Carried Out

As general rule, TBLC needs to be carried out in a centre with experience in interstitial lung diseases (ILDs); in an endoscopic room with standard monitoring that includes oxygen saturation, electrocardiography and non-invasive blood pressure; by trained interventional pulmonologists; and where a prompt management of potential complications is possible.

The list below illustrates the technical points one has to consider in performing TBLC:

– Sedation/anaesthesia
– Airway management
– Patient ventilation
– Bronchial blockers
– Fluoroscopic guidance
– Cryogenic gas
– Cryoprobes and freezing times
– Where to take a TBLC and how many samples should be taken
– How to manage the TBLC samples

For each point, a variability in the technique and in the equipment used could be found, but it has to be underlined that for many of these points, a head-to-head comparison has not been done, so there is no or little evidence regarding clear benefits of an operating method over another one.

5.3 Sedation/Anaesthesia

Deep sedation or general anaesthesia is mandatory in order to improve the tolerance of the procedure, to better manage the patient oxygenation, to reduce potential harmful complications and to improve the working conditions [2].

S. Colella (✉)
Pulmonary Unit, Ascoli Piceno, Italy

© Springer Nature Switzerland AG 2019
V. Poletti (ed.), *Transbronchial cryobiopsy in diffuse parenchymal lung disease*,
https://doi.org/10.1007/978-3-030-14891-1_5

Table 5.1 A summary of the type of sedation/anaesthesia commonly used

Author, year	Type of study	Number of patients	GA/DS/CS (name used in the article)	Agent
Bango-Alvarez, 2017 [11]	Prosp	106	DS	Midazolam + fentanyl
Kronborg-White, 2017 [12]	Retro	38	DS	Propofol + remifentanil
Ravaglia, 2017 [13]	Prosp	46	DS	Propofol + remifentanil
Ravaglia, 2016 [6]	Retro	297	GS	Propofol + remifentanil
Tomassetti, 2016 [14]	Prosp	58	DS	Propofol + remifentanil
Ramasway, 2016 [15]	Retro	56	CS	Midazolam + fentanyl
Hernandez-Gonzalez, 2015 [7]	Retro	33	GA	Propofol + remifentanil
Gershman, 2015 [16]	Retro	300	CS	Midazolam + afentanyl ± Diprivan
Casoni, 2014 [10]	Prosp	69	GA	Propofol + remifentanil
Griff, 2014 [17]	Retro	52	DS	Disoprivan + midazolam
Frutcher, 2014 [18]	Retro	75	DS	Midazolam + alfentanyl
Yarmus, 2013 [9]	Prosp	21	GA/DS	Propofol ± paralytics

Different drugs are used, commonly propofol, midazolam and remifentanil [3]: the use of some of these agents is regulated in different ways since some of them could be used only by anaesthesiologists in some countries whilst in others could be used also by other physicians or even nurses in some protocols [4, 5]. A different terminology is also used across the studies: agents considered for deep sedation by some authors [6, 7] are considered for general anaesthesia by others [8–10]; therefore it is a matter of what agent is used rather than of the name used to indicate the anaesthesiologist support. In Table 5.1 an overview of the agents used in some studies is shown.

Muscle relaxation could be added, but in this case, the patient has to be ventilated, with either mechanical, manual or jet ventilation [9].

The addition of local anaesthesia is important as well, and it is used with the same modalities as in other bronchoscopic procedures [19].

Conscious sedation with the use of midazolam and fentanyl without the need to intubate the patient is described by some authors [11, 15] without reporting a higher complication rate compared to other studies, but apparently there are no clear benefits to prefer conscious sedation over deep sedation or general anaesthesia.

5.4   Airway Management

The majority of the reports in the literature describe the TBLC technique with intubated patient, with either a rigid tracheo-bronchoscope or an endotracheal tube [3]. The choice of a rigid bronchoscope or an endotracheal tube is mainly related to the operator skills.

Supraglottic devices (such as laryngeal mask) were also described and were proven to have also an acceptable safety [8, 20] but may raise some concerns in the management of severe bleeding.

TBLC can be performed also without the need to intubate the patient, with a trans-oral approach: in this case two bronchoscopes are used, one for taking the biopsy and the second one immediately after to manage the bleeding with suction or wedge the bronchoscope in the selected segmental bronchus [8, 16]. Among the studies that used the trans-oral approach, no bleeding complications were reported by some authors [11, 21, 22], whilst a percentage that ranges between 2% [15] and 5.2% was reported by others [16].

Ravaglia et al. [6] analysed the impact of airway management and sedation on the diagnostic yield and on the pneumothorax rate: in comparison with patients non-intubated in conscious sedation, the diagnostic yield was slightly lower in intubated patients in deep sedation (83% versus 81%, respectively), and in this group, the proportion of pneumothorax was higher (1% versus 7%, respectively).

Thus, intubation, with either a rigid bronchoscope or an endotracheal tube, is recommended in TBLC [1], since there are advantages over the trans-oral approach in terms of patient's safety and operator's comfort. Moreover, a better stability of the bronchial blocker is ensured with the intubated patient, since the bronchial blocker can be fixed at the proximal part of the airway device. However, the trans-oral approach could be also possible, apparently without an increased rate of complications.

5.5 Patient Ventilation

A consequent aspect of the choice of sedation rather than anaesthesia is the ventilation of the patient. Whereas in case of conscious sedation a spontaneous breathing is maintained, in case of general anaesthesia or deep sedation, a support in ventilation could be needed.

Three modalities have been described, spontaneous, manual, mechanical and jet ventilation. During spontaneous ventilation, only oxygen supply via nasal or endotracheal cannula is given, and this is the most common ventilation modality reported. Manual and mechanical ventilation is also used, in which the patient is connected, respectively, to a balloon or to a ventilator. Jet ventilation consists in sending small air volumes, manually or mechanically, enriched with O_2 at high speed, and to do so, the induction of a respiratory muscle paralysis is needed: the main advantage is to reduce the possibility of lung barotrauma, but the efficacy decreases when several instruments are introduced into the rigid bronchoscope like forceps or suction catheters [23].

Data from surgical lung biopsy indicates that a higher risk of barotrauma could be observed in case of single lung ventilation [1], but similar data regarding TBLC has never been reported. A summary of ventilation support across the studies is provided in Table 5.2.

Table 5.2 An overview of the sedation/anaesthesia used and the ventilation support across the studies

Author, year	Type of study	Number of patients	GA/DS/CS (name used in the article)	Agent	ETT/RB/ SGD/NI	Ventilation
Almeida, 2017 [24]	Retro	100	GA	–	RB	Manual jet 2 bar
Schmutz, 2017 [25]	Retro	132	GA	–	SGD	–
Bango-Alvarez, 2017 [11]	Prosp	106	DS	Midazolam + fentanyl	NI	Spontaneous
Kronborg-White, 2017 [12]	Retro	38	DS	Propofol + remifentanil	ETT	Spontaneous
Siprasart, 2017 [8]	Retro	74	GA	–	ETT	Spontaneous
Ravaglia, 2017 [13]	Prosp	46	DS	Propofol + remifentanil	RB	Spontaneous
Ussavarungsi, 2017 [26]	Retro	74	DS	–	ETT	Spontaneous
DiBardino, 2017 [20]	Retro	25	CS	–	SGD/ETT	–
Berim, 2017 [27]	Retro	10	GA	–	ETT	–
Marcoa, 2017 [28]	Prosp	90	GA	–	ETT	Jet
Sousa-Neves, 2017 [29]	Retro	3	GA	–	RT	–
Echevarria-Uraga, 2016 [30]	Retro	100	GA	–	ETT	Mechanical
Ravaglia, 2016 [6]	Retro	297	GS	Propofol + remifentanil	ETT	Spontaneous
Hagmeyer, 2016 [31]	Retro	23	DS/GA	–	ETT/RB	–/jet
Tomassetti, 2016 [14]	Prosp	58	DS	Propofol + remifentanil	ETT	Spontaneous
Hagmeyer, 2016 [31]	Prosp	32	DS	–	ETT	–
Ramasway, 2016 [15]	Retro	56	CS	Midazolam + fentanyl	NI	Spontaneous
Pourabdollah, 2016 [32]	Prosp	41	DS	–	–	–
Hernandez-Gonzalez, 2015 [7]	Retro	33	GA	Propofol + remifentanil	ETT	–

(continued)

Table 5.2 (continued)

Author, year	Type of study	Number of patients	GA/DS/CS (name used in the article)	Agent	ETT/RB/ SGD/NI	Ventilation
Gershman, 2015 [16]	Retro	300	CS	Midazolam + afentanyl ± Diprivan	NI	Spontaneous
Pajares, 2014 [33]	RCT	77	DS	–	ETT	Spontaneous
Casoni, 2014 [10]	Prosp	69	GA	Propofol + remifentanil	ETT	Spontaneous
Griff, 2014 [17]	Retro	52	DS	Disoprivan + midazolam	–	–
Frutcher, 2014 [18]	Retro	75	DS	Midazolam + alfentanyl	NI	Spontaneous
Kropski, 2013 [5]	Retro	25	CS	–	ETT	Spontaneous
Fruchter, 2013 [18]	Retro	11	CS	–	ETT	Spontaneous
Fruchter, 2013 [18]	Retro	40	CS	–	NI	Spontaneous
Yarmus, 2013 [9]	Prosp	21	GA/DS	Propofol ± paralytics	RB/LMA	Jet/ spontaneous
Griff, 2011 [34]	Prosp	15	Sedation (?)	–	–	–
Babiak, 2009 [35]	Prosp	41	DS	–	ETT	Spontaneous

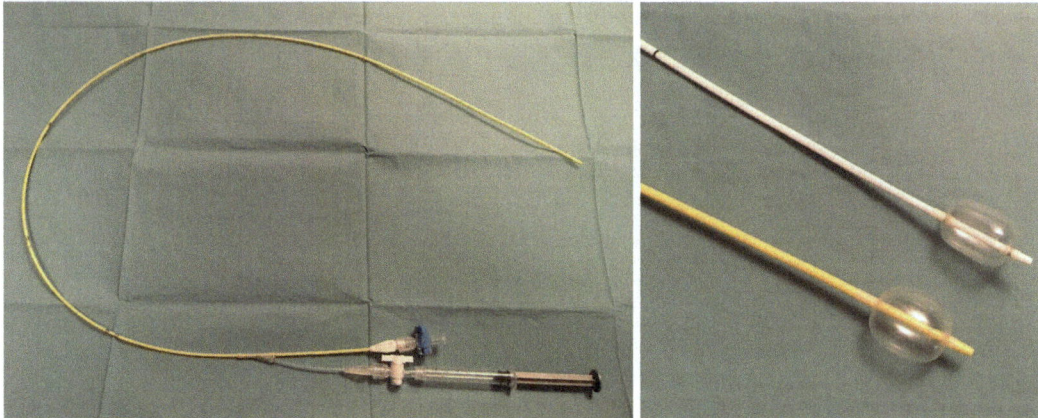

Fig. 5.1 Fogarty catheters

5.6 Bronchial Blockers

Bronchial blockers are positioned in segmental bronchi immediately before the biopsy procedure, and its use is mainly justified to reduce the bleeding. Once in the target place, the blocker has to be fixed to avoid depositioning (e.g. to the endotracheal tube or to the rigid bronchoscope with a sticking plaster).

Two types of bronchial blockers are commonly used in TBLC: the Fogarty catheter (most used, Fig. 5.1) and the Arndt catheter.

The Fogarty balloon (dimensions: 4F, 5F, 6F) consists of a hollow tube with an inflatable bal-

loon attached to its tip. It is available in various dimensions. In its proximal portion, there are two branches, one to inflate balloon with air and the other one for the instillation of fluids, like saline, if necessary.

The Arndt catheter (dimensions: 7F or 9F) has a guide loop in its distal part that has to be tied to the bronchoscope, enabling a more precise placement.

The mechanism of functioning is the same for both devices: they have to be inserted deflated and inflated after the biopsy, immediately after the removal of the cryoprobe, and they have to remain inflated in the biopsy area for 3–5 min. A check of the bleeding before removing the balloon is suggested.

The majority of the studies reported the use of a bronchial blocker with an expected reduction in moderate-to-severe bleeding [36].

However, in some studies, no bronchial blockers are used, and a second bronchoscope was used in place of them: the biopsy is taken with the first bronchoscope, and subsequently a second one is inserted and wedged to stop the bleeding. For example, Sriprasart et al. [8] reported their experience with two scopes and no bronchial blocker: they reported a diagnostic yield of 87.84%, a 7% of pneumothoraces, 1% severe bleeding and a 4% of death.

5.7 Fluoroscopic Guidance

Once the biopsy area is chosen in the computed tomography (CT) scan, the use of the fluoroscope is a further guidance in the biopsy since its use allows to better evaluate the position of the probe and its distance from the pleura.

Indeed, it is suggested that the probe should be placed in the distal part of the lung parenchyma: if too close to the pleura, the risk of pneumothorax is increased, and on the other side, if too proximal, there is a risk of bleeding since the airways are not entirely protected with cartilage plates and vessels could be damaged whilst taking the biopsy.

Some studies reported a distance from the visceral pleura that varies between 1 and 2 cm, and a distance of around 1 cm has been recently suggested [1]. However, biopsy within 1 cm from the pleura could be necessary in the suspicion of idiopathic pulmonary fibrosis/usual interstitial pneumonia (IPF/UIP), and in those cases, a higher rate of pneumothorax has been reported, also due to the more pronounced fibrotic changes [3]. Dhooria et al. [36] found a lower percentage of pneumothorax in case of fluoroscopic use.

Moreover, the fluoroscopic use allows also a prompt evaluation in case of pneumothorax.

In some other studies, the fluoroscope was not used: in the study of Bango-Álvarez et al.

[11], for example, the probe was moved forward until it could not be advanced further and then retracted 1–2 cm following the marks on the probe. They obtained a diagnosis in 86% of patients, and they experienced pneumothorax in 4.7%, no acute exacerbation of IPF and no haemorrhage.

5.8 Cryogenic Gases

Cryogenic gases are the cooling agents that allow the lung tissue to be frozen. They are compressed under high pressure in a tank, and they are released once the probe is activated with the foot-switch (Fig. 5.2). The release of the gases generates a rapid temperature drop with a consequent freeze of the surrounding tissue.

Two cooling gases are used, the carbon dioxide (CO_2) and nitric oxide (N_2O): no difference in the mechanism is observed, but the N_2O reaches lower temperatures, could require an aspiration system in the room to be used and is more expensive than CO_2 (see Chap. 4); therefore, CO_2 is the cooling agent core commonly used.

5.9 Cryoprobes

TBLC is performed by the mean of cryoprobes: they are inserted in the operating channel of the flexible bronchoscope and are pushed forward until the biopsy site, in close contact to the lung tissue.

Cryoprobes are flexible probes, 90 cm in length, available in 2 diameters, 1.9 and 2.4 mm (Fig. 5.3). The 2.4 mm probe provides the largest samples with a fewer activation time since there is a positive correlation between the freezing time, the probe's dimension and the cross-sectional area of the biopsy [37].

A freezing time of 5–6 s has to be used with the 2.4 mm probe, whilst 7–8 s is necessary with the 1.9 mm [13], but when the N_2O is used, this freezing time could be reduced [30].

So far, in terms of complications, no clear data are available proving that a larger dimension of

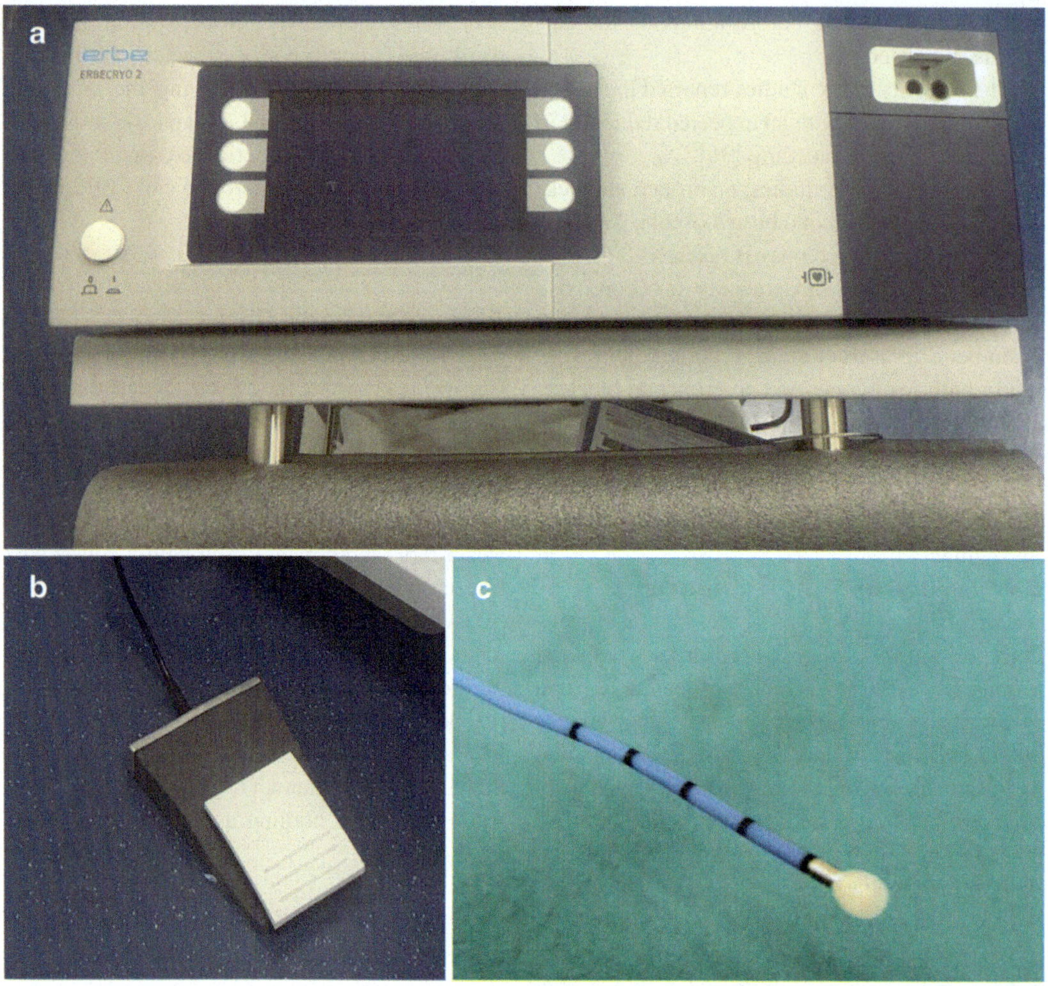

Fig. 5.2 Part of the cryoequipment. (**a**) The console; (**b**) the footswitch; (**c**) the "iceball"

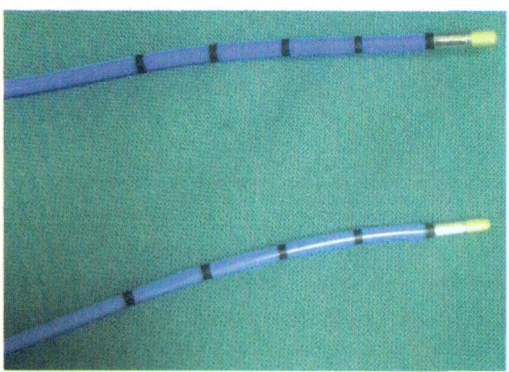

Fig. 5.3 The available cryoprobes

the probe means a higher complication rate; however, a trend towards the rate of pneumothorax was observed in the meta-analysis of Iftikhar and colleagues [38] with the 2.4 mm probe.

5.10 Where to Take a TBLC and How Many Samples Should Be Taken

The choice of the biopsy site is up to the operator, where the most representative radiological abnormalities are present, avoiding the most fibrotic areas. In case where there is a diffuse heterogeneous lung disease, biopsies from different lobes or different segments are preferred.

A significant variability is observed among the studies about this point: some are performed in a single segment, some in more than one segment and in others in different lobes [5, 26], but in most of the cases, no subgroup analyses were performed.

To better evaluate the potential advantages of taking biopsies in different segments rather than in a single segment, Ravaglia et al. [13] conducted a randomized trial in which a significant increase in the diagnostic yield from 69 to 96% was demonstrated when biopsies from a different segment of the same lobe were added. A part from this randomized study, no other data are available that elucidates whether taking biopsy from multiple segments or multiple lobes results in an increase of diagnostic yield; moreover, the impact of this approach on complications is poorly understood.

About the number of biopsies that needs to be taken, in the literature, it ranges from 1 to 7 samples [3]; however, three to five biopsies are the optimal number suggested [1].

5.11 How to Manage the TBLC Samples

Once the tissue is collected, it has to be processed for pathological evaluation.

Comparable to other lung biopsy techniques, TBLC specimens have to be (1) fixed in formalin, (2) embedded in paraffin, (3) orientated in the way to maximize the surface area and finally (4) stained with haematoxylin-eosin (or other stains) or prepared for immunohistochemical analysis.

Attention should be paid in all these phases of tissue manipulation, starting from the removing of the tissue from the probe to the formation of slides in order to minimize tissue damages and artefacts. For example, thawing in hand-warm water may render the tissue removing easier.

Moreover, the TBLC specimens are suitable for investigations such as immunohistochemical and molecular studies [39].

5.12 Learning Curve

The need of standardization is not only expected for technical issues but also for establishing the learning process for TBLC. Nowadays, there is no validated learning protocol for TBLC, and very few studies addressed this point. A relative high complication rate is described with the starting experience of TBLC [20] by unexperienced pulmonologists: out of 25 patients, serious haemorrhage was reported in 3 patients (1 of them life-threatening), pneumothorax in 2 cases and hypercapnic respiratory failure in 1. These results suggest that a high caution should be done with the introduction of TBLC in clinical practice.

Also in the report of Kronborg-White and colleagues [12], the first experience with TBLC was described, and interestingly they specified the learning process of the operator: one of them attended a large experienced centre, and on return, the other two pulmonologists were trained to perform the procedure. Out of 38 patients, complications were seen in 18 cases: 1 has haemoptysis, 6 have moderate bleeding, 10 have pneumothoraces and two has signs of infections on blood tests with fever.

Finally, Almeida et al. performed a retrospective study investigating the diagnostic yield and the complications related to the experience of the operator [24]. Mastering of the procedure was achieved after 70 procedures, in terms of better diagnostic yield, bigger specimens and fewer complications.

Thus, further studies are needed to establish that the learning procedure of TBLC could be with a positive impact on the success and safety of the procedure.

5.13 What Happens After the Biopsy: Writing the Report, Post-procedural Monitoring and Management of Complications

Once the TBLC is performed, there are few more aspects that have to be managed.

First of all, a report of the procedure has to be done, in which the procedure is described.

The description of the technical aspects of TBLC is the responsibility of the operator that has to specify the following details in the report: airway management device (if any), bronchial blocker used (if any), fluoroscopic guidance (if so), probe's size, number of biopsies taken and biopsy site (single/multiple segment(s) or lobe(s)).

Also the pathologist has to write a report to propose the final diagnosis, specifying the specimens' dimension, the percentage of alveolated tissue, the pattern recognition, the immunohistochemical or molecular analyses (if any) and the level of confidence in the proposed diagnosis.

As a second point, after the TBLC, the patient has to be monitored for some hours. The procedure could be performed in both out- [6, 8] and in-patient setting [40]: patients have to be monitored to work off the anaesthesia and to better manage potential complications.

In the literature, a minimum of 2 h of monitoring [8] is suggested to evaluate the possibility of escalation of care or to evaluate if further examinations are needed, such as chest X-ray in the suspicion of pneumothorax. Viglietta et al. [41] found a percentage of pneumothorax of 23% (11/43) diagnosed by concordance of chest X-ray and chest ultrasound in the first 3 h: in 10 cases a diagnosis was made by chest X-ray and in 11 cases with chest ultrasound, thus suggesting a potential role of ultrasound in the detection of pneumothorax after TBLC. Moreover, in one patient, a massive pneumothorax occurred immediately after the TBLC, and in only one case, a pneumothorax was detected after 5 h. Kropski et al. [5] found that among the 33 patients that underwent TBLC in an out-patient setting, only one was readmitted for a mild haemoptysis, and no fatal complications occurred.

Finally, it has to be remembered that TBLC needs to be performed in an endoscopic suite, fully accessorized for the management of the potential complications such as the treatment of bleeding or pneumothorax and even where there is a rapid access to the intensive care unit.

In Table 5.3 a suggestion is provided on how to perform TBLC and which equipment should be used.

In Fig. 5.4 a summary of the procedure is shown.

Table 5.3 Performing TBLC: which technique and which equipment should be used

Topic	Technique	Equipment
Sedation/anaesthesia	Deep sedation or general anaesthesia	Intravenous administration
Airway management	Intubated patient	Rigid trachea—bronchoscope or endotracheal tube
Ventilation	Spontaneous	Oxygen supply
Bronchial blocker	Suggested	Fogarty or Arndt catheter
Fluoroscopic guidance	Distance from the visceral pleura: = or <1 cm; early detection of pneumothorax	Suggested
Cryoprobes and freezing times	2.4 mm → 5–6 s 1.9 mm → 7–8 s	
Where to take TBLC	In the "most affected area"	
How many samples	3–5	
Procedural and post-procedural monitoring	Suggested	SpO_2, heart rate, blood pressure

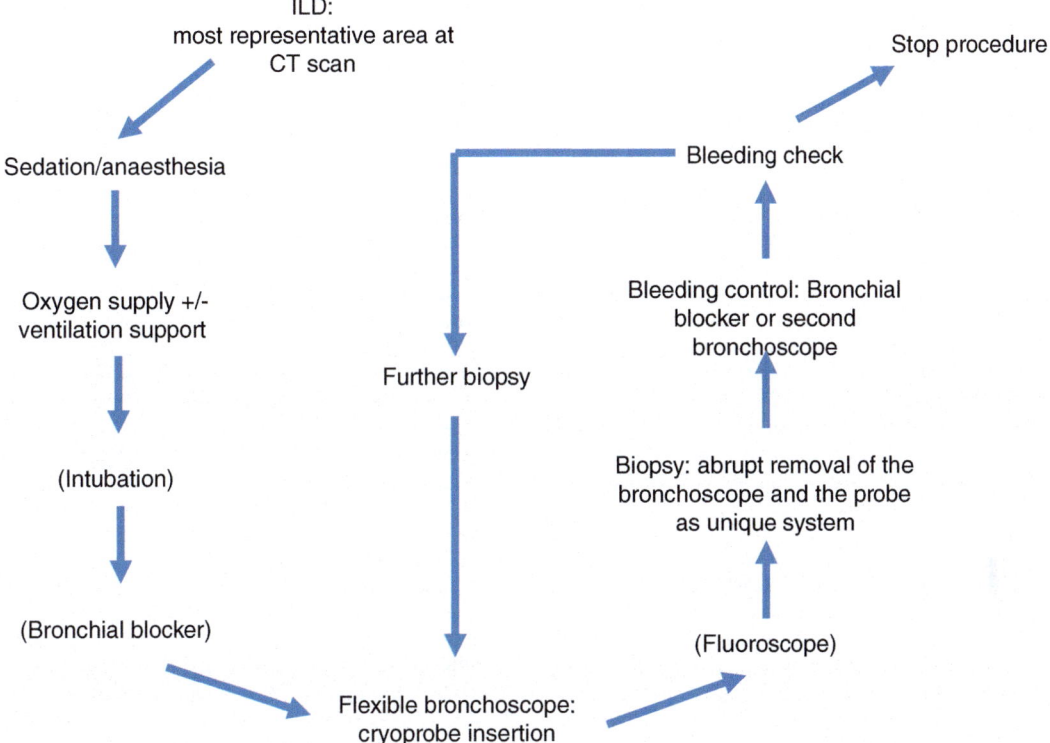

Fig. 5.4 A summary of TBLC technique

References

1. Hetzel J, Maldonado F, Ravaglia C, Wells AU, Colby TV, Tomassetti S, Ryu JH, Fruchter O, Piciucchi S, Dubini A, Cavazza A, Chilosi M, Sverzellati N, Valeyre D, Leduc D, Walsh SLF, Gasparini S, Hetzel M, Hagmeyer L, Haentschel M, Eberhardt R, Darwiche K, Yarmus LB, Torrego A, Krishna G, Shah PL, Annema JT, Herth FJF, Poletti V. Transbronchial cryobiopsies for the diagnosis of diffuse parenchymal lung diseases: expert statement from the cryobiopsy working group on safety and utility and a call for standardization of the procedure. Respiration. 2018;95(3):188–200.
2. Putz L, Mayné A, Dincq AS. Jet ventilation during rigid bronchoscopy in adults: a focused review. Biomed Res Int. 2016;2016:4234861.
3. Lentz RJ, Argento AC, Colby TV, Rickman OB, Maldonado F. Transbronchial cryobiopsy for diffuse parenchymal lung disease: a state-of-the-art review of procedural techniques, current evidence, and future challenges. J Thorac Dis. 2017;9(7):2186–203.
4. Jensen JT, Banning AM, Clementsen P, Hammering A, Hornslet P, Horsted T, Vilmann P. Nurse administered propofol sedation for pulmonary endoscopies requires a specific protocol. Dan Med J. 2012;59(8):A4467.
5. Kropski JA, Pritchett JM, Mason WR, Sivarajan L, Gleaves LA, Johnson JE, Lancaster LH, Lawson WE, Blackwell TS, Steele MP, Loyd JE, Rickman OB. Bronchoscopic cryobiopsy for the diagnosis of diffuse parenchymal lung disease. PLoS One. 2013;8(11):e78674.
6. Ravaglia C, Bonifazi M, Wells AU, Tomassetti S, Gurioli C, Piciucchi S, Dubini A, Tantalocco P, Sanna S, Negri E, Tramacere I, Ventura VA, Cavazza A, Rossi A, Chilosi M, La Vecchia C, Gasparini S, Poletti V. Safety and diagnostic yield of transbronchial lung cryobiopsy in diffuse parenchymal lung diseases: a comparative study versus video-assisted thoracoscopic lung biopsy and a systematic review of the literature. Respiration. 2016;91(3):215–27.
7. Hernández-González F, Lucena CM, Ramírez J, Sánchez M, Jimenez MJ, Xaubet A, Sellares J, Agustí C. Cryobiopsy in the diagnosis of diffuse interstitial lung disease: yield and cost-effectiveness analysis (in English, Spanish). Arch Bronconeumol. 2015;51(6):261–7.
8. Sriprasart T, Aragaki A, Baughman R, Wikenheiser-Brokamp K, Khanna G, Tanase D, Kirschner M, Benzaquen S. A single US center experience of transbronchial lung cryobiopsy for diagnosing interstitial lung disease with a 2-scope technique. J Bronchology Interv Pulmonol. 2017;24(2):131–5.

9. Yarmus L, Akulian J, Gilbert C, Illei P, Shah P, Merlo C, Orens J, Feller-Kopman D. Cryoprobe transbronchial lung biopsy in patients after lung transplantation: a pilot safety study. Chest. 2013;143(3):621–6.

10. Casoni GL, Tomassetti S, Cavazza A, Colby TV, Dubini A, Ryu JH, Carretta E, Tantalocco P, Piciucchi S, Ravaglia C, Gurioli C, Romagnoli M, Gurioli C, Chilosi M, Poletti V. Transbronchial lung cryobiopsy in the diagnosis of fibrotic interstitial lung diseases. PLoS One. 2014;9(2):e86716.

11. Bango-Álvarez A, Ariza-Prota M, Torres-Rivas H, Fernández-Fernández L, Prieto A, Sánchez I, Gil M, Pando-Sandoval A. Transbronchial cryobiopsy in interstitial lung disease: experience in 106 cases—how to do it. ERJ Open Res. 2017;3(1). pii: 00148–2016.

12. Kronborg-White S, Folkersen B, Rasmussen TR, Voldby N, Madsen LB, Rasmussen F, Poletti V, Bendstrup E. Introduction of cryobiopsies in the diagnostics of interstitial lung diseases—experiences in a referral centre. Eur Clin Respir J. 2017;4(1):1274099.

13. Ravaglia C, Wells AU, Tomassetti S, Dubini A, Cavazza A, Piciucchi S, Sverzellati N, Gurioli C, Gurioli C, Costabel U, Tantalocco P, Ryu JH, Chilosi M, Poletti V. Transbronchial lung cryobiopsy in diffuse parenchymal lung disease: comparison between biopsy from 1 segment and biopsy from 2 segments—diagnostic yield and complications. Respiration. 2017;93(4):285–92.

14. Tomassetti S, Wells AU, Costabel U, Cavazza A, Colby TV, Rossi G, Sverzellati N, Carloni A, Carretta E, Buccioli M, Tantalocco P, Ravaglia C, Gurioli C, Dubini A, Piciucchi S, Ryu JH, Poletti V. Bronchoscopic lung cryobiopsy increases diagnostic confidence in the multidisciplinary diagnosis of idiopathic pulmonary fibrosis. Am J Respir Crit Care Med. 2016;193(7):745–52.

15. Ramaswamy A, Homer R, Killam J, Pisani MA, Murphy TE, Araujo K, Puchalski J. Comparison of transbronchial and cryobiopsies in evaluation of diffuse parenchymal lung disease. J Bronchology Interv Pulmonol. 2016;23(1):14–21.

16. Gershman E, Fruchter O, Benjamin F, Nader AR, Rosengarten D, Rusanov V, Fridel L, Kramer MR. Safety of cryo-transbronchial biopsy in diffuse lung diseases: analysis of three hundred cases. Respiration. 2015;90(1):40–6.

17. Griff S, Schönfeld N, Ammenwerth W, Blum TG, Grah C, Bauer TT, Grüning W, Mairinger T, Wurps H. Diagnostic yield of transbronchial cryobiopsy in non-neoplastic lung disease: a retrospective case series. BMC Pulm Med. 2014;14:171.

18. Fruchter O, Fridel L, El Raouf BA, Abdel-Rahman N, Rosengarten D, Kramer MR. Histological diagnosis of interstitial lung diseases by cryo-transbronchial biopsy. Respirology. 2014;19:683–38.

19. Du Rand IA, Blaikley J, Booton R, Chaudhuri N, Gupta V, Khalid S, Mandal S, Martin J, Mills J, Navani N, Rahman NM, Wrightson JM, Munavvar M, British Thoracic Society Bronchoscopy Guideline Group. British Thoracic Society guideline for diagnostic flexible bronchoscopy in adults: accredited by NICE. Thorax. 2013;68(Suppl 1):i1–i44.

20. DiBardino DM, Haas AR, Lanfranco AR, et al. High complication rate after introduction of transbronchial cryobiopsy into clinical practice at an Academic Medical Center. Ann Am Thorac Soc. 2017;14:851–7.

21. Fruchter O, Fridel L, Rosengarten D, et al. Transbronchial cryobiopsy in immunocompromised patients with pulmonary infiltrates: a pilot study. Lung. 2013;191:619–24.

22. Fruchter O, Fridel L, Rosengarten D, et al. Transbronchial cryo-biopsy in lung transplantation patients: first report. Respirology. 2013;18:669–73.

23. Casalini AG, Monica M. La broncoscopia rigida. Pneumologia interventistica. Milan: Springer; 2007. p. 45–58.

24. Almeida LM, Lima B, Mota PC, Melo N, Magalhães A, Pereira JM, Moura CS, Guimarães S, Morais A. Learning curve for transbronchial lung cryobiopsy in diffuse lung disease. Rev Port Pneumol (2006). 2017. pii: S2173–5115(17)30148–3.

25. Schmutz A, Dürk T, Idzko M, Koehler T, Kalbhenn J, Loop T. Feasibility of a supraglottic airway device for transbronchial lung cryobiopsy—a retrospective analysis. J Cardiothorac Vasc Anesth. 2017;31(4):1343–7.

26. Ussavarungsi K, Kern RM, Roden AC, Ryu JH, Edell ES. Transbronchial cryobiopsy in diffuse parenchymal lung disease: retrospective analysis of 74 cases. Chest. 2017;151(2):400–8.

27. Berim IG, Saeed AI, Awab A, Highley A, Colanta A, Chaudry F. Radial probe ultrasound-guided cryobiopsy. J Bronchology Interv Pulmonol. 2017;24(2):170–3.

28. Marçôa R, Linhas R, Apolinário D, Campainha S, Oliveira A, Nogueira C, Loureiro A, Almeida J, Costa F, Wen X, Neves S. Diagnostic yield of transbronchial lung cryobiopsy in interstitial lung diseases. Rev Port Pneumol (2006). 2017;23(5):296–8.

29. Sousa-Neves J, Mota P, Melo N, Santos-Faria D, Bernardes M, Morais A. Transbronchial cryobiopsy: a new way to assess lung disease in rheumatic disorders. Acta Reumatol Port. 2017;42(3):275–6.

30. Echevarria-Uraga JJ, Pérez-Izquierdo J, García-Garai N, Gómez-Jiménez E, Aramburu-Ojembarrena A, Tena-Tudanca L, Miguélez-Vidales JL, Capelastegui-Saiz A. Usefulness of an angioplasty balloon as selective bronchial blockade device after transbronchial cryobiopsy. Respirology. 2016;21(6):1094–9.

31. Hagmeyer L, Theegarten D, Treml M, Priegnitz C, Randerath W. Validation of transbronchial cryobiopsy in interstitial lung disease—interim analysis of a prospective trial and critical review of the literature. Sarcoidosis Vasc Diffuse Lung Dis. 2016;33(1):2–9.

32. Pourabdollah M, Shamaei M, Karimi S, Karimi M, Kiani A, Jabbari HR. Transbronchial lung biopsy: the pathologist's point of view. Clin Respir J. 2016;10(2):211–6.

33. Pajares V, Puzo C, Castillo D, Lerma E, Montero MA, Ramos-Barbón D, Amor-Carro O, Gil De

Bernabé A, Franquet T, Plaza V, Hetzel J, Sanchis J, Torrego A. Diagnostic yield of transbronchial cryobiopsy in interstitial lung disease: a randomized trial. Respirology. 2014;19:900–6.

34. Griff S, Ammenwerth W, Schönfeld N, Bauer TT, Mairinger T, Blum TG, Kollmeier J, Grüning W. Morphometrical analysis of transbronchial cryobiopsies. Diagn Pathol. 2011;6:53.

35. Babiak A, Hetzel J, Krishna G, Fritz P, Moeller P, Balli T, Hetzel M. Transbronchial cryobiopsy: a new tool for lung biopsies. Respiration. 2009;78:203–8.

36. Dhooria S, Mehta RM, Srinivasan A, Madan K, Sehgal IS, Pattabhiraman V, Yadav P, Sivaramakrishnan M, Mohan A, Bal A, Garg M, Agarwal R. The safety and efficacy of different methods for obtaining transbronchial lung cryobiopsy in diffuse lung diseases. Clin Respir J. 2018;12(4):1711–20.

37. Ing M, Oliver RA, Oliver BG, Walsh WR, Williamson JP. Evaluation of transbronchial lung cryobiopsy size and freezing time: a prognostic animal study. Respiration. 2016;92(1):34–9.

38. Iftikhar IH, Alghothani L, Sardi A, Berkowitz D, Musani AI. Transbronchial lung cryobiopsy and video-assisted thoracoscopic lung biopsy in the diagnosis of diffuse parenchymal lung disease. A meta-analysis of diagnostic test accuracy. Ann Am Thorac Soc. 2017;14(7):1197–211.

39. Colby TV, Tomassetti S, Cavazza A, Dubini A, Poletti V. Transbronchial cryobiopsy in diffuse lung disease: update for the pathologist. Arch Pathol Lab Med. 2017;141(7):891–900.

40. Colella S, Massaccesi C, Fioretti F, Panella G, Primomo GL, D'Emilio V, Pela R. Transbronchial lung cryobiopsy in lung diseases: diagnostic yield and safety. Eur Res J. 2017;50:PA3025. https://doi.org/10.1183/1393003.congress-2017.PA3025.

41. Viglietta L, Inchingolo R, Pavano C, Tomassetti S, Piciucchi S, Smargiassi A, Ravaglia C, Dubini A, Gurioli C, Gurioli C, Poletti V. Ultrasonography for the diagnosis of pneumothorax after transbronchial lung cryobiopsy in diffuse parenchymal lung diseases. Respiration. 2017;94(2):232–6.

Complications of Transbronchial Cryobiopsy

6

Claudia Ravaglia

Safety profile of transbronchial lung cryobiopsy has been recently compared to that of the conventional forceps or surgical lung biopsy; however, literature shows a variable incidence of complications, mostly bleeding and pneumothorax (Table 6.1). The significant variability of complications is related to the rapid spread of the technique around the world with variable competency and safety standards in different centers and the consequent variability of the procedure itself, in terms of airway access, ventilation, sedation, use of balloon/endobronchial blockers, probe size and freezing time, distance from the pleura, or sampling strategy.

Unlike conventional transbronchial biopsy, which is more rarely complicated by pneumothorax [39], pneumothorax seems to be the most common complication occurring after transbronchial lung cryobiopsy (TLCB), with a rate that varies considerably between different studies: from less than 1% to almost 30% [2, 3, 5, 6, 9, 11, 12, 15, 40–43]. In a meta-analysis that included 15 studies comprising 994 patients, the average rate was 10% [15], and similar results were confirmed by a more recent meta-analysis of 13 studies with an incidence of post-procedural pneumothorax of 9.5% (5.9–14.9%) [41]. There are very few data regarding chest drain-

age; however Ravaglia et al. showed that out of the pneumothoraces reported, 70% required chest tube drainage, with an overall probability of developing a pneumothorax requiring chest tube drainage of 0.03 (95% CI 0.01–0.08); furthermore, when chest drainage is necessary, time of drainage is usually similar to that of drainage after video-assisted thoracoscopy (VATS) [15]. The risk of pneumothorax can be influenced by patient-related factors (radiological fibrotic score and UIP pattern) or procedure-related factors (type of sedation/airway control, distance from the pleura, size of the probe and freezing time, sampling strategy, skill level of operator) (Table 6.2). Ravaglia et al. showed a higher proportion of events among intubated patients undergoing the procedure under deep sedation compared to those under conscious sedation [15]; this difference could be mainly due to the type of ventilation used, as patients undergoing the procedure under general anesthesia with invasive jet ventilation may develop pneumothorax much more frequently than under conditions of sedation and spontaneous breathing over a bronchoscopy tube [11]. In a large cohort of 699 patients who underwent transbronchial lung cryobiopsy for suspected diffuse parenchymal lung diseases at the Pulmonology Unit of Morgagni Hospital in Forlì (Italy), the risk of pneumothorax appears to be significantly reduced when a 1.9 mm probe is used compared to the 2.4 mm probe (2.7% vs 21.1%,

C. Ravaglia (✉)
Department of Diseases of the Thorax, Pulmonology Unit, GB Morgagni – L Pierantoni Hospital, Forlì, Italy

© Springer Nature Switzerland AG 2019
V. Poletti (ed.), *Transbronchial cryobiopsy in diffuse parenchymal lung disease*,
https://doi.org/10.1007/978-3-030-14891-1_6

Table 6.1 Comparison between transbronchial forceps biopsy, transbronchial cryobiopsy, and surgical lung biopsy (Modified by Hetzel J et al. [1])

	Reference, year	Pneumothorax	Serious bleeding	Mortality due to AE (in 30 days)
Cryobiopsy	Babiak [2], 2009	2 (4.8%)	0	–
	Kropski [3], 2013	0	0	–
	Fruchter [4], 2013	0	0	–
	Yarmus [5], 2013	1 (4.8%)	0	0
	Pajares [6], 2014	3 (8%)	0	–
	Fruchter [7], 2014	2 (2.6%)	3 (4%)	0
	Pourabdollah [8], 2016	–	–	–
	Griff [9], 2014	0	0	0
	Hernández-Gonzáles [10], 2015	4 (12%)	0	0
	Hagmeyer [11], 2016	6 (19%)	2 (6%)	–
	Gershman [12], 2015	15 (5%)	16 (5%)	–
	Ramaswamy [13], 2016	11 (20%)	1 (2%)	0
	Echevarria-Uraga [14], 2016	3 (3%)	10 (10%)	–
	Ravaglia [15], 2016	60 (20%)	0	1 (0.3%)
	Ussavarungsi [16], 2017	1 (1.4%)	9 (12%)	–
	DiBardino [17], 2017	2 (8%)	3 (12%)	–
	Bango-Alvarez [18], 2017	5 (4.7%)	0	0
	Kronborg-White [19], 2017	10 (26%)	3 (8%)	0
	Sriprasart [20], 2017	5 (7%)	1 (1%)	–
	Ravaglia [21], 2017	7 (16%)	0	–
Forceps biopsy	Wall [22], 1981	2/52 (3.8%)	0	0
	O'Brien [23], 1997	10/83 (14.3%)	5/83 (6.0%)	0
	Berbescu [24], 2006	–	–	–
	Casoni [25], 2008	0	0	0
	Facciolongo [26], 2009	22/1660 (1.3%)	21/1660 (1.3%)	0
	Tomassetti [27], 2012	5/64 (8%)	–	0
	Yarmus [5], 2013	1/21 (4.76%)	0	0
	Pajares [6], 2014	2/38 (5.3%)	0	0
	Pourabdollah [8], 2016	–	–	–
	Gershman [12], 2015	9/286 (3.15%)	13/288 (4.4%)	0
	Ramaswamy [13], 2016	–	–	–
	Sheth [28], 2017	–	–	–
Surgical biopsy	Rena [29], 1999	NA	0	0
	Kreider [30], 2007	NA	0	3/68 (4.4%)
	Zhang [31], 2010	NA	0	3/418 (0.7%)
	Fibla [32], 2012	NA	0	–
	Blackhall [33], 2013	NA	0	4/103 (3.9%)
	Morris [34], 2014	NA	0	1/66 (1.5%)
	Rotolo [35], 2015	NA	0	4/161 (2.5%)
	Fibla [32], 2015	NA	0	28 (9%)
	Hutchinson [36], 2016	NA	–	2051/32,022 (6.4%)
	Hutchinson [37], 2016	NA	–	68/2820 (2.4%)
	Ravaglia [15], 2016	NA	0	4/150 (2.7%)
	Sheth [28], 2017	NA	0	–
	Lieberman [38], 2017	NA	0	1 (2.1%)

respectively, p 0.00010). Furthermore, the risk of pneumothorax increases when samples are taken from different sites instead of a unique site (p 0.0005) [21] and if they are taken close to the pleura [15, 25]. Finally, the risk of pneumo-thorax seems to correlate significantly with the presence of histological UIP pattern on biopsy, high-resolution computed tomography (HRCT) fibrosis score of the lower lung zones, and the bronchoscopist's learning curve [15, 25]. Chest

Table 6.2 Factors that can influence the risk of pneumothorax

Procedure-related factors
1. Type of sedation/airway control
2. Distance from the pleura
3. Size of the probe and freezing time
4. Sampling strategy
5. Skill level of operator
Patient-related factors
(a) HRCT fibrotic score
(b) UIP pattern

HRCT high-resolution computed tomography, *UIP* usual interstitial pneumonia

computed tomography (CT) represents currently the gold standard for the diagnosis of pneumothorax; however it is not routinely used, to avoid excess of radiation [37], and it is applicable only to uncertain cases; chest X-ray is used routinely for pneumothorax diagnosis, but with a sensitivity of 46% [44]. In recent years, the use of chest ultrasonography (US) has spread for the diagnosis of pneumothorax as it can reach a pooled sensitivity of 87% (95% CI 81–92%) and a specificity of 99% (95% CI 98–99%) [45] according to a standardized method searching for specific pathognomonic signs [46]. Accuracy of US for the detection of pneumothorax is higher than that of chest X-ray with reference to CT scan as a gold standard, and its use would have some advantages, avoiding exposure to radiation and reducing costs of health care and hospital stay. Chest US in pneumothorax diagnosis after transbronchial lung cryobiopsy has been evaluated for the first time by Viglietta et al. [47]: the analysis showed a sensitivity and a specificity of 90% and 94%, respectively. This approach exploits the ready availability of US that allows the pulmonologist who perform cryobiopsy to detect post-procedural pneumothorax within a short time and optimizes the use of ionizing radiation. A post-procedural chest X-ray or ultrasound examination should be performed to assess for the occurrence of pneumothorax either immediately (if desaturation, persistent cough, and/or thoracic pain are present) or 2–3 h after the end of the procedure if the patient is asymptomatic [47]; this is particularly relevant in the outpatient setting. Patients should be observed in the recovery area as per local institutional guidelines.

Another common complication of cryobiopsy is bleeding [2, 3, 5, 6, 9, 11, 14, 43, 48–51], although is generally readily controlled endoscopically, e.g., by the use of bronchial blockers (Fogarty balloon or other tools) and/or use of rigid bronchoscopy [5, 14, 15, 25, 51, 52]. There is no generally accepted bleeding severity scale, and therefore comparability of different papers is difficult. However, most papers grade on a scale of four steps: no bleeding, mild bleeding (e.g., requiring suction to clear but no other endoscopic procedures), moderate bleeding (e.g., requiring endoscopic procedures like bronchial occlusion-collapse and/or instillation of ice-cold saline), and severe bleeding (e.g., causing hemodynamic or respiratory instability, requiring tamponade or other surgical interventions, transfusions, or admission to the intensive care unit) [53]. In a previous meta-analysis, moderate bleeding after cryobiopsy was observed in 65 cases among 383 patients from 12 studies (16.9%), with an overall pooled probability of developing a moderate bleeding of about 0.12 (CI 0.02–0.25) [15]. No episodes of severe bleeding, as defined above, are reported in literature (in some papers bleeding has been reported as severe, but it was controlled by placement of bronchial blocker or catheter) [49], and no bleeding-related deaths have been reported after cryobiopsy. A recently published report highlights the risk of potentially life-threatening complications when these precautions are not taken [17]. Abnormal coagulation parameters and the use of clopidogrel or other new antiplatelet drugs are considered contraindications; treatment with aspirin is regarded as a relative contraindication. In the absence of more definitive data and given the increased bleeding risk compared to conventional forceps biopsies, a conservative approach would be to hold all medications potentially associated with increased bleeding risk. Thrombocytopenia (<50 × 10/L) is suggested to be a contraindication for biopsies during flexible bronchoscopy [51]. These values may be accepted also for TLCB until data on this topic will become available. Patients with clinical or radiological signs of pulmonary hypertension should have a pre-procedural evaluation of pulmonary artery pressure by echocardiography or right heart catheterization. An estimated systolic pulmonary artery pressure >50 mmHg on echocardiography indicates an increased likelihood of pulmonary hypertension and, in the absence of more definitive data, is considered a relative contraindication to TLCB [51].

Other complications are anecdotal and can comprise transient respiratory failure, neurological manifestations (e.g., seizures), pneumomediastinum, prolonged air leak, and pulmonary abscess [52].

Regarding mortality, current data are showing that TLCB appears to be safer than surgical lung biopsy; a recent meta-analysis has revealed an overall mortality rate with this procedure of about 0.1% among approximately 1000 patients [15]. A more recent analysis of data published in the literature on cryobiopsy documents seven deaths within a month after the procedure: one patient died from respiratory failure due to carcinomatous lymphangitis, one from acute myocardial infarction manifesting weeks later, one from pulmonary edema from newly diagnosed severe aortic stenosis, one with organizing pneumonia and who was on palliative care, one from pulmonary embolism, and two patients from acute exacerbation of idiopathic pulmonary fibrosis (IPF) [14, 20, 25, 49] (in both cases of death from acute exacerbation of IPF, diffuse alveolar damage was the histological background on autopsy and the death developed after significant procedural complications: tension pneumothorax with subsequent ventilation with high positive airway pressures and severe bleeding). A more recent case of acute exacerbation of interstitial lung disease (ILD) as a complication of TLCB has been reported in a patient with nonspecific interstitial pneumonitis (although this case report does not describe the TLCB technique specifically analysis of histology, description of HRCT features, and clinical information documenting the presence of a stable disease or rapid progressive deterioration before the TLCB) [53]. The risk of acute exacerbation needs to be assessed before the procedure, particularly in case of recent worsening [37, 54, 55]: recent onset of patchy ground-glass areas on HRCT scan, functional deterioration and/or increased dyspnea on exertion in the last month, and/or high levels of inflammatory or more specific markers (KL-6) could be predictors of high acute exacerbation risk [56, 57]. Acute deterioration in respiratory status should be considered a relative contraindication, although the decision needs to be individualized based on assessment of benefits and risks [1].

Anecdotal data suggest that complications are more frequent when pulmonary function is severely impaired. Forced expiratory volume in the first second (FEV_1) <0.8 L or <50% predicted, forced vital capacity (FVC) <50% predicted, and diffusing capacity of the lungs for carbon monoxide (DLCO) <35% or <50% predicted have been used to exclude biopsy candidates in some series, though not in all [2, 15, 25]; however, these limitations are drawn from data reported in studies dealing with SLB; additionally, in the subset of patients with severe fibrosing ILD, the risk-benefit analysis is less advantageous, because in these patients it seems that the prognostic significance of an exact histological diagnosis is reduced [58] and data on the efficacy of a specific "anti-fibrotic" drug on patients with severe IPF are still scanty [58–63]. Our large cohort of 699 patients who underwent transbronchial lung cryobiopsy for suspected diffuse parenchymal lung diseases, pneumothorax incidence, was significantly higher when FVC was <50% (p 0.008), but it was not influenced by DLCO (p 0.7842), while bleeding appeared independent by the lung function tests (both FVC and DLCO). We suggest that FVC < 50% should be considered as a relative contraindication to transbronchial lung biopsy on safety grounds while baseline DLCO should be evaluated together with other clinical, radiological, and laboratory features [1]. Significant hypoxemia, defined as PaO_2 < 55–60 mmHg on room air or while receiving 2 L/min of nasal oxygen, has also been considered a contraindication by some but not others [3, 6, 25]. A high body mass index (BMI > 35) can result in failure of the procedure [1, 25], mainly because of desaturation in intubated and spontaneously breathing patients. Additionally, a study evaluated TBCB in mechanically ventilated patients in the intensive care unit, though the experience remains anecdotal at this time [1, 64]. No age limit has been suggested at this time, as TBCB has been performed safely in a wide age range of patients, which need to be carefully evaluated in terms of comorbidities and fitness for anesthesia [1].

References

1. Hetzel J, Maldonado F, Ravaglia C, et al. Transbronchial cryobiopsies for the diagnosis of diffuse parenchymal lung diseases: expert statement from the cryobiopsy working group on safety and utility and a call for standardization of the procedure. Respiration. 2018;95:188–200.
2. Babiak A, Hetzel J, Krishna G, et al. Tranbronchial cryobiopsy: a new tool for lung biopsies. Respiration. 2009;78:203–8.
3. Kropski JA, Pritchett JM, Mason WR, et al. Bronchoscopic cryobiopsy for the diagnosis of diffuse parenchymal lung disease. PLoS One. 2013;12:e78674.
4. Fruchter O, Fridel L, Rosengarten D, et al. Transbronchial cryobiopsy in immunocompromised patients with pulmonary infiltrates: a pilot study. Lung. 2013;91:619–24.
5. Yarmus L, Akulian J, Gilbert C, et al. Cryoprobe transbronchial lung biopsy in patients after lung transplantation: a pilot safety study. Chest. 2013;143:621–6.
6. Pajares V, Puzo C, Castillo D, et al. Diagnostic yield of transbronchial cryobiopsy in interstitial lung disease: a randomized trial. Respirology. 2014;19:900–6.
7. Fruchter O, Fridel L, El Raouf BA, et al. Histological diagnosis of interstitial lung diseases by cryo-transbronchial biopsy. Respirology. 2014;19:683–38.
8. Pourabdollah M, Shamaei M, Karimi S, et al. Transbronchial lung biopsy: the pathologist's point of view. Clin Respir J. 2016;10:211–6.
9. Griff S, Schönfeld N, Ammenwerth W, et al. Diagnostic yield of transbronchial cryobiopsy in non-neoplastic lung disease: a retrospective case series. BMC Pulm Med. 2014;14:171.
10. Hernández-González F, Lucena CM, Ramírez J, et al. Cryobiopsy in the diagnosis of diffuse interstitial lung disease: yield and cost- effectiveness analysis (in English, Spanish). Arch Bronconeumol. 2015;6:261–7.
11. Hagmeyer L, Theegarten D, Wohlschläger J, et al. The role of transbronchial cryobiopsy and surgical lung biopsy in the diagnostic algorithm of interstitial lung disease. Clin Respir J. 2016;10:589–95.
12. Gershman E, Fruchter O, Benjamin F, et al. Safety of cryo-transbronchial biopsy in diffuse lung diseases: analysis of three hundred cases. Respiration. 2015;90:40–6.
13. Ramaswamy A, Homer R, Killam J, et al. Comparison of transbronchial and cryobiopsies in evaluation of diffuse parenchymal lung disease. J Bronchology Interv Pulmonol. 2016;23:14–21.
14. Echevarria-Uraga JJ, Pèerez-Izquierdo J, Garcìa-Garai N, et al. Usefulness of an angioplasty balloon as selective bronchial blockade device after transbronchial cryobiopsy. Respirology. 2016;21:1094–9.
15. Ravaglia C, Bonifazi M, Wells AU, et al. Safety and diagnostic yield of transbronchial lung cryobiopsy in diffuse parenchymal lung diseases: a comparative study versus video-assisted thoracoscopic lung biopsy and a systematic review of the literature. Respiration. 2016;91:215–27.
16. Ussavarungsi K, Kern RM, Roden AC, et al. Transbronchial cryobiopsy in diffuse parenchymal lung disease: retrospective analysis of 74 cases. Chest. 2017;151:400–8.
17. DiBardino DM, Haas AR, Lanfranco AR, et al. High complication rate after introduction of transbronchial cryobiopsy into clinical practice at an Academic Medical Center. Ann Am Thorac Soc. 2017;14:851–7.
18. Bango-Alvarez A, Ariza-Prota M, Torres-Rivas H, et al. Transbronchial cryobiopsy in interstitial lung disease: experience in 106 cases—how to do it. ERJ Open Res. 2017;3:00148-2016.
19. Kronborg-White S, Folkersen B, Rasmussen TR, et al. Introduction of cryobiopsies in the diagnostics of interstitial lung diseases—experiences in a referral center. Eur Clin Respir J. 2017;4:1274099.
20. Sriprasart T, Aragaki A, Baughman R, et al. A single US center experience of transbronchial lung cryobiopsy for diagnosing interstitial lung disease with a 2-scope technique. J Bronchology Interv Pulmonol. 2017;24:131–5.
21. Ravaglia C, Wells AU, Tomassetti S, et al. Transbronchial lung cryobiopsy in diffuse parenchymal lung disease: comparison between biopsy from 1 segment and biopsy from 2 segments—diagnostic yield and complications. Respiration. 2017;93:285–92.
22. Wall CP, Gaensler EA, Carrington CB, et al. Comparison of transbronchial and open biopsies in chronic infiltrative lung diseases. Am Rev Respir Dis. 1981;123:280–5.
23. O'Brien JD, Ettinger NA, Shevlin D, et al. Safety and yield of transbronchial biopsy in mechanically ventilated patients. Crit Care Med. 1997;25:440–6.
24. Berbescu EA, Katzenstein AL, Snow JL, et al. Transbronchial biopsy in usual interstitial pneumonia. Chest. 2006;129:1126–31.
25. Casoni GL, Tomassetti S, Cavazza A, et al. Transbronchial lung cryobiopsy in the diagnosis of fibrotic interstitial lung diseases. PLoS One. 2014;9:e86716.
26. Facciolongo N, Patelli M, Gasparini S, et al. Incidence of complications in bronchoscopy. Multicentre prospective study of 20,986 bronchoscopies. Monaldi Arch Chest Dis. 2009;71:8–14.
27. Tomassetti S, Piciucchi S, Tantalocco P, et al. The multidisciplinary approach in the diagnosis of idiopathic pulmonary fibrosis: a patient case-based review. Eur Respir Rev. 2015;24:69–773.

28. Sheth JS, Belperio JA, Fishbein MC, et al. Utility of transbronchial versus surgical lung biopsy in the diagnosis of suspected fibrotic interstitial lung disease. Chest. 2017;151:389–99.
29. Rena O, Casadio C, Leo F, et al. Videothoracoscopic lung biopsy in the diagnosis of interstitial lung disease. Eur J Cardiothorac Surg. 1999;16:624–7.
30. Kreider ME, Hansen-Flaschen J, Ahmad NN, et al. Complications of video-assisted thoracoscopic lung biopsy in patients with interstitial lung disease. Ann Thorac Surg. 2007;83:1140–4.
31. Zhang D, Liu Y. Surgical lung biopsies in 418 patients with suspected interstitial lung disease in China. Intern Med. 2010;49:1097–102.
32. Fibla JJ, Molins L, Blanco A, et al. Video-assisted thoracoscopic lung biopsy in the diagnosis of interstitial lung disease: a prospective, multi-center study in 224 patients. Arch Bronconeumol. 2012;48:81–5.
33. Blackhall V, Asif M, Renieri A, et al. The role of surgical lung biopsy in the management of interstitial lung disease: experience from a single institution in the UK. Interact Cardiovasc Thorac Surg. 2013;17:253–7.
34. Morris D, Zamvar V. The efficacy of video-assisted thoracoscopic surgery lung biopsies in patients with interstitial lung disease: a retrospective study of 66 patients. J Cardiothorac Surg. 2014;9:45.
35. Rotolo N, Imperatori A, Dominioni L, et al. Efficacy and safety of surgical lung biopsy for interstitial disease. Experience of 161 consecutive patients from a single institution in Italy. Sarcoidosis Vasc Diffuse Lung Dis. 2015;32:251–8.
36. Hutchinson JP, McKeever TM, Fogarty AW, et al. Surgical lung biopsy for the diagnosis of interstitial lung disease in England: 1997–2008. Eur Respir J. 2016;48:1453–61.
37. Hutchinson JP, Fogarty AW, McKeever TM, et al. In-hospital mortality after surgical lung biopsy for interstitial lung disease in the United States. 2000 to 2011. Am J Respir Crit Care Med. 2016;193:1161–7.
38. Lieberman S, Gleason JB, Ilyas MIM, et al. Assessing the safety and clinical impact of thoracoscopic lung biopsy in patients with interstitial lung disease. J Clin Diagn Res. 2017;11:OC57–9.
39. Patel RR, Utz JP. Bronchoscopic lung biopsy. In: Wang K-P, Metha AC, Turner Jr JF, editors. Flexible bronchoscopy. Chichester: Wiley-Blackwell; 2011. p. 117–31.
40. Griff S, Ammenwerth W, Schönfeld N, et al. Morphometrical analysis of transbronchial cryobiopsies. Diagn Pathol. 2011;6:53.
41. Iftikhar IH, Alghothani L, Sardi A, et al. Transbronchial lung cryobiopsy and video-assisted thoracoscopic lung biopsy in the diagnosis of diffuse parenchymal lung disease: a meta-analysis of diagnostic test accuracy. Ann Am Thorac Soc. 2017;14:1197–211.
42. O'Donovan JP, Khan KA, Burke L, et al. Bronchoscopic cryobiopsy: initial experience in an interstitial lung disease centre. Irish J Med Sci. 2014;183(11 Suppl 1):S515–6.
43. Sharp C, McCabe M, Adamali H, et al. Use of transbronchial cryobiopsy in the diagnosis of interstitial lung disease-a systematic review and cost analysis. QJM. 2017;110:207–14.
44. Ball CG, Kirkpatrick AW, Laupland KB, et al. Factors related to the failure of radiographic recognition of occult post traumatic pneumothoraces. Am J Surg. 2005;189:541.
45. Ebrahimi A, Yousefifard M, Mohammad Kazemi H, et al. Diagnostic accuracy of chest ultrasonography versus chest radiography for identification of pneumothorax: a systematic review and meta-analysis. Tanaffos. 2014;13:29–40.
46. Husain LF, Hagopian L, Wayman D, et al. Sonographic diagnosis of pneumothorax. J Emerg Trauma Shock. 2012;5:76–81.
47. Viglietta L, Inchingolo R, Pavano C, et al. Ultrasonography for the diagnosis of pneumothorax after transbronchial lung cryobiopsy in diffuse cryobiopsy in diffuse parenchymal lung diseases. Respiration. 2017;94:232–6.
48. Poletti V, Hetzel J. Transbronchial cryobiopsy in diffuse parenchymal lung disease: need for procedural standardization. Respiration. 2015;90:275–8.
49. Hagmeyer L, Theegarten D, Treml M, et al. Validation of transbronchial cryobiopsy in interstitial lung disease—interim analysis of a prospective trial and critical review of the literature. Sarcoidosis Vasc Diffuse Lung Dis. 2016;33:2–9.
50. Linhas R, Marçôa R, Oliveira A, et al. Transbronchial lung cryobiopsy: associated complications. Rev Port Pneumol (2006). 2017;23:331–7.
51. Chan JWM, Yeung YC, Sin KM, et al. Guidelines of procedural and sedation safety in flexible bronchoscopy and pleuroscopy. Hong Kong Thoracic Society, American College of Chest Physicians (Hong Kong and Macau Chapter), Hong Kong Lung Foundation. 2016.
52. Skalski JH, Kern RM, Midthun DE, et al. Pulmonary abscess as a complication of transbronchial lung cryobiopsy. J Bronchology Interv Pulmonol. 2016;23:63–6.
53. Tomic R, Cortes-Puentes GA, Murugan P, et al. Acute exacerbation of interstitial lung disease after cryobiopsy. J Bronchology Interv Pulmonol. 2017;24:319–22.
54. Ernst A, Eberhardt R, Wahidi M. Effect of routine clopidogrel use on bleeding complications after transbronchial biopsy in humans. Chest. 2006;129:734–7.
55. Utz JP, Ryu JH, Douglas WW, et al. High short-term mortality following lung biopsy for usual interstitial pneumonia. Eur Respir J. 2001;17:175–9.
56. Qiu M, Chen Y, Ye Q. Risk factors for acute exacerbation of idiopathic pulmonary fibrosis: a systematic review and meta-analysis. Clin Respir J. 2018;12:1084–92.

57. Fujimoto K, Taniguchi H, Johkoh T, et al. Acute exacerbation of idiopathic pulmonary fibrosis: high resolution CT scores predict mortality. Eur Radiol. 2012;22:83–92.

58. Latsi PI, du Bois RM, Nicholson AG, et al. Fibrotic idiopathic interstitial pneumonia: the prognostic value of longitudinal functional trends. Am J Respir Crit Care Med. 2003;168:531–7.

59. King TE Jr, Bradford WZ, Castro-Bernardini S, et al. A phase 3 trial of pirfenidone in patients with idiopathic pulmonary fibrosis. N Engl J Med. 2014;370:2083–92.

60. Richeldi L, du Bois RM, Raghu G, et al. Efficacy and safety of nintedanib in idiopathic pulmonary fibrosis. N Engl J Med. 2014;370:2071–82.

61. Harari S, Caminati A, Albera C, et al. Efficacy of pirfenidone for idiopathic pulmonary fibrosis: an Italian real life study. Respir Med. 2015;109:904–13.

62. Martinez FJ, Flaherty KR. Comprehensive and individualized patient care in idiopathic pulmonary fibrosis: refining approaches to diagnosis, prognosis, and treatment. Chest. 2017;151:1173–4.

63. Lee SH, Shim HS, Cho SH, et al. Prognostic factors for idiopathic pulmonary fibrosis: clinical, physiologic, pathologic, and molecular aspects. Sarcoidosis Vasc Diffuse Lung Dis. 2011;28:102–12.

64. Munoz Fernandez AM, Pajares V, Lucena C, et al. Safety of transbronchial lung criobiopsy in mechanically ventilated patients in critical care. Multicenter study. European Respiratory Congress. 2016.

Histology for Transbronchial Lung Cryobiopsy Samples

7

Tamiko Takemura, Tomohisa Baba, Takashi Niwa, and Takashi Ogura

7.1 Introduction

Transbronchial lung cryobiopsy (TBLC) is now recognized as a useful tool for the diagnosis of diffuse interstitial lung diseases [1–5], although surgical lung biopsy (SLB) still remains the standard diagnostic procedure [6, 7].

The lung tissue specimens obtained by TBLC are usually smaller than those obtained by SLB [8]. It is important for pathological diagnosis to recognize the anatomical location of structures in the obtained lung tissue specimens. In this chapter, we present a comparison of normal lung tissue samples and representative specimens obtained by cryobiopsy, in the viewpoint of lung architecture.

7.1.1 Processing of Cryobiopsy Specimens

The frozen lung tissue samples are immersed in saline, and the thawed lung specimens are trans-

ferred into a 20-mL syringe containing a small amount of saline and inflated by slow application of negative pressure for 30–60 s. After this process, the alveoli are well inflated and eligible for histopathological examination. Figure 7.1 shows well-inflated lung tissue specimens measuring up to about 7 mm in diameter, as compared with the specimens containing non-inflated alveoli.

As for the staining, we recommend elastic van Gieson (EVG) staining and Alcian blue staining in addition to hematoxylin-eosin staining. EVG staining is necessary to recognize the normal and remodeled pulmonary architecture. Alcian blue staining is also useful to detect immature fibrosis such as fibroblastic foci containing much glycoprotein.

7.1.2 Normal Structure of the Lobules and Acini in TBLC Specimens

What are the structures that can be obtained by TBLC? Figure 7.2 shows a Softex image of the peripheral lung tissue, indicating the area from which TBLC specimens are obtained. Usually the cryoprobe is inserted into a membranous bronchiole through the bronchus and pulled 1 cm from the chest wall. The area sampled by the cryoprobe includes the membranous and respiratory bronchioles and peribronchiolar alveoli and

T. Takemura (✉)
Department of Pathology, Japanese Red Cross Medical Center, Tokyo, Japan
e-mail: byori@med.jrc.or.jp

T. Baba · T. Niwa · T. Ogura
Department of Respiratory Medicine, Kanagawa Cardiovascular and Respiratory Center,
Yokohama, Japan
e-mail: baba@kanagawa-junko.jp; niwa@kanagawa-junko.jp; ogura@kanagawa-junko.jp

© Springer Nature Switzerland AG 2019
V. Poletti (ed.), *Transbronchial cryobiopsy in diffuse parenchymal lung disease*,
https://doi.org/10.1007/978-3-030-14891-1_7

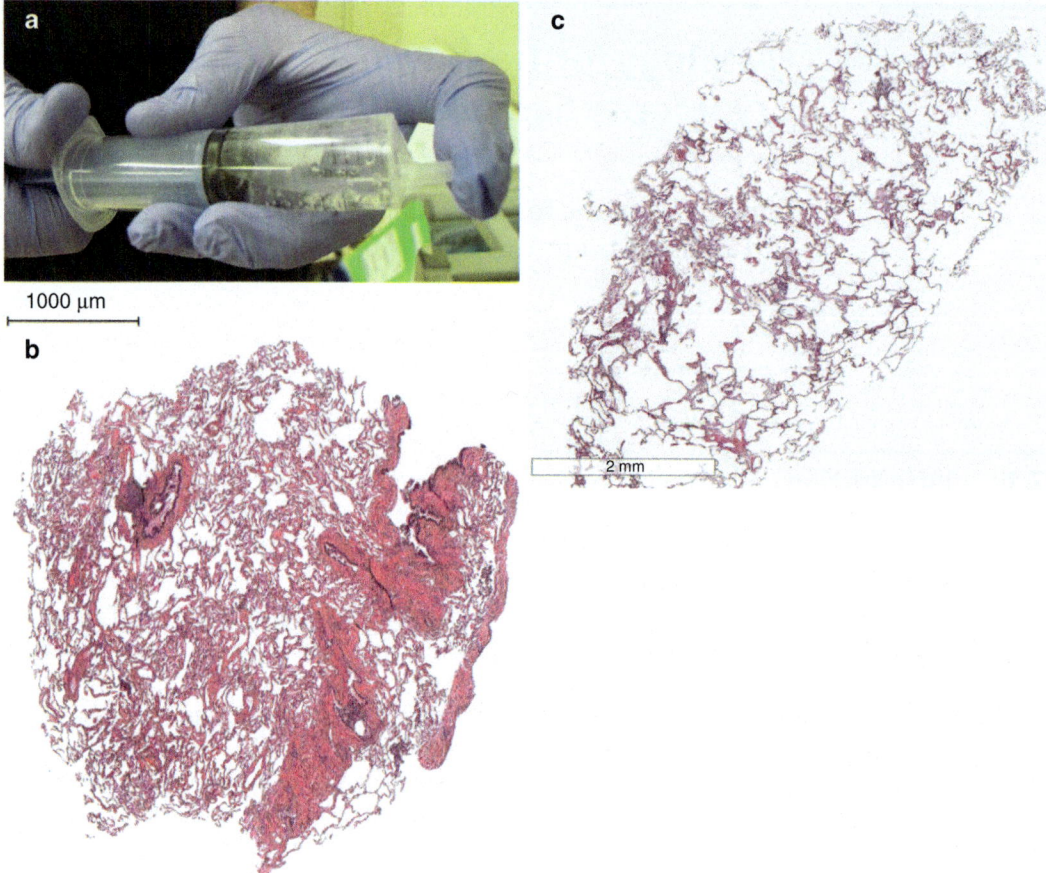

Fig. 7.1 Expansion of the thawed lung specimens. (**a**) Expansion of a thawed specimen in a 20-mL syringe by negative pressure before fixation with buffered formalin. (**b**) Poorly aerated alveoli in an uninflated specimen (HE, ×1). (**c**) Inflated alveoli obtained by application of negative pressure before fixation (HE, ×1)

pulmonary arteries and veins. Figure 7.3 reveals a more detailed three-dimensional scheme of a pulmonary lobule [9]. A pulmonary lobule measures 8–10 mm in diameter and is encircled by interlobular veins. One lobule contains about 3–5 acini, and a terminal bronchiole is located at the entrance to the acinus; respiratory bronchioles are located in the subacinar level. Red circle area may be sampled by TBLC.

The area encircled in green in the paraffin-embedded tissue is sampled by TBLC; it contains the terminal bronchiole, respiratory bronchioles, interlobular (interacinar) septa, and alveoli (Fig. 7.4). Pathological diagnosis is based on a clear understanding of the normal lung architecture, especially in view of the patchy distribution

of some diseases, e.g., usual interstitial pneumonia (UIP)/idiopathic pulmonary fibrosis (IPF).

7.1.3 Pathological Diagnosis of UIP Based on the Pulmonary Architecture

7.1.3.1 UIP Diagnosed in SLB Specimens

Pathology of UIP is characterized by dense fibrosis with architectural distortion, predominant subpleural and/or paraseptal distribution of fibrosis, patchy involvement of the lung parenchyma by fibrosis, fibroblastic foci, and absence of features to suggest an alternate diagnosis [7, 10].

Fig. 7.2 Peripheral lung tissue. Softex image of normal peripheral lung tissue containing several lobules. The area encircled in green reveals the area possibly sampled by cryobiopsy and includes a membranous bronchiole, interlobular septa, veins, and arteries (Courtesy of Dr. H. Itoh, Fukui University)

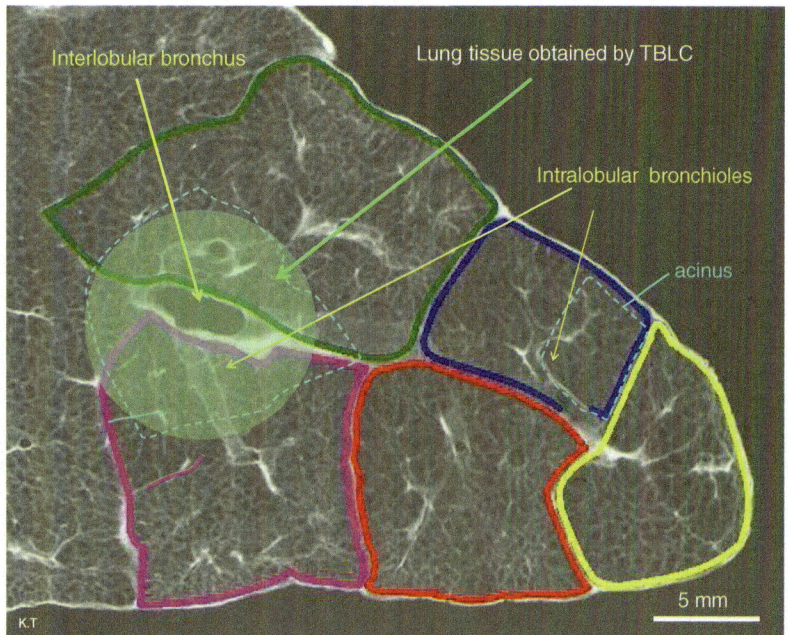

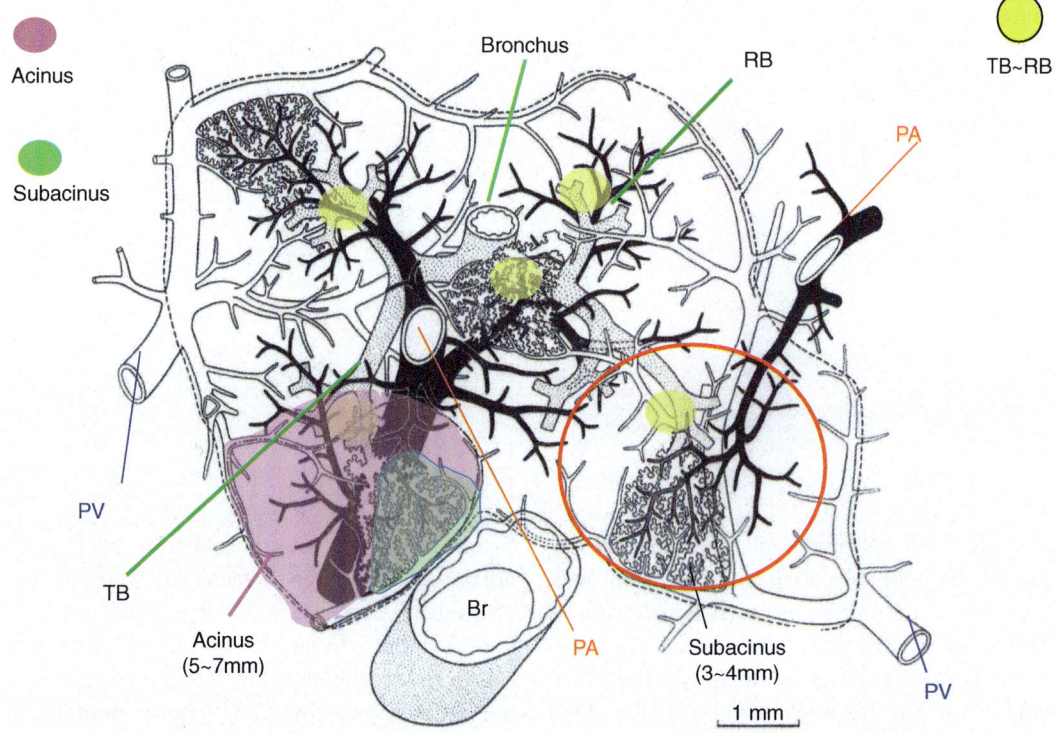

Fig. 7.3 Scheme of a pulmonary lobule. Scheme of a pulmonary lobule measuring 8–10 mm in diameter encircled by interlobular veins. Each lobule contains 3–5 acini (Permission from Iwanami Publisher, Tokyo, Japan). Area encircled in red may be sampled by cryobiopsy. *TB* terminal bronchiole, *RB* respiratory bronchiole

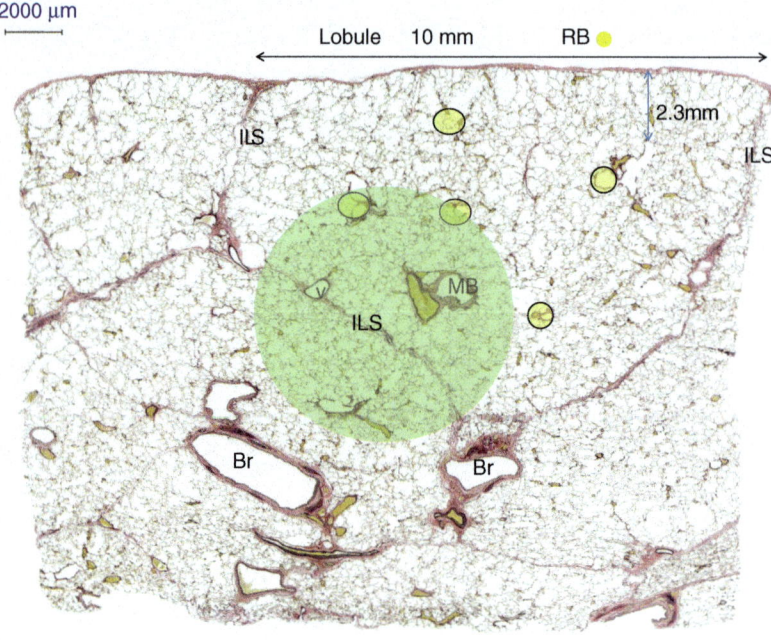

Fig. 7.4 Paraffin-embedded normal pulmonary lobule. Area encircled in green indicates the area sampled by cryobiopsy (EVG, ×1)

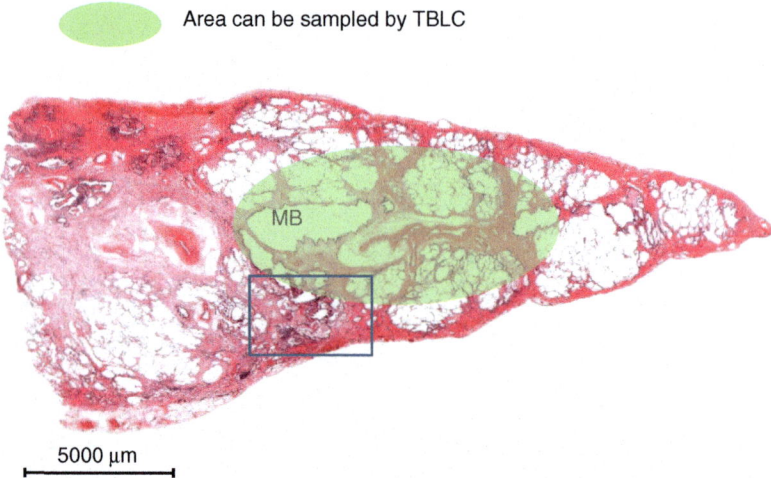

Fig. 7.5 Surgical lung biopsy specimen of UIP/IPF. Surgical lung biopsy specimen from the lower lobe with UIP/IPF, showing subpleural and paraseptal fibrosis alternating with normal alveoli. A square area shows microscopic honeycombing (HE, ×1)

Figure 7.5 reveals subpleural and paraseptal fibrosis with normal alveoli, consistent with the typical UIP pattern, in an SLB specimen. If TBLC were performed, structures in the area encircled in green can be obtained. The encircled area in Fig. 7.6, if obtained by TBLC, shows paraseptal fibrosis and peribronchiolar fibrosis with fibroblastic foci and alternating normal alveoli, consistent with UIP, even without pleural or subpleural fibrosis.

In TBLC specimens, honeycomb lesions cannot be easily observed, as seen in SLB specimens. The square area in Fig. 7.5 reveals microscopic honeycombing. Figure 7.7 reveals the structures shown in the square of Fig. 7.5 in greater detail; the area stained by EVG shows perilobular alveolar collapse, bronchiolar epithelialization of dilated alveoli, and traction bronchiolectasis. The area encircled may be sampled by TBLC is corresponding to microscopic honeycombing.

Fig. 7.6 A part of lobule of UIP. Paraseptal and peribronchiolar fibrosis with fibroblastic foci (arrows) are the hallmarks of UIP. This area is a part of Fig. 7.5 (EVG ×2.5). The circled area may be sampled by cryobiopsy, even in the absence of pleural and subpleural fibrosis

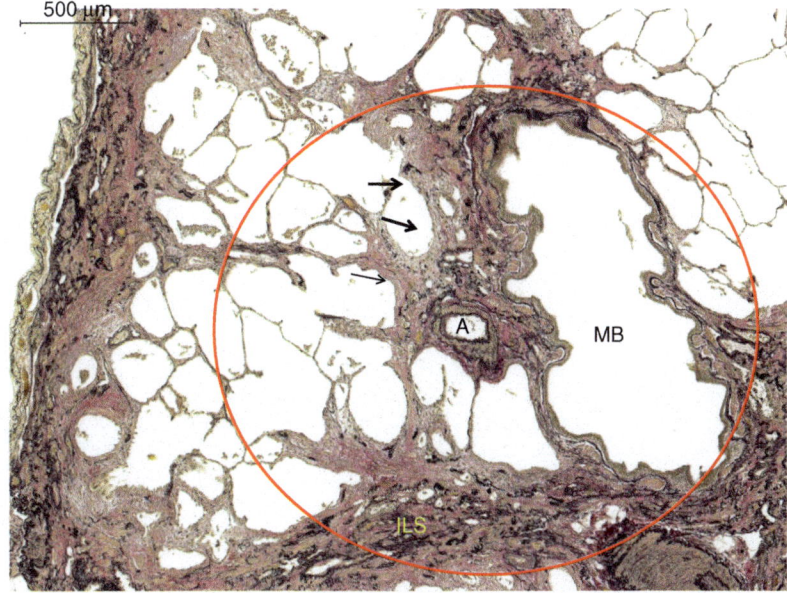

Fig. 7.7 Microscopic honeycombing. Microscopic honeycombing shows perilobular collapsed alveoli, bronchiolar epithelization, and traction bronchiolectasis. The encircled area, i.e., a part of microscopic honeycombing, may be sampled by cryobiopsy (EVG, ×2.5). *MB* membranous bronchiole, *TB* terminal bronchiole, *ILS* interlobular septum

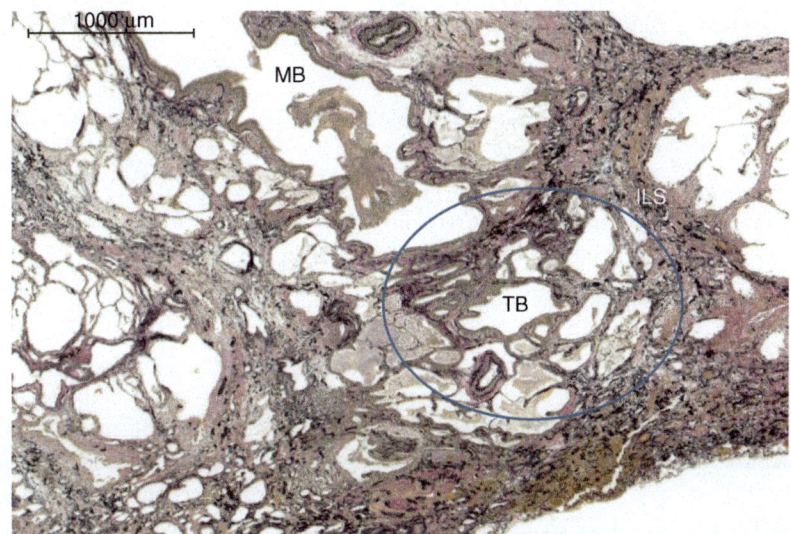

7.1.3.2 UIP Diagnosed in TBLC Specimens

Figure 7.8a shows dense patchy fibrosis alternating with normal alveoli, containing two subacini, which are more clearly demonstrated by EVG staining, because of interlobular septum in the center (Fig. 7.8b) and fibroblastic foci (Fig. 7.8b, c).

Thus, pathological diagnosis of UIP by TBLC can be made with some degree of confidence [3, 5]. However, the histologic features in a small area of the lung cannot represent the entire pathological events. Thus, care must be ensured to avoid overdiagnosis. Patchy fibrosis in the pulmonary lobule can be observed in many clinical settings. Fibrosis apposed to the bronchovascular sheath or in the periacinar region is diagnostic of UIP. Microscopic honeycombing can be detected by TBLC. However, peribronchiolar

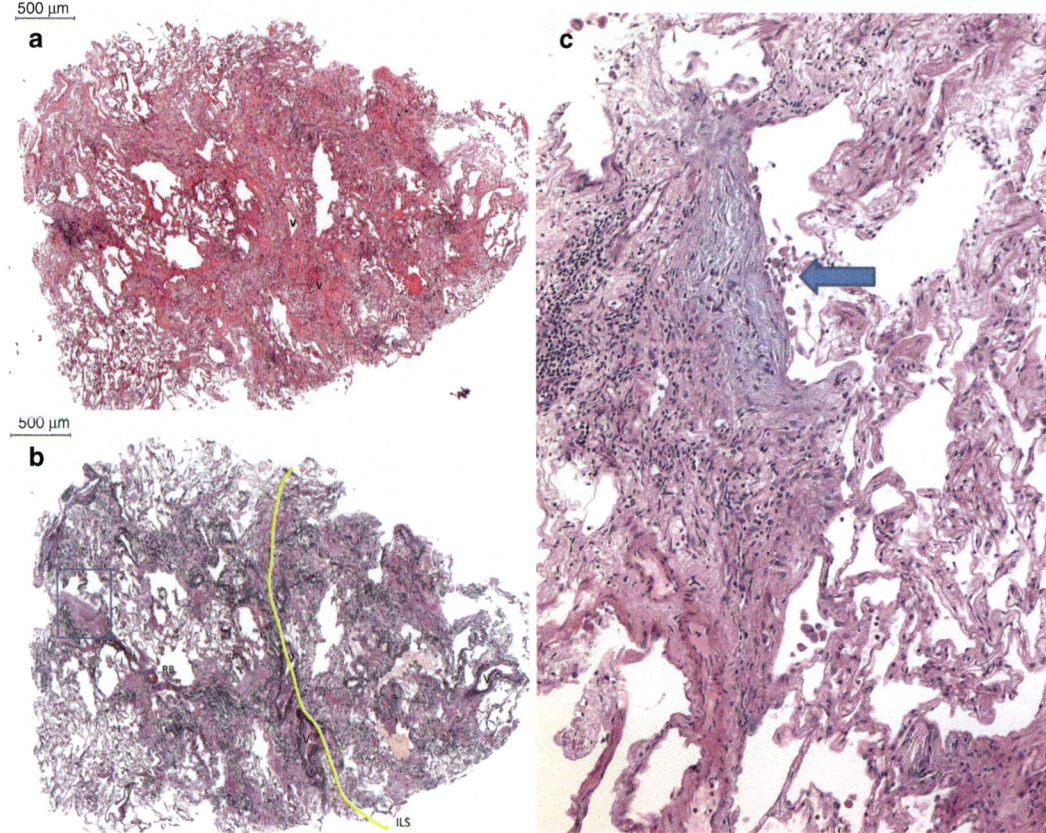

Fig. 7.8 UIP in cryobiopsy. (**a**) Cryobiopsy from the lower bronchus shows dense patchy fibrosis alternating normal alveoli (HE, ×4). *V* interlobular vein. (**b**) Fibrosis is mainly apposed to the interlobular septum and perivenular area (EVG, ×4). (**c**) Fibroblastic focus (*arrow*) is located on the old fibrosis (square of **b**), clearly demonstrated by Alcian blue staining (PAS-Alcian blue, ×10)

metaplasia, which is usually observed around bronchioles, must be differentiated from microscopic honeycombing.

7.2 Conclusion

TBLC can be safely performed for the diagnosis of diffuse interstitial lung disease (ILD) and provides reliable pathological diagnosis, potentially enabling prompt decision on the appropriate therapy.

However, there are still limitations of TBLC, as compared to SLB, for the pathological diagnosis of ILD, because of the limitation of the area from which samples can be obtained (more central area) and a high frequency of discordance with the radiological diagnosis. Further studies of correlations between diagnoses by TBLC and SLB are needed to determine the degree of diagnostic confidence that can be obtained with TBLC.

References

1. Poletti V, Hetzel J. Transbronchial cryobiopsy in diffuse parenchymal lung disease: need for procedural standardization. Respiration. 2015;90:275–8.
2. Hetzel J, Maldonado F, Ravaglia C, Wells AU, Colby TV, Tomassetti S, Ryu JH, Fruchter O, Piciucchi S, Dubini A, Cavazza A, Chilosi M, Sverzellati N, Valeyre D, Leduc D, Walsh SLF, Gasparini S, Hetzel M, Hagmeyer L, Haentschel M, Eberhardt R,

Darwiche K, Yarmus LB, Torrego A, Krishna G, Shah PL, Annema JT, Herth FJF, Poletti V. Transbronchial cryobiopsies for the diagnosis of diffuse parenchymal lung diseases: expert statement from the cryobiopsy working group on safety and utility and a call for standardization of the procedure. Respiration. 2018;95:188–200.

3. Ravaglia C, Wells AU, Tomassetti S, Dubini A, Cavazza A, Piciucchi S, Sverzellati N, Gurioli C, Gurioli C, Costabel U, Tantalocco P, Ryu JH, Chilosi M, Poletti V. Transbronchial lung cryobiopsy in diffuse parenchymal lung disease: comparison between biopsy from 1 segment and biopsy from 2 segments-diagnostic yield and complications. Respiration. 2017;93:285–92.

4. Colby TV, Tomassetti S, Cavazza A, Dubini A, Poletti V. Transbronchial cryobiopsy in diffuse lung disease. Update for the pathologist. Arch Pathol Lab Med. 2017;141:891–900.

5. Tomassetti S, Wells AU, Costabel U, Cavazza A, Colby TV, Rossi G, Sverzellati N, Carloni A, Carretta E, Buccioli M, Tantalocco P, Ravaglia C, Gurioli C, Dubini A, Piciucchi S, Ryu JH, Poletti V. Bronchoscopic lung cryobiopsy increases diagnostic confidence in the multidisciplinary diagnosis of idiopathic pulmonary fibrosis. Am J Respir Crit Care Med. 2016;193:745–52.

6. Lynch DA, Sverzellati N, Travis WD, Brown KK, Colby TV, Galvin JR, Goldin JG, Hansell DM, Inoue Y, Johkoh T, Nicholson AG, Knight SL, Raoof S, RIcheldi L, Ryerson CJ, Ryu JH, Wells AU. Diagnostic criteria for idiopathic pulmonary fibrosis: a Fleischner Society White Paper. Lancet Respir Med. 2018;6:138–53.

7. Raghu G, Remy-Jardin M, Myers JL, Richeldi R, Ryerson CJ, Ledere DJ, Behr J, Cottin V, Danoff SK, Morell F, Flaherty KR, Wells A, Martinez FJ, Azuma A, Bice TJ, Bouros D, Brown KK, Collard HR, Duggal A, Galvin L, Inoue Y, Jenkins RG, Johkoh T, Kazerooni EA, Kitaichi M, Knight SL, Mansour G, Nicholson AG, Pipavath SNJ, Buendia-Roldan I, Selman M, Travis WD, Walsh S, Wilson KC, On behalf of the American Thoracic Society, European Respiratory Society, Japanese Respiratory Society, and Latin American Thoracic Society. Diagnosis of idiopathic pulmonary fibrosis. An official ATS/ERS/JRS/ALAT clinical practice guideline. Am J Respir Crit Care Med. 2018;198(5):e44–68.

8. Pajares V, Puzo C, Castillo D, Lerma E, Montero MA, Ramos-Barbon D, Amor-Carro O, Gil de Bernabe A, Franquet T, Plaza V, Hetzel J, Sanchis J, Torrego A. Diagnostic yield of transbronchial cryobiopsy in interstitial lung disease: a randomized trial. Respirology. 2014;19:900–6.

9. Matsumoto T. Lung. Chapter 10 in tissue and organ. In: Modern biology course 10. Tokyo: Iwanami Publisher; 1977. p. 315–72.

10. Raghu G, Collard HR, Egan JJ, et al. An official ATS/ERS/JRS/ALAT statement: idiopathic pulmonary fibrosis: evidence-based guidelines for diagnosis and management. Am J Respir Crit Care Med. 2011;183:788–214.

Pathologic Considerations in Transbronchial Cryobiopsy

8

Alberto Cavazza, Maria Cecilia Mengoli,
Alessandra Dubini, Giulio Rossi, Rita Bianchi,
and Thomas V. Colby

Technical recommendations. Cryobiopsy specimens should be processed in the same way as other pathology specimens [1, 2], with minimal manipulation both in the bronchoscopy suite and in the laboratory to minimize artifacts. The tissue should be embedded in paraffin along the long axis to maximize the cut surface area, and histologic sections should be obtained at different levels and stained with hematoxylin-eosin. Leaving about 40% of residual tissue in the block allows one to obtain additional slides, if they are needed for further study, special stains, immunohistochemistry, etc.

Optimum size of the specimens. Cryobiopsy specimens should be at least 5 mm in diameter; if smaller they provide little more information than traditional transbronchial forceps biopsies. The

technique of cryobiopsy is operator-dependent, and good samples require a skilled and experience operator.

Artifacts and tissues other than lung encountered in cryobiopsies. Cryobiopsies are easier to interpret than traditional transbronchial forceps biopsies because they are generally bigger and without appreciable crush artifact, a typical finding in the latter. The main artifacts and nonpulmonary tissues that can be found with cryobiopsies are shown in Figs. 8.1 and 8.2.

Pathologist's interpretation. Cryobiopsies should be interpreted like any other biopsy performed for diffuse parenchymal lung diseases [1, 3]: the pathologist should try to identify histologic pattern, anatomic distribution, and any histologic findings which may be specific for a single disease (i.e., neoplastic cells, microorganisms) or nonspecific but useful to narrow the differential diagnosis (i.e., granulomas). Although cryobiopsies are significantly smaller than surgical lung biopsies and the histologic diagnosis rate is lower (75–80% vs >95%), in many cases cryobiopsies are "large enough" to reach a specific diagnosis including a pattern diagnosis such as usual interstitial pneumonia. We have found it useful to give a level of confidence (high vs low) for the pathologic interpretation that is then discussed in the context of the multidisciplinary team [4]. In this setting cryobiopsy histologic diagnosis both informs and is informed by the

A. Cavazza (✉) · M. C. Mengoli
Pathology Unit, Azienda USL/IRCCS,
Reggio Emilia, Italy
e-mail: cavazza.alberto@ausl.re.it

A. Dubini
Pathology Unit, Ospedale Morgagni/Pietrantoni,
Forlì, Italy

G. Rossi
Pathology Unit, Ospedale S. Croce, Ravenna, Italy

R. Bianchi
Pathology Unit, Policlinico S. Martino, Genova, Italy

T. V. Colby
Pathology Unit, Mayo Clinic, Phoenix, AZ, USA

© Springer Nature Switzerland AG 2019
V. Poletti (ed.), *Transbronchial cryobiopsy in diffuse parenchymal lung disease*,
https://doi.org/10.1007/978-3-030-14891-1_8

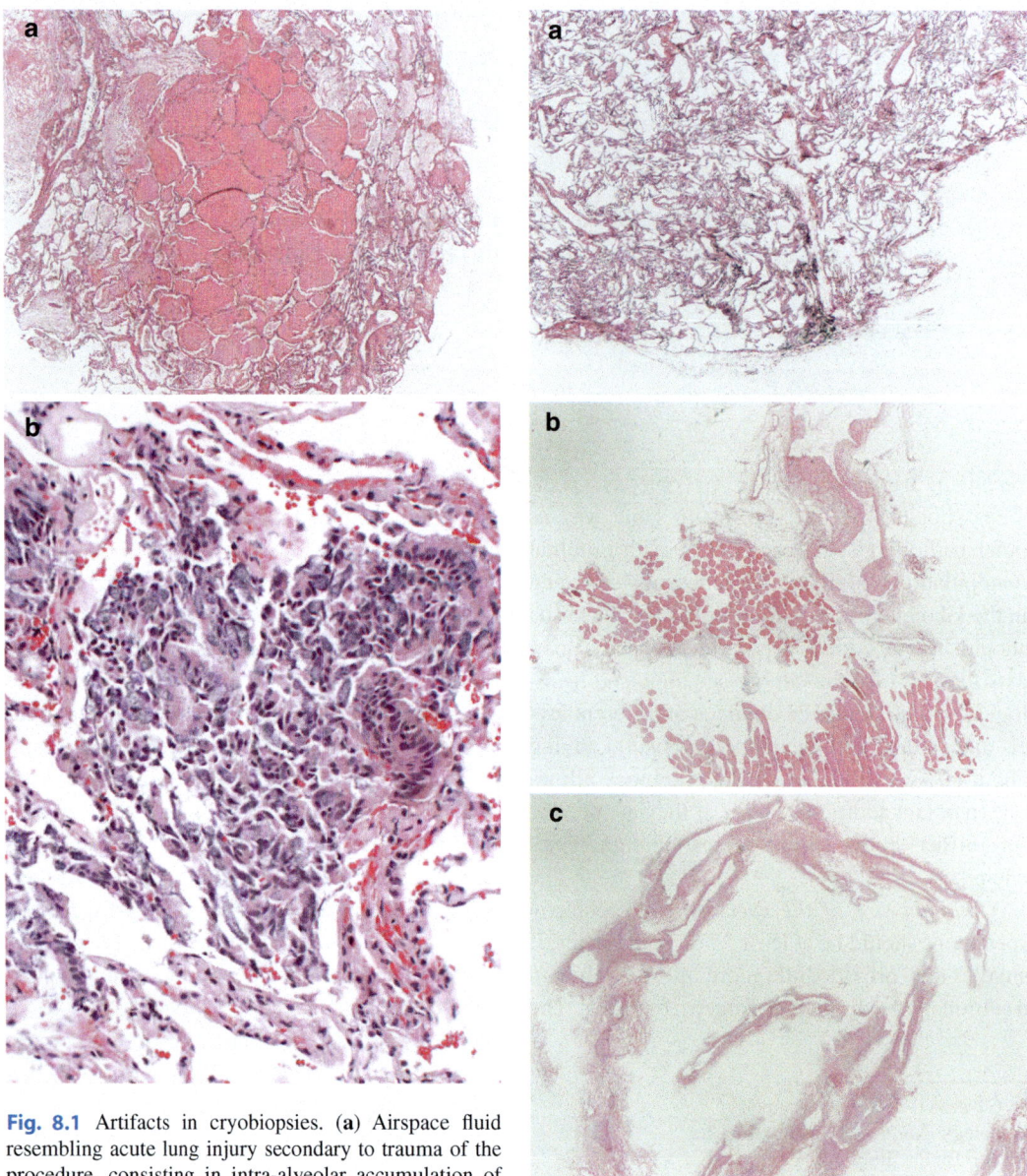

Fig. 8.1 Artifacts in cryobiopsies. (**a**) Airspace fluid resembling acute lung injury secondary to trauma of the procedure, consisting in intra-alveolar accumulation of blood and fibrin/proteinaceous material. Note the normal alveolar walls. This finding appears to be more common when multiple specimens from the same region are taken. (**b**) Intraparenchymal displacement of bronchiolar epithelium by the cryoprobe

Fig. 8.2 The main non-pulmonary tissues that can be found in cryobiopsies include visceral pleura (**a**), fragments of parietal pleura/thoracic wall (**b**), and medium-sized vessels (**c**). Visceral/parietal pleura was present in about 30% of the cases in the large series from Forlì (Italy)

multidisciplinary discussion, and it becomes an integral part of patient management. In diffuse parenchymal lung diseases, interobserver agreement between expert pathologists in cryobiopsies appears similar to that of surgical lung biopsies. Some examples of cryobiopsies are illustrated in Figs. 8.3, 8.4, 8.5, 8.6, 8.7, 8.8, 8.9, 8.10, 8.11, 8.12, and 8.13.

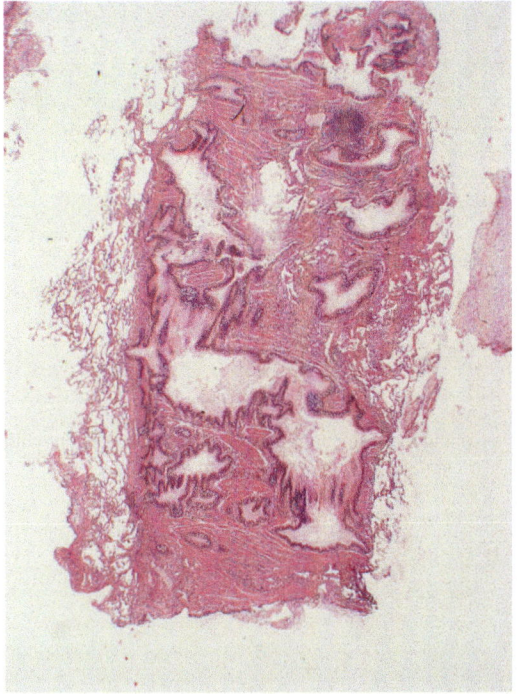

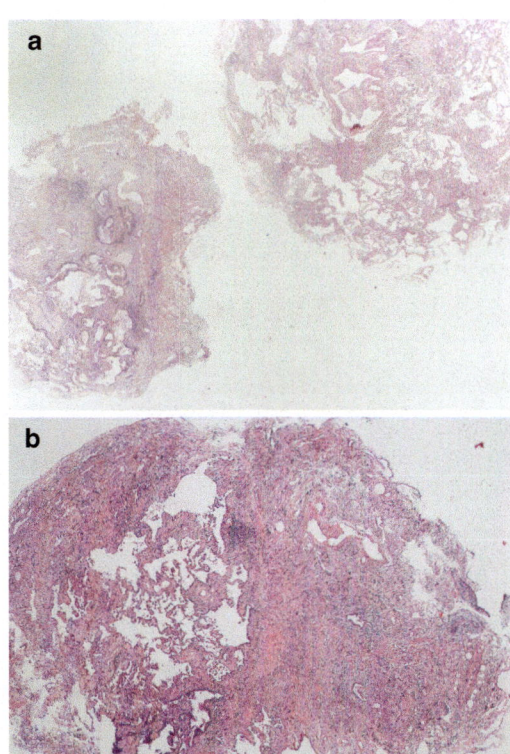

Fig. 8.3 An inadequate cryobiopsy, mainly consisting in bronchial wall with only a minimal amount of peribronchial parenchyma, showing mild nonspecific changes. Specimens comprising primarily airway wall are the result of inadequate penetration of the probe into alveolar tissue and are relatively common when the operator is inexperienced

Fig. 8.4 Two different cryobiopsies (**a**, **b**), both showing UIP in IPF consisting in the combination of patchy fibrosis and fibroblastic foci. In (**a**) microscopic honeycombing is present. Note the absence of ancillary findings suggestive of secondary UIP (significant cellularity, bronchiolocentricity, granulomas, pleuritis, etc.). In these cases the level of diagnostic confidence is high, similar to surgical lung biopsies

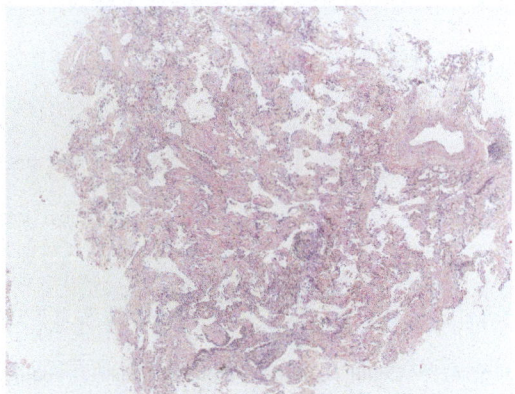

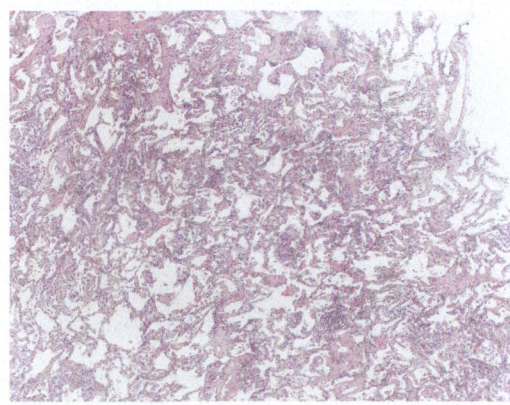

Fig. 8.5 Fibrotic NSIP consisting of uniform interstitial fibrosis without fibroblastic foci

Fig. 8.6 Cellular NSIP with mild diffuse lymphocytic interstitial infiltrate

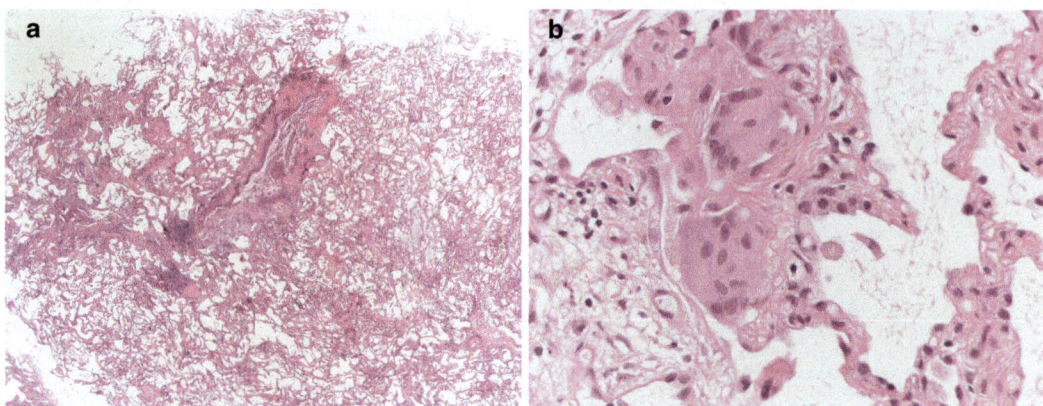

Fig. 8.7 Cellular bronchiolocentric process with mild fibrosis (**a**) and inconspicuous granulomas (**b**), consistent with hypersensitivity pneumonitis

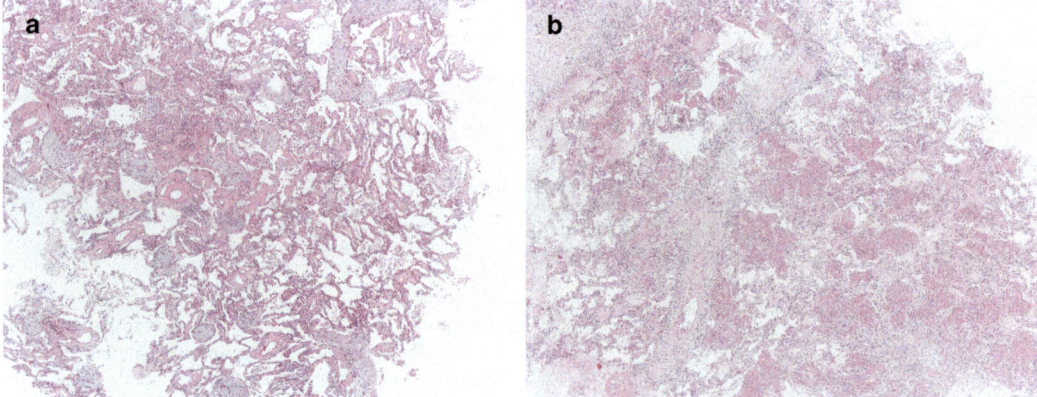

Fig. 8.8 Intra-alveolar buds of granulation tissue of organizing pneumonia (**a**) and airspace fibrin balls in acute fibrinous and organizing pneumonia (AFOP, **b**)

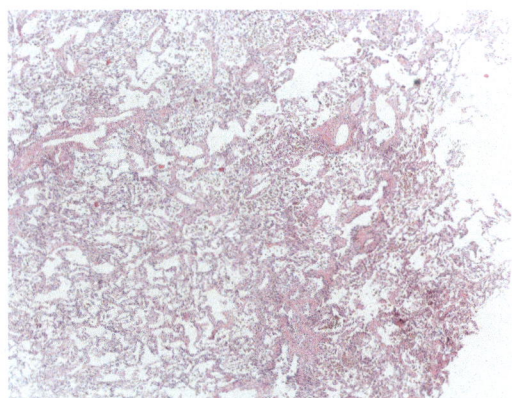

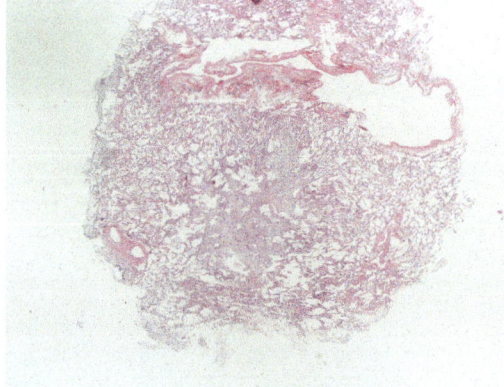

Fig. 8.9 Smoking-related changes with respiratory bronchiolitis and mild fibrosis. This sort of histologic finding can be incidental or clinically significant (smoking-related interstitial lung disease), depending on the clinical context

Fig. 8.10 Cellular stellate bronchiolocentric nodule diagnostic of Langerhans cell histiocytosis (immunohistochemically confirmed)

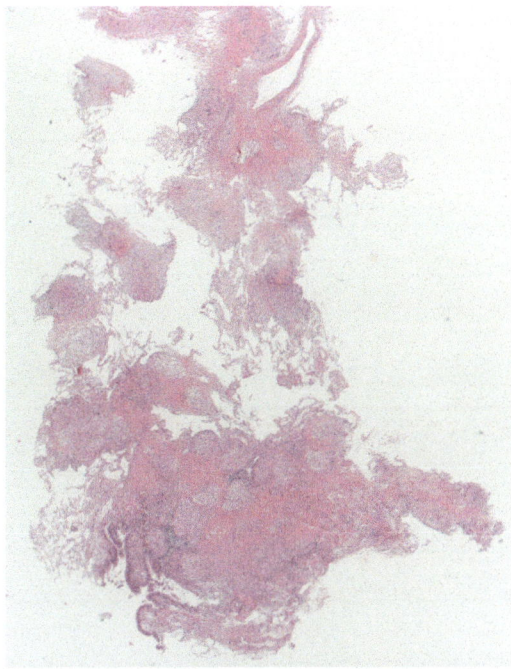

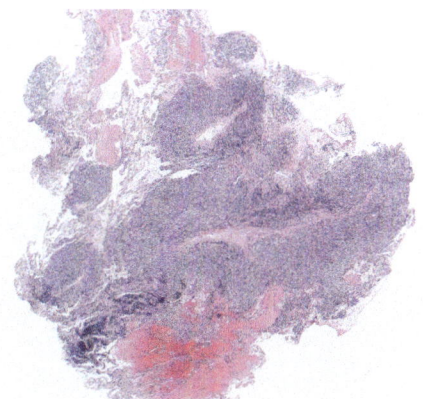

Fig. 8.13 Dense mature lymphoid aggregate in a case of MALT lymphoma (immunohistochemically confirmed)

Fig. 8.11 Non-necrotizing granulomas embedded in dense fibrosis along lymphatic routes, characteristic of sarcoidosis

References

1. Colby TV, Tomassetti S, Cavazza A, et al. Transbronchial cryobiopsy in diffuse lung disease. Update for the pathologist. Arch Pathol Lab Med. 2017;141:891–900.
2. Lentz RJ, Argento AC, Colby TV, et al. Transbronchial cryobiopsy for diffuse parenchymal lung disease: a state-of-the-art review of procedural techniques, current evidence, and future challenges. J Thorac Dis. 2017;9:2186–203.
3. Poletti V, Tomassetti S, Ravaglia C, et al. Histopathology and cryobiopsy. ERS Monogr. 2016;71:1–17.
4. Tomassetti S, Wells AU, Costabel U, et al. Bronchoscopic lung cryobiopsy increases diagnostic confidence in the multidisciplinary diagnosis of idiopathic pulmonary fibrosis. Am J Respir Crit Care Med. 2016;193:745–52.

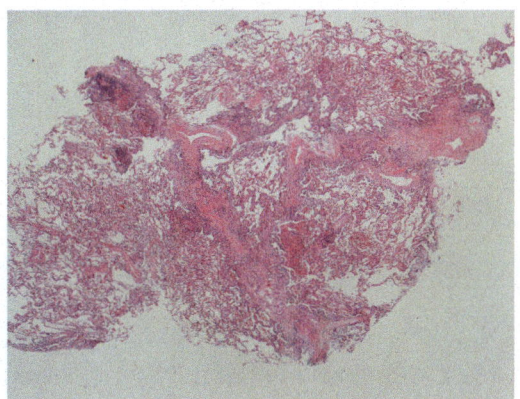

Fig. 8.12 Fibro-inflammatory expansion along lymphatic routes, suggestive of Erdheim-Chester disease (clinically/radiologically confirmed)

Immunohistochemistry and Molecular Biology in Transbronchial Cryobiopsies

9

Marco Chilosi, Lisa Marcolini, Anna Caliò, and Venerino Poletti

9.1 Introduction

Invasive procedures are frequently needed in the diagnostic workflow of pulmonary pathology, in both neoplastic and nonneoplastic cases. Precise diagnoses, complete of all molecular and immunophenotypic data, are requested by updated WHO tumor classifications and precision-medicine criteria, but this need has to be reconciled with the emerging requests of minimally invasive methods for obtaining tissue samples aimed to minimize patients' risks and discomfort [1]. In this scenario, pathologists are faced by the contradictory demands for maximal data and minimal tissue availability. The morphological (histological) analysis of a tissue sample still remains the most informative and economic diagnostic tool, usually performed on hematoxylin- and eosin-stained slides (H&E), and this approach still represents the first step in pulmonary pathology. Nevertheless, morphology alone is not sufficient to provide all the diagnostic, prognostic, and predictive information needed by updated protocols in pulmonary oncology.

Immunohistochemistry represents a widely utilized method to provide relevant information on the antigenic/proteomic profile of atypical cells, allowing the precise definition of the "cell of origin" of a tumor (e.g., squamous cell carcinoma versus adenocarcinoma, poorly differentiated lung carcinoma versus epithelioid mesothelioma, etc.), and also details on the expression of molecules with prognostic and/or predictive significance, such as ALK, ROS, PDL1, p53, and others [2–7] (Table 9.1). Molecular tests (EGFR mutation status and others) are also necessary in the managing of oncologic patients, and the availability of these tests is nowadays a major issue when either cytological samples or small biopsies are only accessible [1, 8–12].

Diffuse parenchymal lung diseases (DPLD) are a wide group of disorders with heterogeneous clinical presentation, prognosis, and pathogenesis. The diagnosis of these diseases is generally obtained by the coordinated evaluation of labora-

M. Chilosi (✉)
Department of Pathology, P. Pederzoli Hospital, Peschiera del Garda, Italy

Verona University, Verona, Italy
e-mail: marco.chilosi@univr.it

L. Marcolini
Department of Pathology, P. Pederzoli Hospital, Peschiera del Garda, Italy
e-mail: lmarcolini@ospedalepederzoli.it

A. Caliò
Department of Diagnostics and Public Health, Anatomic Pathology, University and Hospital Trust, Verona, Italy
e-mail: anna.calio@univr.it

V. Poletti
Department of Diseases of the Thorax, Ospedale Morgagni-Pierantoni, Forlì, Italy

Department of Respiratory Diseases and Allergy, Aarhus University Hospital, Aarhus, Denmark

© Springer Nature Switzerland AG 2019
V. Poletti (ed.), *Transbronchial cryobiopsy in diffuse parenchymal lung disease*,
https://doi.org/10.1007/978-3-030-14891-1_9

Table 9.1 Suggested immunohistochemical markers in lung pathology

Pathology	Suggested immunostains
Lung carcinoma (general)	CK7, CK5/6, ΔN-p63, MUC5AC, TTF1, Napsin-A, CDX2, CD56, Synaptophysin, ALK, p53, *others*
Squamous	CK5/6, ΔN-p63, p53
Adenocarcinoma	CK7, TTF1, Napsin-A, MUC5AC, CDX2, p53
Small cell	CD56, Synaptophysin, Chromogranin, p53, CK7
Mesothelioma	Calretinin, WT1, Podoplanin, CK5/6, BerEP4, BAP1
Lymphoma	CD20, CD3, EBV/EBER, CD30, kappa, lambda, granzyme, p53, *others*
Langerhans' cell hystiocytosis	CD1a, S100, CD68, Langerin, BRAF
Lymphangioleyomiomatosis	HMB45, α-SMA, Cathepsin-K
Erdheim-Chester disease	CD68, S100, BRAF
Infections	EBV/EBER, HHV8, Pneumocystis J, CMV, *others*
Hypersensitivity pneumonitis	Cathepsin-K
PPFE	Elastin, Podoplanin
IPF and other ILD	CK8/18, CK5/6, Tenascin, α-SMA, hsp27, Laminin-5-γ-2, β-catenin, p16, p21

tory, imaging, and clinical data, but frequently a histological evaluation on lung biopsies is needed to substantiate the diagnosis. Large surgical biopsies (SLB, generally obtained by VATS—video-assisted thoracic surgery) are usually considered the gold standard for histological examination, but the risks related to this procedure have suggested that alternative, less invasive, techniques should be performed [13, 14].

Transbronchial lung biopsies, especially transbronchial cryobiopsies (TCB), have been recently described as an alternative to SLB, since they allow a good sensitivity with minor risks and costs [15–17]. The clinical applications of TCB are increasing, with experiences available in the diagnosis and characterization of endobronchial tumor lesions [18–20], pleural lesions [21, 22],

infections [20], and DPLD [15, 17, 23, 24]. Nevertheless, since TCB provide less tissue for morphological analysis than SLB and about 20% TCB are nondiagnostic [24], some concerns have been recently raised on the opportunity to change [25]. In a series of previous publications, we have suggested that the diagnostic sensitivity and specificity on transbronchial biopsies can be significantly increased by utilizing a limited number of immunohistochemical markers related to the different pathogenesis of DPLD [26–28]. This approach, which can be also applied to TCB, may potentially increase the yield of morphologic analysis, thus reconciling the need of both more safe procedures and high sensitivity [29].

According to different studies, immunohistochemical markers can be successfully demonstrated on TCB, as can be molecular tests carried out on nucleic acids extracted from cryobiopsies [16, 29], without any specific problem related to this new procedure (Fig. 9.1). The minimal artifacts that can at times be observed on TCB [30] do not affect the staining quality of all tested nuclear-, cytoplasmic-, and membrane-located antigens [29].

9.2 Immunohistochemistry in Neoplastic Pulmonary Pathology

Immunohistochemistry is a non-expensive methodology that is widely available in most histological laboratories and is broadly applied in the characterization and diagnosis of tumors according to WHO guidelines. Specific immunophenotypic profiles are available for different types of human malignancies (e.g., lymphomas and leukemias, lung carcinoma, breast carcinoma, renal cell carcinoma, etc.). In lung carcinoma, well-established sets of immunohistochemical markers have been introduced in clinical practice that allow the precise characterization of tumor cell differentiation (e.g., adenocarcinoma versus squamous cell carcinoma, versus small-cell carcinoma), as well as markers helping in the differential diagnosis between primary lung carcinomas and either mesothelioma or metastatic spread from other sites [2, 31, 32].

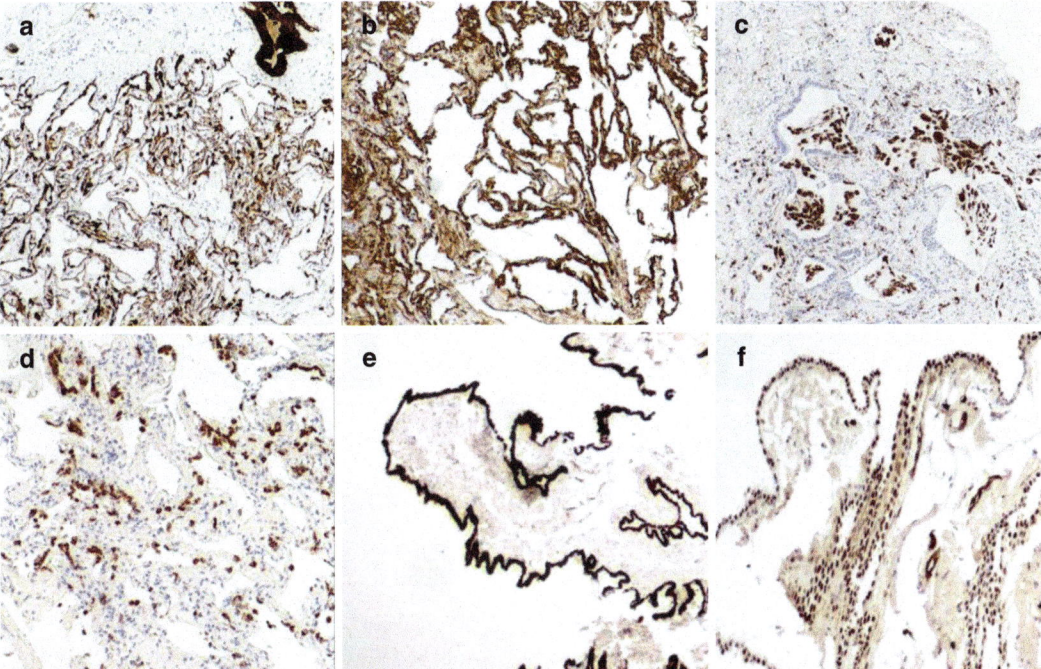

Fig. 9.1 Good quality immunohistochemical stains can be obtained on transbronchial cryobiopsies fixed and paraffin embedded following standard histology protocols: (**a**) cytokeratin 8/18 in alveolar and bronchiolar epithelia; (**b**) CD34 in interstitial vessels; (**c**) CD68 in alveolar macrophages; (**d**) ABCA3 in type II pneumocytes; (**e**) calretinin in mesothelial cells; (**f**) WT1 in mesothelial cells

9.2.1 Immunohistochemical Markers in the Diagnosis of Lung Carcinomas

9.2.1.1 Markers of Pulmonary Epithelial Differentiation
(Fig. 9.2)

Cytokeratins (CK) are a large family of proteins, mainly present in intermediate filaments, that are expressed in all epithelial tissues [33]. The biochemical properties of cytokeratins allow their subdivision into two major groups: acidic (n. CK9–CK28) and basic (CK1–CK8) [33]. Within the lung, pneumocytes mainly express low-molecular-weight (LMW) cytokeratins (e.g., CK7, CK8, CK18), whereas airway basal cells express high-molecular-weight (HMW) cytokeratins (e.g., CK5, CK6). Interestingly, during their differentiation into goblet cells and ciliated columnar cells, the airway epithelial precursors loose the HMW cyto-keratins that can be re-expressed in "squamous" metaplasia.

Pneumocytes type II (AECII that represent precursors of alveolar epithelium) express a range of proteins that can be successfully demonstrated by immunohistochemistry, including the transcription factor TTF1, the serine protease Napsin A [31, 34], surfactant proteins (especially SP-A), DC-LAMP/CD208, and others [35–38].

TTF-1 belongs to the family of mammalian *NKx2* homeobox genes and encodes for a nuclear transcription factor required for normal development of the thyroid gland and lung epithelial cells, regulating early morphogenesis and branching, as well as inducing later surfactant protein expression by type II pneumocytes. In alveolar pneumocytes, TTF1 is expressed at higher levels when compared to bronchiolar cells, paralleling the expression of several products of TTF1-responsive genes including surfactant proteins A, B, C, ABCA3, and DC-LAMP/CD208 [35–38].

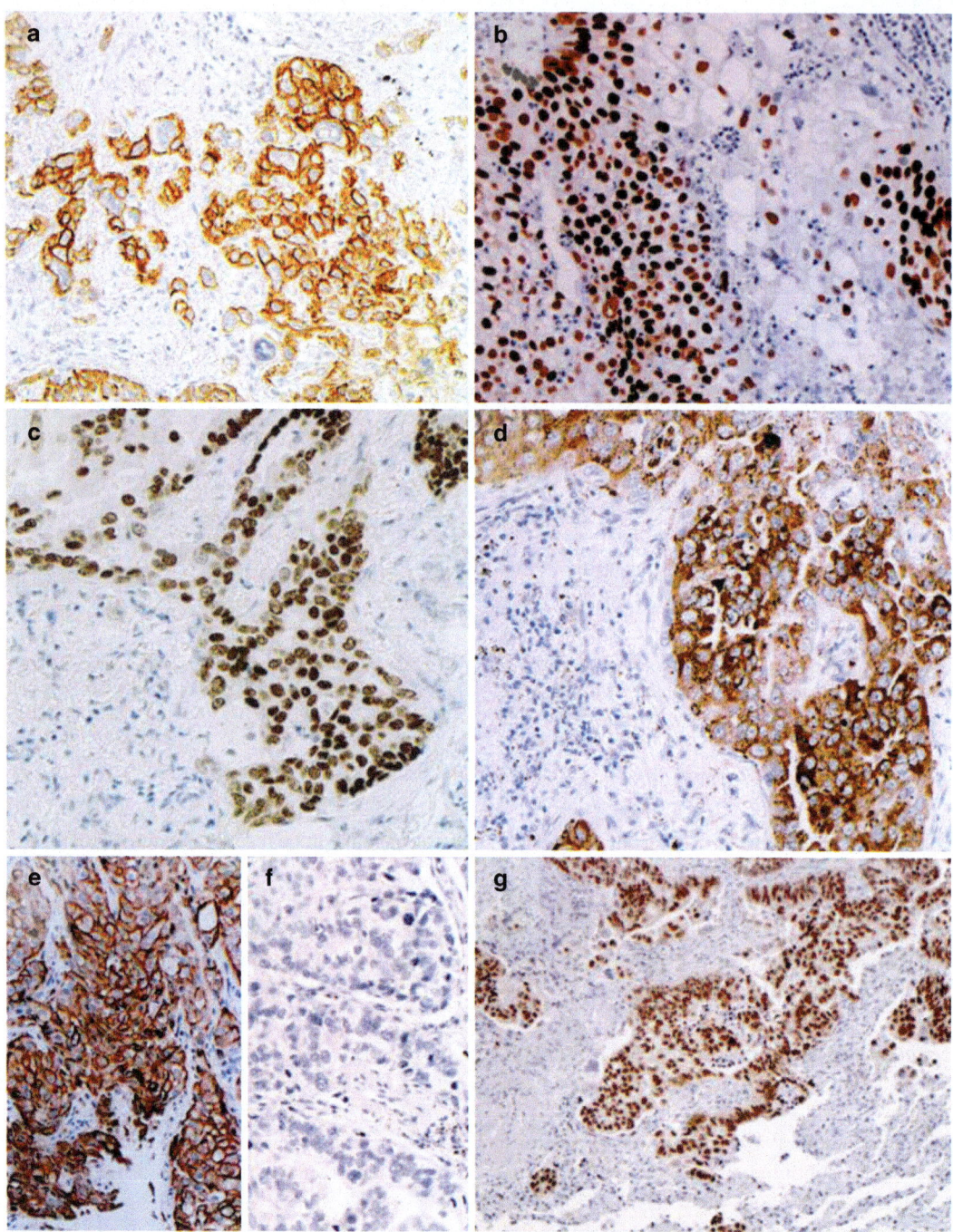

Fig. 9.2 Immunohistochemical characterization of lung carcinomas: (**a**) high-molecular-weight CK5/6 expression in a poorly differentiated squamous cell lung carcinoma; (**b**) p53 overexpression in the same case; (**c**) TTF1 expres- sion in a case of lung adenocarcinoma; (**d**) Napsin A expression in the same case; (**e**) CK7 expression in a case of TTF1-negative (**f**), CDX2 positive (**g**), adenocarcinoma with enteric differentiation

All these markers have been described as useful to positively characterize lung epithelial tumors [34–40]. Lack of expression of these proteins in a proportion of lung carcinomas has been generally considered as a negative feature which decreases markers' sensitivity or specificity. Nevertheless, these molecules can be of value as differentiation markers, since invasive mucinous adenocarcinomas mostly lack their expression, but express the goblet cell-related mucin MUC5AC, and sometimes markers of enteric differentiation (MUC2, CK20, CDX2) [41–45]. This observation can be considered as evidence of a divergent histogenetic derivation (bronchiolar/goblet versus alveolar). The availability of a growing array of "pulmonary," "alveolar," and "bronchiolar" markers can highly improve our understanding of tumor diversity and can be used to better diagnose and classify lung adenocarcinomas [46]. In addition, the decrease or loss of pneumocyte markers is related to the grade of differentiation of conventional adenocarcinomas and can have diagnostic and prognostic value [45, 47].

9.2.1.2 MUC5AC a Marker of Airway Goblet Cells

Goblet cells are increased in the airways as consequence of chronic stimulation (e.g., in smokers). MUC5AC is a secretory mucin typically expressed in bronchial and bronchiolar goblet cells. This mucin is expressed in invasive mucinous adenocarcinoma and is an optimal marker to distinguish this tumor from non-mucinous histotypes [46, 48]. The expression of this mucin in an adenocarcinoma can be considered as an evidence of its "bronchiolar" derivation. MUC5AC is also expressed in adenocarcinomas showing enteric/intestinal differentiation. Interestingly, this entity is highly overrepresented in patients with IPF and carcinoma, and this finding can be considered as evidence of a derivation of these tumors from bronchiolar honeycomb lesions [49].

9.2.1.3 p63 Truncated Isoforms: A Marker of Squamous Metaplasia

The p63 gene is a member of the p53 tumor suppressor gene family playing an important role in the physiological maintenance of different specialized epithelia [50, 51]. Its gene functions are heterogeneous and complex since it undergoes splicing by alternative transcription from two different promoters, producing as many as six distinct isoforms which exert potentially contrasting effects on the same molecular and cellular targets [51]. Transactivating isoforms (the TA-p63 class) maintain a sequence corresponding to the transactivating domain of p53 and have in fact functions similar to p53 in inducing cell cycle arrest and apoptosis. The second class, on the other hand, includes forms lacking the NH_2-terminal domain (ΔN-p63), produced when the p63 gene is transcribed from the cryptic promoter in intron 3. ΔN-p63 forms act as dominant-negative agents toward transactivation by p53 and p63 itself, inhibiting the activity of p53 [52]. When overexpressed, these molecular p63 variants can thus behave as oncogenic molecules. Accordingly, p63 gene amplification and overexpression of ΔN-p63 have been demonstrated in primary lung squamous cell carcinomas [53]. ΔN-p63 (also known as p40) is considered one of the best markers for distinguishing adenocarcinomas from squamous cell carcinomas, together with high-molecular-weight cytokeratins (CK5/6) [10, 54, 55]. ΔN-p63 is also expressed in all cases of thymoma, but not in mesotheliomas [56]. The use of antibodies recognizing all isoforms of p63 (e.g., 4A4) should be used cautiously since the TA-p63 isoform is also expressed by mediastinal B-cell lymphomas [57].

Other IHC tests that should be available for lung cancer diagnosis and characterization include markers of "endocrine" differentiation and proliferation (CD56, chromogranin, synaptophysin, Ki67). These markers are useful for the diagnosis of neuroendocrine lung tumors and also for rare conditions such as endocrine cell hyperplasia [58, 59].

9.2.1.4 Predictive Markers

Intense investigation is currently devoted to find molecular targets for updated therapies in lung carcinoma that need a predictive evaluation of their efficacy, based on the presence of genetic abnormalities and/or the intensity of specific gene product expression. ALK, ROS1, HER2, and others are the best known among the predictive tests validated for immunohistochemical analysis [60–65]. FISH (fluorescence in situ hybridization) analyses, detecting gene amplifications, deletions, or translocations can be also applied to better define the molecular abnormalities of the neoplastic clones [60, 66–68]. Immunohistochemical analysis has also recently investigated as a predictive tool to maximize the efficacy of immunotherapies [6, 69].

9.2.2 Pleural Pathology (Fig. 9.3)

The differential diagnosis of mesothelial malignancies has been the object of intense investiga-

tion, and the use of immunohistochemistry has become a fundamental tool in clinical practice. All international and national guidelines include a panel of immunohistochemical markers that can allow consistent distinction between mesotheliomas and metastatic tumors (mainly lung carcinomas) in order to validate the diagnosis for both clinical and legal issues [70–73].

Immunohistochemical markers can be roughly divided into (1) those confirming the mesothelial origin of a pleural malignancy (e.g., calretinin, WT1, podoplanin/D2–40, and others) [74–76], (2) molecules expressed by pulmonary epithelial carcinomas (BER-EP4, TTF1, CEA, CD15, and others) [77–79], and (3) markers specific for

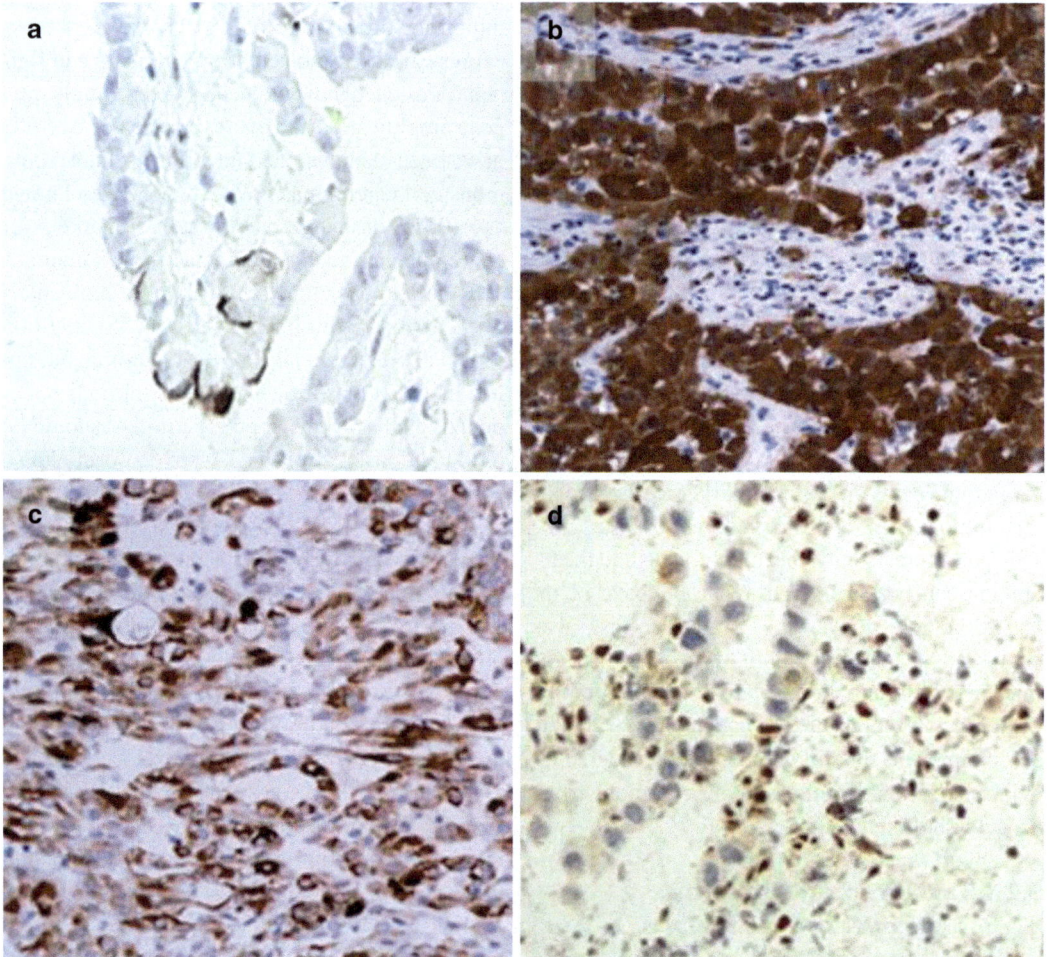

Fig. 9.3 Immunohistochemical characterization of mesothelioma: (**a**) BER-EP4 negative; (**b**) calretinin positive; (**c**) podoplanin positive; (**d**) BAP1 negative (positive internal control is evident)

extrapulmonary metastases of carcinomas (e.g., GATA3, PAX8, CDX2, and others) [32].

In some cases, the distinction between malignant mesothelioma and reactive mesothelial proliferation can be problematic. Advances on the pathogenic mechanisms occurring in mesothelioma development have provided reliable tests for this crucial differential diagnosis, such as the detection of abnormalities affecting p16 and BAP1 genes [73, 80–82]. Loss of the BAP1 nuclear immunoreactivity in mesothelial cells can be considered a robust evidence of malignancy [80–82].

9.2.3 Immunohistochemical Markers in the Diagnosis of Pulmonary Lymphomas

Immunohistochemical analysis is strongly recommended for the characterization of lymphoproliferative disorders occurring in the lung. Among the rare pulmonary lymphomas, the most common subtype is represented by low-grade mucosa-associated lymphoid tissue (MALT) lymphoma, whose immune profile includes the demonstration of the B-cell-specific antigen CD20, the lack of markers specific for other B-cell lymphomas (CD5, cyclin-D1, CD23, etc.), and also the loss of TCL1 expression [83, 84]. A plasma cell differentiation is frequent in MALT lymphoma, and the restricted expression of Ig light chains can represent a reliable diagnostic feature. Lymphomatoid granulomatosis (LYG) is an angiocentric and angiodestructive extranodal lymphoproliferative disease. The histologic presentation of LYG is heterogenous, with variable proportions of large and atypical EBV-infected B cells admixed with reactive T lymphocytes. T-/NK-cell lymphomas can rarely occur in the lungs, and the differential diagnosis between nasal-type T/NK lymphomas and LYG can be difficult, since they share many morphological and immunophenotypic features as angioinvasion, expression of markers of EBV infection, necrosis, and a rich T-cell infiltrate exhibiting cytotoxic immunophenotype, (positivity for CD8, TIA-1, granzyme-B) [83]. Cryobiopsy can be successfully utilized for the diagnosis of pulmonary lymphomas, including the rare endovascular large B-cell lymphomas [85–87].

9.3 Immunohistochemistry in Nonneoplastic Pulmonary Pathology

9.3.1 Immunohistochemical Markers in the Diagnosis of Lung Infections (Fig. 9.4)

A limited number of immunohistochemical markers recognizing infectious organisms (mainly viral) can be applied to paraffin-embedded routine histological samples and can have a diagnostic role in pulmonary pathology. The reagents' panel includes antibodies recognizing polyomavirus, adenovirus, various herpes viruses (herpes simplex virus, cytomegalovirus, human herpesvirus 8, and Epstein-Barr virus). *Pneumocystis jirovecii* can be demonstrated either by Grocott stain or specific antibody [88, 89]. High analytical specificity and sensitivity for mycobacterial detection can be obtained by molecular analysis [90].

9.3.2 Immunohistochemical Markers in the Diagnosis of Interstitial Lung Diseases

The pulmonary microenvironment. When morphological details cannot be easily recognized by H&E staining, some immunohistochemical markers can be useful to precisely define the nature of cells, including epithelial, mesenchymal, and inflammatory cells, as well as extracellular matrix proteins. The epithelial component of the lung tissue can be precisely characterized using cytokeratin subsets, allowing a better evaluation of minimal interstitial changes, pneumocyte hyperplasia, and cell damage or loss (Fig. 9.1). Focal foci of squamous metaplasia can be demonstrated either by ΔN-p63 or high-molecular-weight cytokeratins [91–95]. Surprisingly, CK14 is expressed on type II pneumocytes in focal or diffuse alveolar damage, and

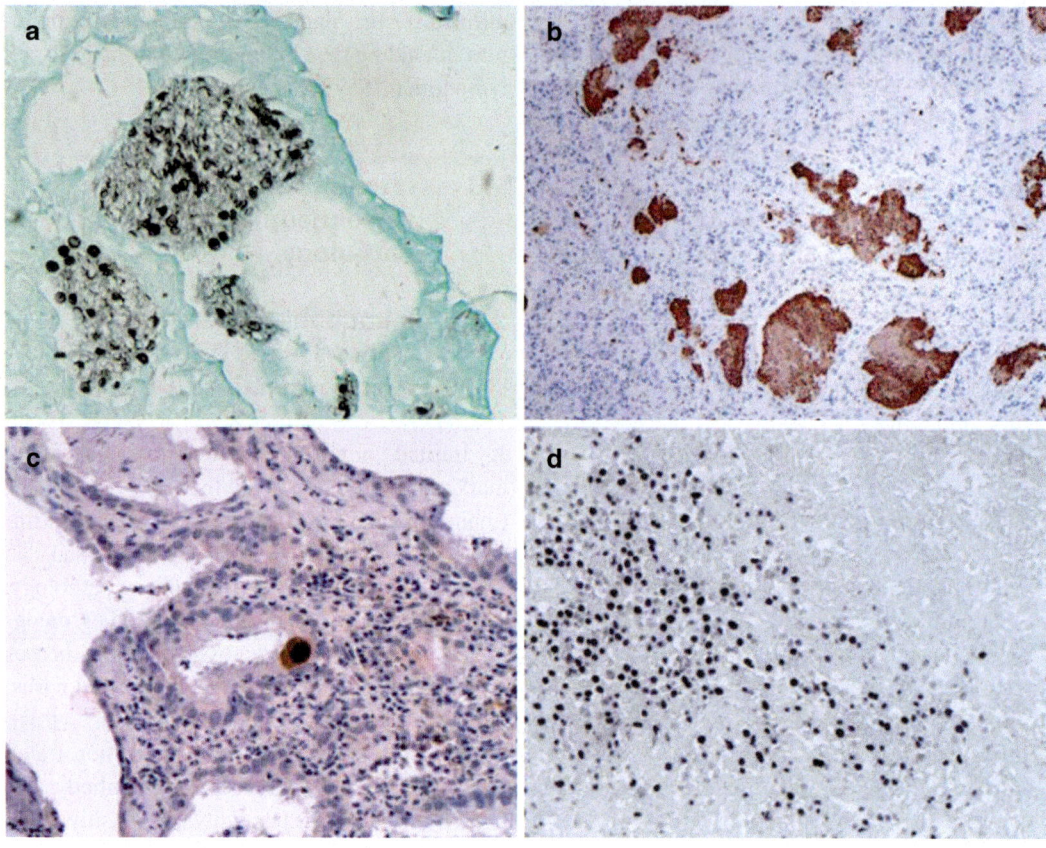

Fig. 9.4 Immunohistochemical characterization of infectious organisms: (**a**) pneumocystis J. (Grocott stain); (**b**) anti-pneumocystis J. immunostaining; (**c**) Cytomegalovirus; (**d**) EBV (EBER in situ hybridization) in a case of pulmonary nasal-type T cell lymphoma

this may be considered a sign of abnormal activation [96]. Different mesenchymal cells can be characterized by markers such as alpha-smooth-muscle actin for smooth muscle and myofibroblasts, tenascin and tubulin beta-3 for myofibroblasts, CD34 for endothelial cells, podoplanin/D2–40 for lymphatic vessels, and others [92, 97, 98].

Increasing information is available regarding the complexity of the immune system. A large number of markers can be applied by immunohistochemical on lung tissue that can precisely detect biologically relevant subsets of lymphoid and inflammatory cells. The classical T-cell lymphoid heterogeneity, based on the expression of membrane antigens such as CD4 and CD8, can now be analyzed in more detail using markers such as GATA3, T-BET, FOXP3, and others, associated to relevant T-cell functional profiles (TH1, TH2, TH17, Treg, etc.), in experimental and clinical studies [99, 100]. Although little evidence has been so far provided on the possible clinical relevance of in situ analyses of these markers, cryobiopsies can provide the samples to better investigate their potential (Fig. 9.5).

9.3.3 Macrophage Markers and Pathology

Macrophages represent a major cell component within the pulmonary microenvironment and exert fundamental roles in maintaining respiratory functions by regulating the surfactant turnover and eliminating infective agents, foreign particles, mucus, dead cell remnants, etc. The majority of macrophages in the normal lung home the alveolar spaces (then they are named alveolar macrophages) and changes of their number, morphology,

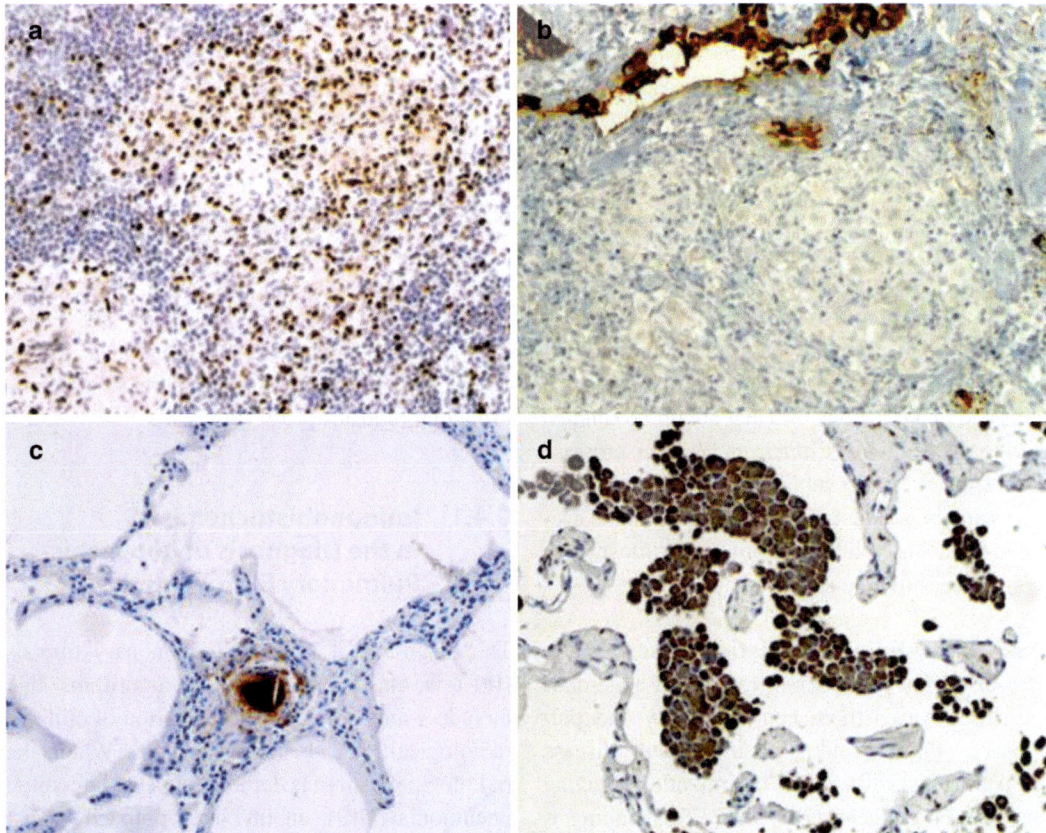

Fig. 9.5 Immunohistochemical characterization of immune-response in situ: (**a**) TH1 T-Bet positive T cells within a sarcoid granuloma; (**b**) sarcoid granuloma macrophages are negative for surfactant-A protein, whereas positive alveolar macrophages show the ingested antigen; (**c**) a small interstitial granuloma evidenced by cathepsin-K immunoreactivity in hypersensitivity pneumonitis; (**d**) clusters of CD68-positive macrophages in Desquamative Interstitial Pneumonia

and/or distribution can provide useful diagnostic information in different pulmonary diseases.

Several markers of alveolar macrophages are available, including *CD68*, *CD11c*, and others. Calgranulins (recognized by the antibody MAC387) are expressed by "young" macrophages, being also expressed by neutrophils [101]. Some antigenic proteins that can be demonstrated by IHC within the cytoplasm of alveolar macrophages are in fact derived by other cell types that are ingested by macrophages, such as the epithelial aspartic peptidase Napsin A and surfactant protein A (Fig. 9.5).

Diseases characterized by abnormalities of alveolar macrophages. Focal or diffuse accumulations of alveolar macrophages characterize smoking-related interstitial lung diseases such as respiratory bronchiolitis-ILD and desquamative interstitial pneumonia. Clusters of foamy macrophages (engulfing surfactant proteins and lipids) can be related to diseases of disturbed surfactant turnover (e.g., diffuse panbronchiolitis or in amiodarone lung disease).

Diseases characterized by accumulation of extrapulmonary macrophages. In some pulmonary lesions, the accumulation of macrophages is due to the recruitment of circulating monocytes that eventually differentiate in the lung interstitial spaces. These include a variety of inflammatory diseases and can be divided in granulomatous and non-granulomatous.

Granulomatous diseases. A particular type of macrophage activation leads to the formation of epithelioid granulomas. This reaction is triggered by TH1 lymphocytes and characterizes different pulmonary granulomatous diseases including immunological (sarcoidosis, berylliosis, hypersensitivity pneumonitis) and infective diseases (mycobacteriosis, etc.). Epithelioid and giant cells in granulomas are not modified alveolar macrophages but directly derive from circulating monocytes. The phenotype of epithelioid cells is different from that exerted by alveolar macrophages (negative for ZAP 70, Napsin A), and these markers can occasionally be used to help in difficult cases. Epithelioid macrophages are activated cells and express molecules that are up-modulated during activation. *Cathepsin K*, a protease expressed at high levels in bone marrow osteoclasts and in granuloma macrophages, can be useful in detecting small granulomas as in most cases of hypersensitivity pneumonitis [102] (Fig. 9.5).

9.3.3.1 BRAF-Related Histiocytoses

Recently, it has been demonstrated that Langerhans cell histiocytosis (both non-pulmonary and pulmonary—PLCH) and Erdheim-Chester disease are pathogenetically related to a mutation affecting the BRAF oncogene [103, 104]. This finding is relevant since it can be considered as evidence of the "clonal/neoplastic" nature of these histiocytoses (previously considered as "inflammatory") and also provides a robust diagnostic tool, either utilizing immunohistochemistry or molecular analysis [105, 106]. Interestingly, in both these diseases, oncogene-induced cell senescence (OIS) has been suggested as a pathogenic feature, this explaining the SASP (senescence-associated secretory phenotype)-related secondary inflammatory features of the diseases [106, 107]. Demonstration of senescence-related markers such as $p21^{waf1}$ and p16 can provide in this context prognostic information [106]. Pulmonary Langerhans cell histiocytosis is characterized by accumulation of CD1a-positive and CD68-negative cells, whereas Erdheim-Chester histiocytes are typically CD68 positive and CD1a negative.

9.4 Lymphangioleiomyomatosis

Lymphangioleiomyomatosis (LAM) is a rare disease that affects the lungs of women, usually in premenopausal age. The disease is progressive and potentially fatal. The LAM cells, which harbor mutations in tuberous sclerosis genes, progressively infiltrate the perilymphatic spaces of the lung parenchyma. The phenotype of LAM cells is peculiar, since they express alpha-smooth muscle actin and desmin, together with melanocytic markers such as HMB45, HMSA-1, MelanA/Mart1, microphthalmia transcription factor (MITF), and cathepsin k [28, 108]. This distinctive phenotypic profile can be useful to precisely characterize the disease on small transbronchial biopsies [109] (Fig. 9.6).

9.4.1 Immunohistochemistry in the Diagnosis of Idiopathic Pulmonary Fibrosis and DPLD

The diagnosis of idiopathic pulmonary fibrosis (IPF) is classically based on algorithms that include a multidisciplinary evaluation of clinical, radiological, and histological data. When the radiological pattern is definite for usual interstitial pneumonia (UIP), an invasive approach is discouraged in the consensus protocols. The introduction of TCB can help in providing a definite diagnosis of UIP in those cases where the data are dubious or not consistent for UIP, thus avoiding either SLB or renounce to a certain diagnosis. The use of some markers related to the pathogenesis of IPF can help in some difficult cases. To date, there is a wide consensus on the assumption that IPF is not an inflammatory disease, but its pathogenesis is related to an accelerated senescence affecting pneumocytes that progressively reach a status of stem cell insufficiency at particular sites [110–113]. The causes of this intrinsic and irreversible defect are multifactorial, including age-related telomere attrition, a genetic predisposition (that is predominant in familiar cases), together with the chronic exposure to toxic substances (e.g., cigarette smoke), and also an anatomic component related to mechanical stress [114]. Immunohistochemistry can be useful in detecting early evidence of pneumocyte senescence. The expression of cell senescence-related markers such as p16, p21, and beta-galactosidase [111, 115–117] in hyperplastic type II pneumocytes

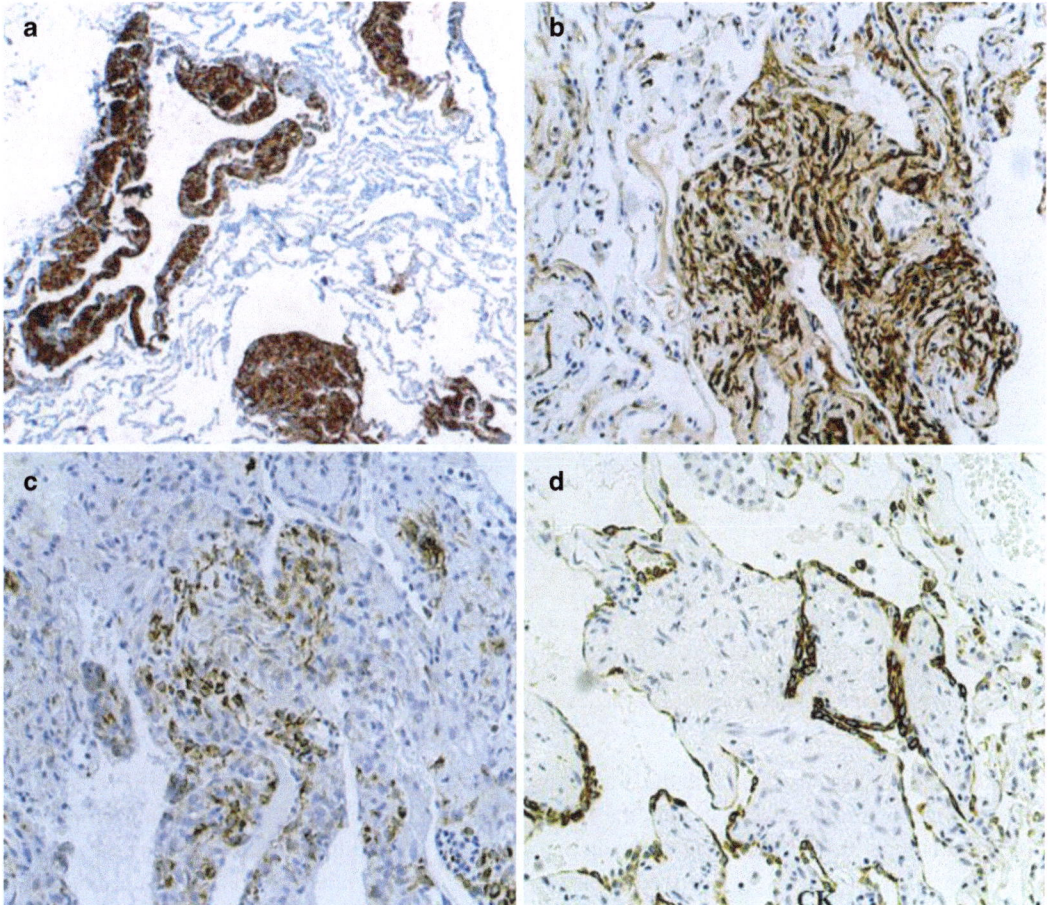

Fig. 9.6 Immunohistochemical characterization of lymphangioleyomiomatosis (LAM) cells: (**a**) cathepsin-K positive; (**b**) alpha-smooth muscle actin positive; (**c**) HMB45 positive; (**d**) cytokeratin 8/18 negative

represents the evidence of focal alveolar damage in IPF and also on small TCB (Fig. 9.7).

The use of other markers can help to better visualize small fibrotic lesions that can be missed on H&E morphology, together with details demonstrating abnormalities, including epithelial-mesenchymal transition (EMT) and abnormal angiogenesis, occurring in microenvironmental organization of the normal parenchyma [118]. Several myofibroblastic markers have been described, including the extracellular matrix protein tenascin, and its immunohistochemical evaluation can have prognostic significance in pulmonary fibrosis [98, 119]. Tubulin beta-3 has been recently proposed as a reliable immunohistochemical marker of myofibroblast foci in IPF [120]. This marker in fact is expressed in both myofibroblasts and epithelial cells exhibiting

EMT in fibroblast foci, together with a variety of molecules aberrantly expressed within the fibrotic lung tissue (ZEB1, TWIST, beta-catenin, and others) [118, 120–124]. A useful immunohistochemical finding is observed within honeycomb lesions that we named "sandwich foci" because of the peculiar three-layer structure formed by myofibroblasts, basal cells expressing laminin-5 γ-2 chain, and heat shock protein hsp27 [122] (Fig. 9.7). Although these findings appear useful diagnostic features in the differential diagnosis of IPF and other DPLD, they need to be validated on large case series.

9.4.1.1 Microscopic Honeycomb Lesions
Micro-honeycombing is a major morphological feature of IPF, although it is not requested by consensus statements for its histological diagno-

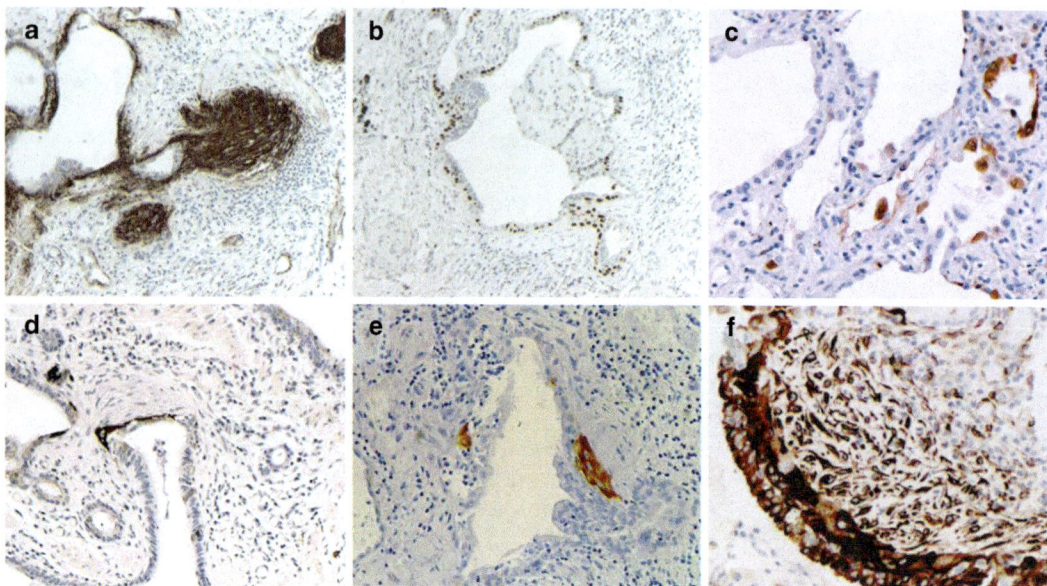

Fig. 9.7 Immunohistochemical features in IPF: (**a**) strong tenascin expression in fibroblast foci; (**b**) abnormal distribution of ΔN-p63 basal cells in bronchiolar honeycombing; (**c**) focal expression of the cell senescence-asso- ciated marker p16 in type II pneumocytes; (**d**) laminin-5 γ-2 chain expression in "sandwich" fibroblast foci; (**e**) heat shock protein 27 in sandwich foci; (**f**) strong tubulin beta-3 in both luminal epithelium and fibroblast foci

sis when imaging is consistent with the diagnosis of UIP pattern. In honeycomb lesions the bronchiolar structures that are close to parenchymal fibrotic area are progressively changed showing distortion, enlargement, mucous accumulation, and abnormal proliferation. Fibroblast foci are frequently observed within these lesions, showing a three-layered *sandwich* structure (see above). The mucous accumulation within these lesions always contains the mucin MUC5B, regardless of the occurrence of the MUC5B polymorphism (a well-known predisposing genetic feature of IPF) [125–127]. This finding is typical of IPF micro-honeycombing. In addition, micro-honeycomb lesions in IPF show several abnormalities that can be demonstrated by immunohistochemistry, including increased expression of WNT/beta-catenin targets such as MMP7, cyclin-D1, and MYC, as well increased expression of senescence-related markers p16 and p21 [111, 117, 121]. These abnormal features are likely related to the development of epithelial malignancies with bronchiolar phenotypes in IPF [49].

9.4.1.2 Molecular Analysis in IPF

The demonstration of an increasing number of gene abnormalities (affecting genes involved in surfactant synthesis, telomerase functions, MUC5B polymorphisms, telomere length, etc.) in familiar and sporadic IPF is crucial for the understanding of the pathogenesis of these devastating diseases and may provide a new perspective for their classification, diagnosis, and prognostication [128–131].

9.5   Diffuse Alveolar Damage (DAD)

In diffuse alveolar damage (DAD), the morphological pattern characterizing acute respiratory distress syndrome, the pneumocyte type II hyperplasia is generalized and diffuse, and markers of EMT are easily demonstrated, including nuclear beta-catenin, slug, tubulin beta-3, CK14, and others (Fig. 9.8) [96, 120–123].

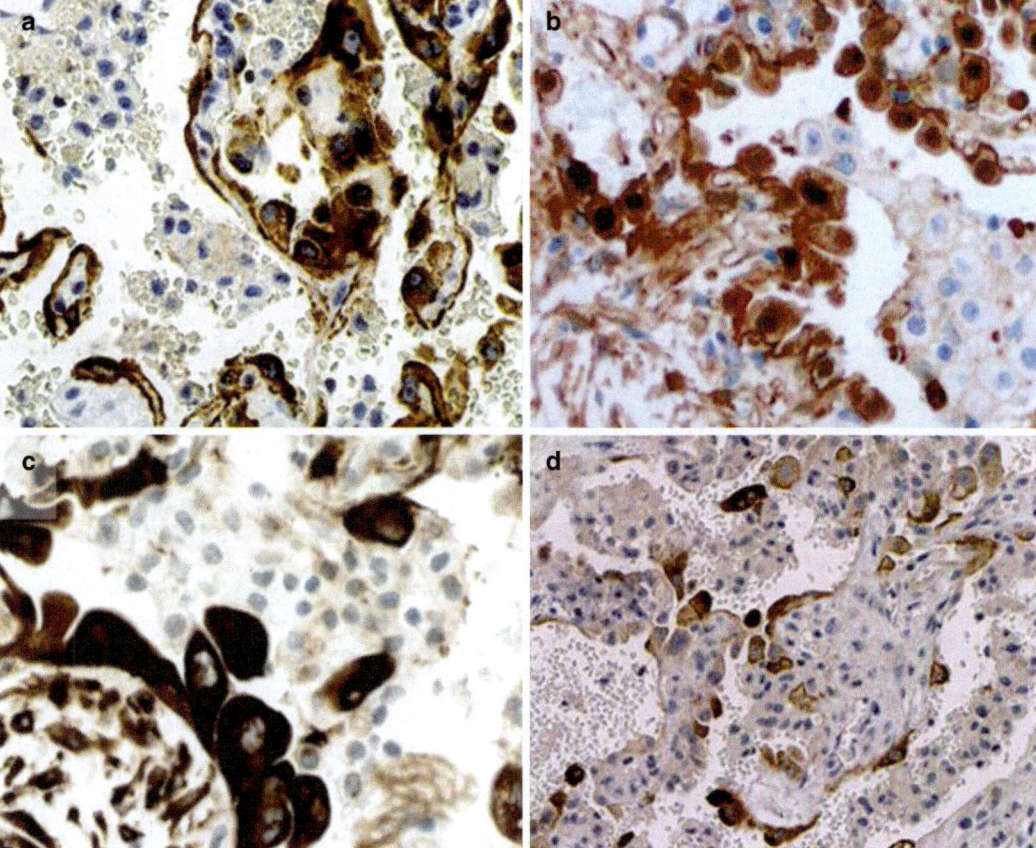

Fig. 9.8 Immunohistochemical characterization of hyperplastic type II pneumocytes in diffuse alveolar damage: (**a**) cytokeratin 8/18; (**b**) nuclear and cytoplasmic accumulation of beta-catenin; (**c**) strong immunoreactivity for tubulin beta-3 in both epithelial cells and myofibroblasts; (**d**) laminin-5 γ-2 chain expression in activated pneumocytes

9.6 Pleuroparenchymal Fibroelastosis (PPFE)

PPFE is a severe interstitial disease characterized by progressive effacement of the pulmonary parenchyma with pleural/subpleural fibroelastosis often accompanied by interstitial thickening and remodeling. Although PPFE has been included within the idiopathic interstitial pneumonias [132], its identity is still matter of debate [133, 134]. Relevant to diagnosis is the demonstration of abnormal interstitial accumulation of elastic fibers that can be evidenced either using elastic Van Gieson's stain or, more precisely, with elastin-specific monoclonal antibodies. Recently, the occurrence of podoplanin-reactive myofibroblasts has been proposed as a specific immunohistochemical staining to distinguish between PPFE and IPF abnormal remodeling of the lung parenchyma [135].

References

1. Khan J, Pritchard CC, Martins RG. Tissue is the issue for diagnosis of EGFR T790M mutation. J Thorac Oncol. 2016;11:e91–2.
2. Kaufmann O, Dietel M. Thyroid transcription factor-1 is the superior immunohistochemical marker for pulmonary adenocarcinomas and large cell

carcinomas compared to surfactant proteins A and B. Histopathology. 2000;36:8–16.

3. Kargi A, Gurel D, Tuna B. The diagnostic value of TTF-1, CK 5/6, and p63 immunostaining in classification of lung carcinomas. Appl Immunohistochem Mol Morphol. 2007;15:415–20.

4. Koivunen JP, Mermel C, Zejnullahu K, et al. EML4-ALK fusion gene and efficacy of an ALK kinase inhibitor in lung cancer. Clin Cancer Res. 2008;14:4275–83.

5. Aguiar PN Jr, De Mello RA, Hall P, Tadokoro H, Lima Lopes G. PD-L1 expression as a predictive biomarker in advanced non-small-cell lung cancer: updated survival data. Immunotherapy. 2017;9:499–506.

6. Carbognin L, Pilotto S, Milella M, Vaccaro V, Brunelli M, Caliò A, et al. Differential activity of nivolumab, pembrolizumab and MPDL3280A according to the tumor expression of programmed death-ligand-1 (PD-L1): sensitivity analysis of trials in melanoma, lung and genitourinary cancers. PLoS One. 2015;10:e0130142.

7. Huang CL, Taki T, Adachi M, Konishi T, Higashiyama M, Kinoshita M, et al. Mutations of p53 and K-ras genes as prognostic factors for non-small cell lung cancer. Int J Oncol. 1998;12:553–63.

8. Lynch TJ, Bell DW, Sordella R, Gurubhagavatula S, Okimoto RA, Brannigan BW, et al. Activating mutations in the epidermal growth factor receptor underlying responsiveness of non-small-cell lung cancer to gefitinib. N Engl J Med. 2004;350:2129–39.

9. Marchetti A, Martella C, Felicioni L, Barassi F, Salvatore S, Chella A, et al. EGFR mutations in non-small-cell lung cancer: analysis of a large series of cases and development of a rapid and sensitive method for diagnostic screening with potential implications on pharmacologic treatment. J Clin Oncol. 2005;23:857–65.

10. Pelosi G, Fabbri A, Bianchi F, Maisonneuve P, Rossi G, Barbareschi M, et al. ΔNp63 (p40) and thyroid transcription factor-1 immunoreactivity on small biopsies or cellblocks for typing non-small cell lung cancer: a novel two-hit, sparing-material approach. J Thorac Oncol. 2012;7:281–90.

11. Doxtader EE, Cheng YW, Zhang Y. Molecular testing of non-small cell lung carcinoma diagnosed by endobronchial ultrasound-guided transbronchial fine-needle aspiration. Arch Pathol Lab Med. 2018.

12. Cai G, Wong R, Chhieng D, Levy GH, Gettinger SN, Herbst RS, et al. Identification of EGFR mutation, KRAS mutation, and ALK gene rearrangement in cytological specimens of primary and metastatic lung adenocarcinoma. Cancer Cytopathol. 2013;121:500–7.

13. Kondoh Y, Taniguchi H, Kitaichi M, Yokoi T, Johkoh T, Oishi T, et al. Acute exacerbation of interstitial pneumonia following surgical lung biopsy. Respir Med. 2006;100:1753–9.

14. Park IN, Kim DS, Shim TS, Lim CM, Lee SD, Koh Y, et al. Acute exacerbation of interstitial pneumonia other than idiopathic pulmonary fibrosis. Chest. 2007;132:214–20.

15. Babiak A, Hetzel J, Krishna G, Fritz P, Moeller P, Balli T, et al. Transbronchial cryobiopsy: a new tool for lung biopsies. Respiration. 2009;78:203–8.

16. Hetzel J, Hetzel M, Hasel C, Moeller P, Babiak A. Old meets modern: the use of traditional cryoprobes in the age of molecular biology. Respiration. 2008;76:193–7.

17. Casoni GL, Tomassetti S, Cavazza A, Colby TV, Dubini A, Ryu JH, et al. Transbronchial lung cryobiopsy in the diagnosis of fibrotic interstitial lung diseases. PLoS One. 2014;9:e86716.

18. Schumann C, Hetzel J, Babiak AJ, Merk T, Wibmer T, Möller P, et al. Cryoprobe biopsy increases the diagnostic yield in endobronchial tumor lesions. J Thorac Cardiovasc Surg. 2010;140:417–21.

19. Hetzel J, Eberhardt R, Herth FJ, Petermann C, Reichle G, Freitag L, et al. Cryobiopsy increases the diagnostic yield of endobronchial biopsy: a multicentre trial. Eur Respir J. 2012;39:685–90.

20. Sánchez-Cabral O, Martínez-Mendoza D, Fernandez-Bussy S, López-González B, Perea-Talamantes C, Rivera-Rosales RM, et al. Utility of transbronchial lung cryobiopsy in non-interstitial diseases. Respiration. 2017;94:285–92.

21. Pathak V, Shepherd RW, Hussein E, Malhotra R. Safety and feasibility of pleural cryobiopsy compared to forceps biopsy during semi-rigid pleuroscopy. Lung. 2017;195:371–5.

22. Tousheed SZ, Manjunath PH, Chandrasekar S, Murali Mohan BV, Kumar H, Hibare KR, et al. Cryobiopsy of the pleura: an improved diagnostic tool. J Bronchology Interv Pulmonol. 2018;25:37–41.

23. Tomassetti S, Wells AU, Costabel U, Cavazza A, Colby TV, Rossi G, et al. Bronchoscopic lung cryobiopsy increases diagnostic confidence in the multidisciplinary diagnosis of idiopathic pulmonary fibrosis. Am J Respir Crit Care Med. 2016;193:745–52.

24. Hetzel J, Maldonado F, Ravaglia C, Wells AU, Colby TV, Tomassetti S, et al. Transbronchial cryobiopsies for the diagnosis of diffuse parenchymal lung diseases: expert statement from the cryobiopsy working group on safety and utility and a call for standardization of the procedure. Respiration. 2018;95:188–200.

25. Raparia K, Aisner DL, Allen TC, Beasley MB, Borczuk A, Cagle PT, et al. Transbronchial lung cryobiopsy for interstitial lung disease diagnosis: a perspective from members of the Pulmonary Pathology Society. Arch Pathol Lab Med. 2016;140(11):1281–4.

26. Menestrina F, Lestani M, Mombello A, Cipriani A, Pomponi F, Adami F, et al. Transbronchial biopsy in sarcoidosis: the role of immunohistochemical analysis for granuloma detection. Sarcoidosis. 1992;9:95–100.

27. Poletti V, Chilosi M, Olivieri D. Diagnostic invasive procedures in diffuse infiltrative lung diseases. Respiration. 2004;71:107–19.

28. Chilosi M, Pea M, Martignoni G, Brunelli M, Gobbo S, Poletti V, et al. Cathepsin-k expression in pulmonary lymphangioleiomyomatosis. Mod Pathol. 2009;22:161–6.

29. Poletti V, Tomassetti S, Ravaglia C, Dubini A, Piciucchi S, Cavazza A, et al. Histopathology and cryobiopsy. In: ERS Monograph. Idiopathic pulmonary fibrosis. ERS Monograph. 2016; p. 57–73.

30. Colby TV, Tomassetti S, Cavazza A, Dubini A, Poletti V. Transbronchial cryobiopsy in diffuse lung disease: update for the pathologist. Arch Pathol Lab Med. 2017;141:891–900.

31. Dejmek A, Naucler P, Smedjeback A, Kato H, Maeda M, Yashima K, et al. Napsin A (TA02) is a useful alternative to thyroid transcription factor-1 (TTF-1) for the identification of pulmonary adenocarcinoma cells in pleural effusions. Diagn Cytopathol. 2007;35:493–7.

32. Ordóñez NG. Value of PAX8, PAX2, napsin A, carbonic anhydrase IX, and claudin-4 immunostaining in distinguishing pleural epithelioid mesothelioma from metastatic renal cell carcinoma. Mod Pathol. 2013;26:1132–43.

33. Moll R, Franke WW, Schiller DL, Geiger B, Krepler R. The catalog of human cytokeratins: patterns of expression in normal epithelia, tumors and cultured cells. Cell. 1982;31:11–24.

34. Hirano T, Gong Y, Yoshida K, Kato Y, Yashima K, Maeda M, et al. Usefulness of TA02 (napsin A) to distinguish primary lung adenocarcinoma from metastatic lung adenocarcinoma. Lung Cancer. 2003;41:155–62.

35. Kolla V, Gonzales LW, Gonzales J, Wang P, Angampalli S, Feinstein SI, et al. Thyroid transcription factor in differentiating type II cells: regulation, isoforms, and target genes. Am J Respir Cell Mol Biol. 2007;36:213–25.

36. Zhu LC, Yim J, Chiriboga L, Cassai ND, Sidhu GS, Moreira AL. DC-LAMP stains pulmonary adenocarcinoma with bronchiolar Clara cell differentiation. Hum Pathol. 2007;38:260–8.

37. Tsutahara S, Shijubo N, Hirasawa M, Honda Y, Satoh M, Kuroki Y, et al. Lung adenocarcinoma with type II pneumocyte characteristics. Eur Respir J. 1993;6:135–7.

38. Mizutani Y, Nakajima T, Morinaga S, Gotoh M, Shimosato Y, Akino T, et al. Immunohistochemical localization of pulmonary surfactant apoproteins in various lung tumors. Special reference to non-mucus producing lung adenocarcinomas. Cancer. 1988;61:532–7.

39. Pelosi G, Fraggetta F, Pasini F, Maisonneuve P, Sonzogni A, Iannucci A, et al. Immunoreactivity for thyroid transcription factor-1 in stage I non-small cell carcinomas of the lung. Am J Surg Pathol. 2001;25:363–72.

40. Fabbro D, di Loreto C, Stamerra O, Beltrami CA, Lonigro R, Damante G. TTF-1 gene expression in human lung tumours. Eur J Cancer. 1996;32A:512–7.

41. Inamura K, Satoh Y, Okumura S, Nakagawa K, Tsuchiya E, Fukayama M, et al. Pulmonary adenocarcinomas with enteric differentiation: histologic and immunohistochemical characteristics compared with metastatic colorectal cancers and usual pulmonary adenocarcinomas. Am J Surg Pathol. 2005;29:660–5.

42. Mazziotta RM, Borczuk AC, Powell CA, Mansukhani M. CDX2 immunostaining as a gastrointestinal marker: expression in lung carcinomas is a potential pitfall. Appl Immunohistochem Mol Morphol. 2005;13:55–60.

43. Shah RN, Badve S, Papreddy K, Schindler S, Laskin WB, Yeldandi AV. Expression of cytokeratin 20 in mucinous bronchioloalveolar carcinoma. Hum Pathol. 2002;33:915–20.

44. Nottegar A, Tabbò F, Luchini C, Brunelli M, Bria E, Veronese N, et al. Pulmonary adenocarcinoma with enteric differentiation: immunohistochemistry and molecular morphology. Appl Immunohistochem Mol Morphol. 2018;26:383–7.

45. Tabbò F, Nottegar A, Guerrera F, Migliore E, Luchini C, Maletta F, et al. Cell of origin markers identify different prognostic subgroups of lung adenocarcinoma. Hum Pathol. 2018;75:167–78.

46. Chilosi M, Murer B. Mixed adenocarcinomas of the lung: place in new proposals in classification, mandatory for target therapy. Arch Pathol Lab Med. 2010;134:55–65.

47. Puglisi F, Barbone F, Damante G, Bruckbauer M, Di Lauro V, Beltrami CA, et al. Prognostic value of thyroid transcription factor-1 in primary, resected, non-small cell lung carcinoma. Mod Pathol. 1999;12:318–24.

48. Tsuta K, Ishii G, Nitadori J, Murata Y, Kodama T, Nagai K, et al. Comparison of the immunophenotypes of signet-ring cell carcinoma, solid adenocarcinoma with mucin production, and mucinous bronchioloalveolar carcinoma of the lung characterized by the presence of cytoplasmic mucin. J Pathol. 2006;209:78–87.

49. Calió A, Lever V, Rossi A, Gilioli E, Brunelli M, Dubini A, et al. Increased frequency of bronchiolar histotypes in lung carcinomas associated with idiopathic pulmonary fibrosis. Histopathology. 2017;71:725–35.

50. Mills AA, Zheng B, Wang XJ, Vogel H, Roop DR, Bradley A. p63 is a p53 homologue required for limb and epidermal morphogenesis. Nature. 1999;398:708–13.

51. Yang A, Schweitzer R, Sun D, Kaghad M, Walker N, Bronson RT, et al. p63 is essential for regenerative proliferation in limb, craniofacial and epithelial development. Nature. 1999;398:714–8.

52. Yang A, McKeon F. P63 and P73: P53 mimics, menaces and more. Nat Rev Mol Cell Biol. 2000;1:199–207.

53. Hibi K, Trink B, Patturajan M, Westra WH, Caballero OL, Hill DE, et al. AIS is an oncogene amplified in squamous cell carcinoma. Proc Natl Acad Sci U S A. 2000;97:5462–7.

54. Wang BY, Gil J, Kaufman D, Gan L, Kohtz DS, Burstein DE. P63 in pulmonary epithelium, pulmonary squamous neoplasms, and other pulmonary tumors. Hum Pathol. 2002;33:921–6.

55. Tatsumori T, Tsuta K, Masai K, Kinno T, Taniyama T, Yoshida A, et al. p40 is the best marker for diagnosing pulmonary squamous cell carcinoma: comparison with p63, cytokeratin 5/6, desmocollin-3, and sox2. Appl Immunohistochem Mol Morphol. 2014;22:377–82.

56. Chilosi M, Zamò A, Brighenti A, Malpeli G, Montagna L, Piccoli P, et al. Constitutive expression of DeltaN-p63alpha isoform in human thymus and thymic epithelial tumours. Virchows Arch. 2003;443:175–83.

57. Zamò A, Malpeli G, Scarpa A, Doglioni C, Chilosi M, Menestrina F. Expression of TP73L is a helpful diagnostic marker of primary mediastinal large B-cell lymphomas. Mod Pathol. 2005;18:1448–53.

58. Pelosi G, Sonzogni A, Harari S, Albini A, Bresaola E, Marchiò C, et al. Classification of pulmonary neuroendocrine tumors: new insights. Transl Lung Cancer Res. 2017;6:513–29.

59. Mengoli MC, Rossi G, Cavazza A, Franco R, Marino FZ, Migaldi M, et al. Diffuse idiopathic pulmonary neuroendocrine cell hyperplasia (DIPNECH) syndrome and carcinoid tumors with/without NECH: a clinicopathologic, radiologic, and immunomolecular comparison study. Am J Surg Pathol. 2018;42:646–55.

60. Rossi G, Jocollé G, Conti A, Tiseo M, Zito Marino F, Donati G, et al. Detection of ROS1 rearrangement in non-small cell lung cancer: current and future perspectives. Lung Cancer (Auckl). 2017;8:45–55.

61. Rossi G, Ragazzi M, Tamagnini I, Mengoli MC, Vincenzi G, Barbieri F, et al. Does immunohistochemistry represent a robust alternative technique in determining drugable predictive gene alterations in non-small cell lung cancer? Curr Drug Targets. 2017;18:13–26.

62. Boyle TA, Masago K, Ellison KE, Yatabe Y, Hirsch FR. ROS1 immunohistochemistry among major genotypes of non-small-cell lung cancer. Clin Lung Cancer. 2015;16:106–11.

63. Selinger CI, Li BT, Pavlakis N, Links M, Gill AJ, Lee A, et al. Screening for ROS1 gene rearrangements in non-small-cell lung cancers using immunohistochemistry with FISH confirmation is an effective method to identify this rare target. Histopathology. 2017;70:402–11.

64. Kim EK, Kim KA, Lee CY, Shim HS. The frequency and clinical impact of HER2 alterations in lung adenocarcinoma. PLoS One. 2017;12:e0171280.

65. Ko YS, Kim NY, Pyo JS. Concordance analysis between HER2 immunohistochemistry and in situ hybridization in non-small cell lung cancer. Int J Biol Markers. 2018;33:49–54.

66. Wu YC, Chang IC, Wang CL, Chen TD, Chen YT, Liu HP, et al. Comparison of IHC, FISH and RT-PCR methods for detection of ALK rearrangements in 312 non-small cell lung cancer patients in Taiwan. PLoS One. 2013;8:e70839.

67. Peretti U, Ferrara R, Pilotto S, Kinspergher S, Caccese M, Santo A, et al. ALK gene copy number gains in non-small-cell lung cancer: prognostic impact and clinico-pathological correlations. Respir Res. 2016;17:105.

68. Caliò A, Bria E, Pilotto S, Gilioli E, Nottegar A, Eccher A, et al. ALK gene copy number in lung cancer: Unspecific polyploidy versus specific amplification visible as double minutes. Cancer Biomark. 2017;18:215–20.

69. Lan B, Ma C, Zhang C, Chai S, Wang P, Ding L, Wang K. Association between PD-L1 expression and driver gene status in non-small-cell lung cancer: a meta-analysis. Oncotarget. 2018;9:7684–99.

70. Yaziji H, Battifora H, Barry TS, Hwang HC, Bacchi CE, McIntosh MW, et al. Evaluation of 12 antibodies for distinguishing epithelioid mesothelioma from adenocarcinoma: identification of a three-antibody immunohistochemical panel with maximal sensitivity and specificity. Mod Pathol. 2006;19: 514–23.

71. Kushitani K, Amatya VJ, Okada Y, Katayama Y, Mawas AS, Miyata Y, et al. Utility and pitfalls of immunohistochemistry in the differential diagnosis between epithelioid mesothelioma and poorly differentiated lung squamous cell carcinoma. Histopathology. 2017;70:375–84.

72. Marchevsky AM, LeStang N, Hiroshima K, Pelosi G, Attanoos R, Churg A, et al. The differential diagnosis between pleural sarcomatoid mesothelioma and spindle cell/pleomorphic (sarcomatoid) carcinomas of the lung: evidence-based guidelines from the International Mesothelioma Panel and the MESOPATH National Reference Center. Hum Pathol. 2017;67:160–8.

73. Husain AN, Colby TV, Ordóñez NG, Allen TC, Attanoos RL, Beasley MB, et al. Guidelines for pathologic diagnosis of malignant mesothelioma 2017 update of the consensus statement from the International Mesothelioma Interest Group. Arch Pathol Lab Med. 2018;142:89–108.

74. Amin KM, Litzky LA, Smythe WR, Mooney AM, Morris JM, Mews DJ, et al. Wilms' tumor 1 susceptibility (WT1) gene products are selectively expressed in malignant mesothelioma. Am J Pathol. 1995;146:344–56.

75. Doglioni C, Dei Tos AP, Laurino L, Iuzzolino P, Chiarelli C, Celio MR, Viale G. Calretinin: a novel immunocytochemical marker for mesothelioma. Am J Surg Pathol. 1996;20:1037–46.

76. He C, Wang B, Wan C, Yang T, Shen Y. Diagnostic value of D2-40 immunostaining for malignant mesothelioma: a meta-analysis. Oncotarget. 2017;8:64407–16.

77. Sheibani K, Shin SS, Kezirian J, Weiss LM. Ber-EP4 antibody as a discriminant in the differential diagnosis of malignant mesothelioma versus adenocarcinoma. Am J Surg Pathol. 1991;15:779–84.

78. Comin CE, Novelli L, Boddi V, Paglierani M, Dini S. Calretinin, thrombomodulin, CEA, and CD15: a useful combination of immunohistochemical markers for differentiating pleural epithelial mesothelioma from peripheral pulmonary adenocarcinoma. Hum Pathol. 2001;32:529–36.

79. Ordóñez NG. Application of immunohistochemistry in the diagnosis of epithelioid mesothelioma: a review and update. Hum Pathol. 2013;44:1–19.

80. Wu D, Hiroshima K, Matsumoto S, Nabeshima K, Yusa T, Ozaki D, et al. Diagnostic usefulness of p16/CDKN2A FISH in distinguishing between sarcomatoid mesothelioma and fibrous pleuritis. Am J Clin Pathol. 2013;139:39–46.

81. Cigognetti M, Lonardi S, Fisogni S, Balzarini P, Pellegrini V, Tironi A, et al. BAP1 (BRCA1-associated protein 1) is a highly specific marker for differentiating mesothelioma from reactive mesothelial proliferations. Mod Pathol. 2015;28:1043–57.

82. Churg A, Sheffield BS, Galateau-Salle F. New markers for separating benign from malignant mesothelial proliferations: are we there yet? Arch Pathol Lab Med. 2016;140:318–21.

83. Chilosi M, Zinzani PL, Poletti V. Lymphoproliferative lung disorders. Semin Respir Crit Care Med. 2005;26:490–501.

84. Munari E, Rinaldi M, Ambrosetti A, Bonifacio M, Bonalumi A, Chilosi M, et al. Absence of TCL1A expression is a useful diagnostic feature in splenic marginal zone lymphoma. Virchows Arch. 2012;461:677–85.

85. Poletti V, Gurioli C, Piciucchi S, Rossi A, Ravaglia C, Dubini A, et al. Intravascular large B cell lymphoma presenting in the lung: the diagnostic value of transbronchial cryobiopsy. Sarcoidosis Vasc Diffuse Lung Dis. 2015;31:354–8.

86. Schiavo D, Batzlaff C, Maldonado F. Pulmonary parenchymal lymphoma diagnosed by bronchoscopic cryoprobe lung biopsy. J Bronchology Interv Pulmonol. 2016;23:174–6.

87. Yap E, Low I. Bronchoscopic transbronchial cryobiopsy diagnosis of recurrent diffuse large B-cell lymphoma in the lung: a promising new tool? J Bronchology Interv Pulmonol. 2017;24:e22–3.

88. Chilosi M, Lestani M, Baruzzi G, Poletti V. Histopathological and immunohistological findings in AIDS-associated lung disorders. Eur Respir Mon. 1995;2:150–203.

89. Troxell ML, Lanciault C. Practical applications in immunohistochemistry: evaluation of rejection and infection in organ transplantation. Arch Pathol Lab Med. 2016;140:910–25.

90. Hofmann-Thiel S, Turaev L, Hoffmann H. Evaluation of the hyplex TBC PCR test for detection of *Mycobacterium tuberculosis* complex in clinical samples. BMC Microbiol. 2010;10:95.

91. Chilosi M, Doglioni C. Constitutive p63 expression in airway basal cells. A molecular target in diffuse lung diseases. Sarcoidosis Vasc Diffuse Lung Dis. 2001;18:23–6.

92. Chilosi M, Poletti V, Murer B, Lestani M, Cancellieri A, Montagna L, et al. Abnormal re-epithelialization and lung remodeling in idiopathic pulmonary fibrosis: the role of deltaN-p63. Lab Investig. 2002;82:1335–45.

93. Sheikh HA, Fuhrer K, Cieply K, Yousem S. p63 expression in assessment of bronchioloalveolar proliferations of the lung. Mod Pathol. 2004;17:1134–40.

94. Romano RA, Ortt K, Birkaya B, Smalley K, Sinha S. An active role of the DeltaN isoform of p63 in regulating basal keratin genes K5 and K14 and directing epidermal cell fate. PLoS One. 2009;4:e5623.

95. Ficial M, Antonaglia C, Chilosi M, Santagiuliana M, Tahseen AO, Confalonieri D, et al. Keratin-14 expression in pneumocytes as a marker of lung regeneration/repair during diffuse alveolar damage. Am J Respir Crit Care Med. 2014;189:1142–5.

96. Confalonieri M, Buratti E, Grassi G, Bussani R, Chilosi M, Farra R, et al. Keratin14 mRNA expression in human pneumocytes during quiescence, repair and disease. PLoS One. 2017;12:e0172130.

97. Wallace WA, Howie SE, Lamb D, Salter DM. Tenascin immunoreactivity in cryptogenic fibrosing alveolitis. J Pathol. 1995;175:415–20.

98. Kuhn C, Mason RJ. Immunolocalization of SPARC, tenascin, and thrombospondin in pulmonary fibrosis. Am J Pathol. 1995;147:1759–69.

99. Greenberger PA. 7. Immunologic lung disease. J Allergy Clin Immunol. 2008;121(2 Suppl):S393–7.

100. Lu Y, Malmhäll C, Sjöstrand M, Rådinger M, O'Neil SE, Lötvall J, et al. Expansion of CD4(+) CD25(+) and CD25(−) T-Bet, GATA-3, Foxp3 and RORγt cells in allergic inflammation, local lung distribution and chemokine gene expression. PLoS One. 2011;6:e19889.

101. Chilosi M, Mombello A, Montagna L, Benedetti A, Lestani M, Semenzato G, et al. Multimarker immunohistochemical staining of calgranulins, chloroacetate esterase, and S100 for simultaneous demonstration of inflammatory cells on paraffin sections. J Histochem Cytochem. 1990;38:1669–75.

102. Reghellin D, Poletti V, Tomassett S, Dubini A, Cavazza A, Rossi G, et al. Cathepsin-K is a sensitive immunohistochemical marker for detection of micro-granulomas in hypersensitivity pneumonitis. Sarcoidosis Vasc Diffuse Lung Dis. 2010;27:57–63.

103. Badalian-Very G, Vergilio JA, Degar BA, MacConaill LE, Brandner B, Calicchio ML, et al. Recurrent BRAF mutations in Langerhans cell histiocytosis. Blood. 2010;116:1919–23.

104. Haroche J, Charlotte F, Arnaud L, von Deimling A, Hélias-Rodzewicz Z, Hervier B, et al. High prevalence of BRAF V600E mutations in Erdheim-Chester disease but not in other non-Langerhans cell histiocytoses. Blood. 2012;120:2700–3.

105. Roden AC, Hu X, Kip S, Parrilla Castellar ER, Rumilla KM, et al. BRAF V600E expression in Langerhans cell histiocytosis: clinical and immunohistochemical study on 25 pulmonary and 54 extrapulmonary cases. Am J Surg Pathol. 2014;38:548–51.

106. Chilosi M, Facchetti F, Caliò A, Zamò A, Brunelli M, Martignoni G, et al. Oncogene-induced senescence distinguishes indolent from aggressive forms of pulmonary and non-pulmonary Langerhans cell histiocytosis. Leuk Lymphoma. 2014;55:2620–6.

107. Cangi MG, Biavasco R, Cavalli G, Grassini G, Dal-Cin E, Campochiaro C, et al. BRAFV600E-mutation is invariably present and associated to oncogene-induced senescence in Erdheim-Chester disease. Ann Rheum Dis. 2015;74:1596–602.

108. Martignoni G, Pea M, Reghellin D, Gobbo S, Zamboni G, Chilosi M, et al. Molecular pathology of lymphangioleiomyomatosis and other perivascular epithelioid cell tumors. Arch Pathol Lab Med. 2010;134:33–40.

109. Bonetti F, Chiodera PL, Pea M, Martignoni G, Bosi F, Zamboni G, et al. Transbronchial biopsy in lymphangiomyomatosis of the lung. HMB45 for diagnosis. Am J Surg Pathol. 1993;17:1092–102.

110. Chilosi M, Doglioni C, Murer B, Poletti V. Epithelial stem cell exhaustion in the pathogenesis of idiopathic pulmonary fibrosis. Sarcoidosis Vasc Diffuse Lung Dis. 2010;27:7–18.

111. Chilosi M, Carloni A, Rossi A, Poletti V. Premature lung aging and cellular senescence in the pathogenesis of idiopathic pulmonary fibrosis and COPD/emphysema. Transl Res. 2013;162:156–73.

112. Selman M, Pardo A. Revealing the pathogenic and aging-related mechanisms of the enigmatic idiopathic pulmonary fibrosis. An integral model. Am J Respir Crit Care Med. 2014;189:1161–72.

113. Thannickal VJ, Murthy M, Balch WE, Chandel NS, Meiners S, Eickelberg O, et al. Blue journal conference. Aging and susceptibility to lung disease. Am J Respir Crit Care Med. 2015;191:261–9.

114. Carloni A, Poletti V, Fermo L, Bellomo N, Chilosi M. Heterogeneous distribution of mechanical stress in human lung: a mathematical approach to evaluate abnormal remodeling in IPF. J Theor Biol. 2013;332:136–40.

115. Minagawa S, Araya J, Numata T, Nojiri S, Hara H, Yumino Y, et al. Accelerated epithelial cell senescence in IPF and the inhibitory role of SIRT6 in TGF-β-induced senescence of human bronchial epithelial cells. Am J Physiol Lung Cell Mol Physiol. 2011;300:L391–401.

116. Yanai H, Shteinberg A, Porat Z, Budovsky A, Braiman A, Zeische R, et al. Cellular senescence-like features of lung fibroblasts derived from idiopathic pulmonary fibrosis patients. Aging (Albany NY). 2015;7:664–72.

117. Schafer MJ, White TA, Iijima K, Haak AJ, Ligresti G, Atkinson EJ, et al. Cellular senescence mediates fibrotic pulmonary disease. Nat Commun. 2017;8:14532.

118. Yamaguchi M, Hirai S, Tanaka Y, Sumi T, Miyajima M, Mishina T, et al. Fibroblastic foci, covered with alveolar epithelia exhibiting epithelial-mesenchymal transition, destroy alveolar septa by disrupting blood flow in idiopathic pulmonary fibrosis. Lab Investig. 2017;97:232–42.

119. Kaarteenaho-Wiik R, Tani T, Sormunen R, Soini Y, Virtanen I, Pääkkö P. Tenascin immunoreactivity as a prognostic marker in usual interstitial pneumonia. Am J Respir Crit Care Med. 1996;154:511–8.

120. Chilosi M, Caliò A, Rossi A, Gilioli E, Pedica F, Montagna L, et al. Epithelial to mesenchymal transition-related proteins ZEB1, β-catenin, and β-tubulin-III in idiopathic pulmonary fibrosis. Mod Pathol. 2017;30:26–38.

121. Chilosi M, Poletti V, Zamò A, Lestani M, Montagna L, Piccoli P, et al. Aberrant Wnt/beta-catenin pathway activation in idiopathic pulmonary fibrosis. Am J Pathol. 2003;162:1495–502.

122. Chilosi M, Zamò A, Doglioni C, Reghellin D, Lestani M, Montagna L, et al. Migratory marker expression in fibroblast foci of idiopathic pulmonary fibrosis. Respir Res. 2006;7:95.

123. Chilosi M, Murer B, Poletti V. Usual interstitial pneumonia. In: Zander S, Popper HH, Jagirdar J, Haque AK, Cagle PT, Barrios R, editors. Molecular pathology of lung diseases. Berlin: Springer; 2008. p. 607–15.

124. Willis BC, Liebler JM, Luby-Phelps K, Nicholson AG, Crandall ED, du Bois RM, et al. Induction of epithelial-mesenchymal transition in alveolar epithelial cells by transforming growth factor-beta1: potential role in idiopathic pulmonary fibrosis. Am J Pathol. 2005;166:1321–32.

125. Seibold MA, Wise AL, Speer MC, Steele MP, Brown KK, Loyd JE, et al. A common MUC5B promoter polymorphism and pulmonary fibrosis. N Engl J Med. 2011;364:1503–12.

126. Seibold MA, Smith RW, Urbanek C, Groshong SD, Cosgrove GP, Brown KK, et al. The idiopathic pulmonary fibrosis honeycomb cyst contains a mucociliary pseudostratified epithelium. PLoS One. 2013;8:e58658.

127. Plantier L, Crestani B, Wert SE, Dehoux M, Zweytick B, Guenther A, et al. Ectopic respiratory epithelial cell differentiation in bronchiolised distal airspaces in idiopathic pulmonary fibrosis. Thorax. 2011;66:651–7.

128. Alder JK, Chen JJ, Lancaster L, Danoff S, Su SC, Cogan JD, et al. Short telomeres are a risk factor for idiopathic pulmonary fibrosis. Proc Natl Acad Sci U S A. 2008;105:13051–6.

129. Mathai SK, Yang IV, Schwarz MI, Schwartz DA. Incorporating genetics into the identification and treatment of idiopathic pulmonary fibrosis. BMC Med. 2015;13:191.

130. Kaur A, Mathai SK, Schwartz DA. Genetics in idiopathic pulmonary fibrosis pathogenesis, prognosis, and treatment. Front Med (Lausanne). 2017;4:154.

131. Schwartz DA. Idiopathic pulmonary fibrosis is a complex genetic disorder. Trans Am Clin Climatol Assoc. 2016;127:34–45.

132. Travis WD, Costabel U, Hansell DM, King TE Jr, Lynch DA, Nicholson AG, et al. An official American Thoracic Society/European Respiratory Society statement: update of the international

multidisciplinary classification of the idiopathic interstitial pneumonias. Am J Respir Crit Care Med. 2013;188:733–48.

133. Rosenbaum JN, Butt YM, Johnson KA, Meyer K, Batra K, Kanne JP, et al. Pleuroparenchymal fibroelastosis: a pattern of chronic lung injury. Hum Pathol. 2015;46:137–46.

134. Oda T, Ogura T, Kitamura H, Hagiwara E, Baba T, Enomoto Y, et al. Distinct characteristics of pleuroparenchymal fibroelastosis with usual interstitial pneumonia compared with idiopathic pulmonary fibrosis. Chest. 2014;146:1248–55.

135. Enomoto Y, Matsushima S, Meguro S, Kawasaki H, Kosugi I, Fujisawa T, et al. Podoplanin-positive myofibroblasts: a pathologic hallmark of pleuroparenchymal fibroelastosis. Histopathology. 2018;72:1209–15.

Part III

Clinical Role of Transbronchial Cryobiopsy

Clinical Meaning of Transbronchial Cryobiopsy

10

Silvia Puglisi, Claudia Ravaglia, Antonella Arcadu, Sara Tomassetti, and Venerino Poletti

Transbronchial lung cryobiopsy (TLCB) has recently been proposed as a new approach in the diagnosis of diffuse parenchymal lung diseases (DPLDs). The diagnostic workup of diffuse lung disease includes medical history, physical examination, lung function tests, high-resolution computed tomography, and bronchoalveolar lavage; however, often these elements can be insufficient. When the clinical-radiological picture is nondiagnostic, the histology becomes a key element for the multidisciplinary diagnosis (MDD). Since 2014, with the licensing of the new anti-fibrotic drugs (pirfenidone and nintedanib) as important medication for IPF, to secure an accurate diagnosis has become of critical importance [1, 2]. In the half of patients in which UIP pattern (usual interstitial pneumonia) is not detected radiologically, diagnosis rests on histology obtained by lung biopsy [3]. Recently, TLCB has proven to be a safe alternative to surgery in a large group of DPLDs, and the use of TLCB is rapidly changing the approach to DPLD diagnosis in many expert centers.

10.1 Surgical Lung Biopsy and TBB in DPLDs

When tissue sampling is needed, surgical lung biopsy (SLB) is still considered by guidelines the gold standard to obtain sufficient histological information to distinguish UIP pattern from other fibrotic DPLDs [4]. However, two important points need to be considered. Firstly, SLB represents only a small sample of the whole lung, and the minimal quantity of the lung necessary to guarantee the maximum morphological information compared with the whole lung or lungs remains unknown [5]. Secondly, SLB is characterized by appreciable risks and costs. Adverse events related to surgery include chronic chest pain, prolonged air leakage, and infections. Most notably, mortality rate can be 1.7% for elective procedures and 16% for nonelective procedures [5]; mortality can be even higher when the patient conditions are worsening, and there is evidence of significant and rapid decline in pulmonary function [6]. An increase in in-hospital mortality has also been linked to male gender, open rather

S. Puglisi · C. Ravaglia · A. Arcadu
S. Tomassetti (✉)
Department of Diseases of the Thorax,
Ospedale Morgagni-Pierantoni, Forlì, Italy

V. Poletti
Department of Diseases of the Thorax,
Ospedale Morgagni-Pierantoni, Forlì, Italy

Department of Respiratory Diseases and Allergy,
Aarhus University Hospital, Aarhus, Denmark

© Springer Nature Switzerland AG 2019
V. Poletti (ed.), *Transbronchial cryobiopsy in diffuse parenchymal lung disease*,
https://doi.org/10.1007/978-3-030-14891-1_10

than video-assisted thoracoscopic surgery, and a suspected diagnosis of IPF or connective tissue related—DPLD [6]. Balancing the risk/benefit ratio, SLB is often not performed in elderly subjects, in patients with a significant burden of comorbidities and with severe respiratory impairment [7–10]. Furthermore, in common clinical practice, SLB is also not offered to asymptomatic patients with minimal HRCT changes, because the risks and costs of SLB do not appear to be sufficiently counterbalanced by the advantage of an early diagnosis of DPLDs. For these reasons, SLB is usually performed in less than 50% of the cases in which, according to guidelines, histology is necessary [11, 12]. Another practical issue that should be considered is the waiting list for planned admissions for thoracic surgery and the relatively limited number of cases that thoracic surgeons are able to take in charge.

To overcome all the obstacles related to thoracic surgery in the diagnosis of DPLDs, some expert centers have started to search for a less invasive method to collect lung tissue samples. It has been shown that the conventional transbronchial lung biopsy (TBB) captures tissue that is representative mainly of the centrilobular zone [13–15] and that crush artifacts can be an important limiting factor [16]. The disorders that are centered around terminal and respiratory bronchioles or significantly involve these structures or are distributed along the lymphatic routes may be easily sampled by the conventional forceps (e.g., organizing pneumonia, sarcoidosis, carcinomatous lymphangitis). TBB lung specimens may contain specific and informative lesions that are diagnostic by themselves (e.g., carcinomatous lymphangitis and other neoplasms, alveolar proteinosis, Langerhans cell histiocytosis) or can show characteristic features that are diagnostic if combined with the clinical and radiological context (e.g., organizing pneumonia, sarcoidosis, hypersensitivity pneumonitis); however TBB may not be informative when morphologic findings are completely incongruous with the clinical and radiological context and can be more challenging and complex in idiopathic fibrotic interstitial pneumonias such as idiopathic pulmonary fibrosis (IPF), nonspecific interstitial pneumonia

(NSIP), and desquamative interstitial pneumonia (DIP) [13, 14, 17–21]. In fact, negative predictive value of TBB for UIP diagnosis is described between 46 and 55% [20, 21], and in a retrospective analysis, Tomassetti et al. reported that TBB specimens interpreted by expert pathologists can show features of UIP pattern in 30% of cases, with a high specificity (above 80%) for UIP pattern but a very low specificity and sensitivity for other pathological diagnoses (NSIP, CHP, DIP) [20]. In a more recent study, Sheth and coworkers evaluated the diagnostic utility of TBB combined with clinical and HRCT data, and the results were similar, with TBB leading to a diagnosis in approximately 20–30% of patients suspected for DPLDs with a better diagnostic value in identifying the UIP pattern. To obtain a final multidisciplinary diagnosis, 64% of patients underwent a SLB after a nondiagnostic TBB [9].

The gap existing between SLB and TBB is wide and underlines the need for a new minimal invasive approach to provide a specific and confident diagnosis. The search for a minimally invasive alternative to SLB is motivated by the need to reduce not only the complications related to SLB but also to reduce the prevalence of "unclassifiable interstitial lung diseases" [22].

10.2 Clinical Considerations About the Role of TLCB in the Diagnosis of DPLDs

In recent years, transbronchial lung cryobiopsy, used initially for therapeutic purposes, has achieved a relevant role in the diagnostic approach of DPLDs. As any innovative diagnostic method, patient's safety was the main concern, and a correct patient selection process has emerged to be of crucial importance [22]. In fact, anecdotal data suggest that complications (which are described in detail in the specific chapter on this book) are more frequent when pulmonary function is severely impaired. Forced expiratory volume in the first second (FEV1) <0.8 L or <50% predicted, forced vital capacity (FVC) <50% predicted, and diffusing capacity of the lungs for carbon monoxide (DLCO) <35% predicted have been used to exclude biopsy candidates in some series, though not in all [17, 22, 23]; however, these limitations are drawn from data reported in studies dealing with SLB. Additionally, in the subset of patients with severe fibrosing ILDs, the risk-benefit analysis is less advantageous, because in these patients it seems that the prognostic significance of an exact histological diagnosis is reduced, and data on the efficacy of a specific "anti-fibrotic" drug on patients with severe IPF are still scanty [24]. Another important issue is the risk of acute exacerbation which needs to be assessed: recent onset of ground glass areas on HRCT scan, functional impairment and worsening of symptoms and high levels of inflammatory markers could predict the risk of acute exacerbation [22, 25, 26].

Indications for transbronchial lung cryobiopsy in the diagnosis of diffuse parenchymal lung diseases within the context of a multidisciplinary discussion are currently under evaluation, as well as the comparison of its risk/benefit ratio with that of surgical lung biopsy. However, reported diagnostic yields (50–100%) and observed complications of the procedure (e.g., rate of pneumothorax 0–30%) vary widely in different centers [27–29], and the TLCB technique has not yet been standardized. After the rapid spread of the technique in the absence of verified competency and safety standards, in 2018 a statement by experts in the field has been published, proposing some recommendations (requisite equipment, personnel, indications/contraindications, risks and training requirements) with the aim of facilitating uniform practice and providing a guide for those wishing to introduce this technique [22]. Series reporting experience of cryobiopsy in the diagnosis of diffuse parenchymal lung diseases (DPLDs) include a limited number of patients, and it is difficult to compare different series in terms of sampling strategies, procedural technical details, diagnostic yield, and complications. Compared to conventional TBB, cryobiopsy has demonstrated a superior diagnostic yield in interstitial lung diseases, as samples obtained through cryoprobes are many times greater than that obtained by regular forceps (usually 40–50 mm² in size) [16, 20, 30–33], have usually better quality, and contain peripheral

structures of the secondary pulmonary lobules [34]. Improved results are seen in "intubated patients" and when biopsies are taken within 1 cm of the pleura [23, 30, 32, 35, 36].

Our experience involves currently a large cohort of 699 patients who underwent transbronchial lung cryobiopsy for suspected diffuse parenchymal lung diseases; in 630 cases (90.1%) lung tissue obtained from cryobiopsy, combined with clinical and radiographic information, was sufficient to establish a final multidisciplinary diagnosis for patient management (unpublished data) (Table 10.1) [36].

Recognition of the UIP pattern on these large specimens has a good inter-observer variability index and may be recognized by pathologists with high confidence. In a prospective study of 69 cases of TLCB, pathologists identified histopathologic criteria sufficient to define a characteristic pattern in 63 patients (93%), including 47 UIP (36 with high confidence and 11 with low confidence); therefore, TLCB in patients with f-DPLD could identify UIP with high confidence level in 52% of cases and with low confidence level in 16% of cases. Inter-observer agreement between the two pathologists for the recognition of UIP was very good, with a kappa coefficient of 0.83 (95% CI 0.69–0.97); weighted kappa coefficient of agreement for the identification of UIP

Table 10.1 Clinical characteristics, diagnostic yield, and complications in a cohort of 699 patients submitted to transbronchial lung cryobiopsy (TLCB)

Patient characteristic (n = 699)	No. (% or SD)
Median age (SD), years	61 (11)
Male, No. (%)	413 (59.1%)
Mean FVC percent predicted (SD)	85.4 (19.7)
Mean DLCO percent predicted (SD)	61.2 (17.5)
Pathological diagnosis, No. (%)	614 (87.8)
Multidisciplinary diagnosis, No. (%)	630 (90.1)
Pneumothorax, No. (%)	134 (19.2)
Drained pneumothorax (among those with pneumothorax), No. (%)	94 (70.1)
Mild bleeding, No. (%)	29 (4.1)
Moderate bleeding, No. (%)	53 (7.6)
Severe bleeding, No. (%)	5 (0.7%)

FVC forced vital capacity, *DLCO* diffusing capacity of the lungs for carbon monoxide

with high or low confidence was good at 0.70 (95% CI 0.57–0.83) [23].

Moreover, the value of TLCB, in combination with other clinical findings in the context of a multidisciplinary discussion, was found to be similar to that reported for SLB [37]; both the procedures had similar impact on the MDD process, showing similar changes in diagnostic impression, diagnostic confidence, and inter-observer agreement after integration into the MDD discussion, resulting also in a similar distribution of final MDD diagnosis. For ethical reasons, there are no trials describing patients undergoing consecutive TLCB and SLB, and for the high diagnostic yield and low complication rate of TLCB compared to SLB, they seem unlikely to be proposed in the future [21]. Finally, immunohistochemical analysis also may be carried out easily in samples obtained by cryobiopsy [5].

The strategies used to collect samples are not yet standardized [34], with the majority of studies to date having retrieved lung tissue from one segment and only a minority having collected lung samples from different segments of the same lobe [38]. Multiple biopsies are usually taken to reduce sampling error, as we know that diagnosis can be influenced by the heterogeneity of the disease and by the distribution of the parenchymal pathology. The optimal number of biopsies has not been established for cryobiopsy, and different strategies adopted to sample lung tissue are still missing in literature. In our large series (699 patients), diagnostic yield was significantly influenced by the number of samples and the sampling strategy, improving dramatically when ≥2 samples were performed (instead of only one) and when biopsy was obtained in two different sites (instead of only one site), either from the same lobe or from different lobes. This is particularly important for fibrotic lung diseases, in which pathological variability is more challenging, and differential diagnosis could be more difficult; we observed discordant samples between different sites in almost 30% of cases, with a significant increase in diagnostic yield between one site and two sites. Our findings confirm and quantify the frequency of interlobar and intralobar histologic variability in fibrotic ILDs and confirm the adequacy of cryobiopsy in identifying this histologic heterogeneity. Prior data on interlobar heterogeneity of DPLDs support the practice to obtain tissue from two different sites; however, histologic heterogeneity has been evaluated in the literature until now only in surgical lung biopsy (SLB) and not in cryobiopsy [39–42]. It is very important to obtain tissue from two different sites, either from the same lobe or from different lobes when HRCT scan does not show a clear gradient profusion of the pattern or when different patterns are present in different lobes. Significant sampling errors may result from strategies that obtain only one biopsy specimen for ILD.

10.3   The Paradigm Shift

The data published on TLCB in DPLDs lead the clinics to a paradigm shift as a new intriguing mini-invasive method to obtain lung samples is now available, in which peripheral structures of the secondary pulmonary lobule are identifiable (visceral pleura, interlobular septa) and allow to diagnose with high confidence complex morphologic patterns (UIP, pleuroparenchymal fibroelastosis, NSIP, DIP, smoking-related ILDs), with an inter-observer variability value similar to that observed in SLB. The good clinical impact associated with less side effects and lower economic charges is also all elements in favor of this technique [12].

In the last years, it has been observed an increased number of cryobiopsy procedures as compared to a similar number of surgical biopsies. In our clinical experience, the number of SLB performed in the last decades hasn't changed, whereas there has been a stinking growing trend in the number of TLCB that in 2017 has reached a number 20 times higher compared to SLB (Fig. 10.1). This trend suggests that the cryobiopsy is helping in the final multidisciplinary diagnosis in a higher number of patients with DPLDs, leading to an early diagnosis and patient's specific treatment. In this context,

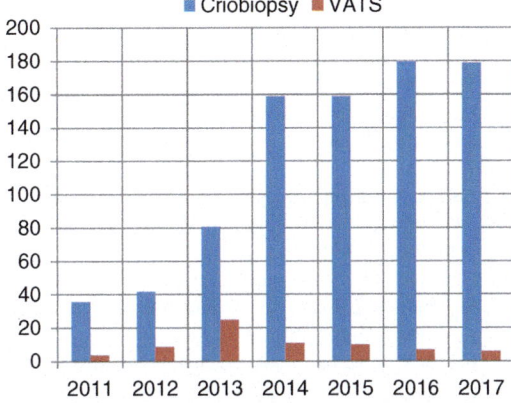

Fig.   10.1 TBCB   and   VATS   at   the G.B. Morgagni—L. Pierantoni Hospital, Forlì (2011–2017)

TLCB and SLB could be integrated in a complementary diagnostic algorithm, with a first diagnostic approach for obtaining tissue with cryobiopsy, reserving the surgical approach for only the minority of cases in which TLCB is not adequate or not diagnostic [27, 35]; TLCB will increase the number of diagnoses in DPLDs with atypical features, avoiding surgical approach in many patients (especially in old people and in those with comorbidity) [43]. The availability of cryobiopsy and its lower morbidity could potentially broaden the indication for lung biopsy such as in DPLD patients with equivocal exposures or suspicion of an occult collagen vascular disease who may exhibit histopathological clues to alternative diagnoses (e.g., small granulomas, foci of organizing pneumonia, lymphoid follicles, pulmonary and pleural chronic inflammation) on cryobiopsy that might add weight to other diagnosis [22]. TLCB could sometimes be proposed in patients with a typical radiological UIP pattern, with the aim of collecting more definite data suggesting occult exposure or collagen vascular diseases; the detection of areas of organizing pneumonia or diffuse alveolar damage in a context of UIP pattern could be a marker of rapid progression of the disease [12] and in some subsets it could suggest a combination of anti-fibrotic and anti-inflammatory drugs [44] or it may implement research on molecular markers in order to reach a target therapy [12].

References

1. King TE Jr, Bradford WZ, Castro-Bernardini S, et al. A phase 3 trial of pirfenidone in patient with idiopathic pulmonary fibrosis. N Engl J Med. 2014;370:2083–92.
2. Richeldi L, du Bois RM, Raghu G, et al. Efficacy and safety of nintedanib in idiopathic pulmonary fibrosis. N Engl J Med. 2014;370:2071–82.
3. ATS/ERS&JRS/ALAT Committee on Idiopathic Pulmonary Fibrosis. An official ATS/ERS/JRS/ALAT statement: idiopathic pulmonary fibrosis: evidence-based guidelines for diagnosis and management. Am J Respir Crit Care Med. 2011;183:788–824.
4. Raghu G, Collard HR, Egan JJ, et al.; ATS/ERS/JRS/ALAT Committee on Idiopathic Pulmonary Fibrosis. An official ATS/ERS/JRS/ALAT statement: idiopathic pulmonary fibrosis: evidence-based guidelines for diagnosis and management. Am J Respir Crit Care Med. 2011;183:788–824.
5. Poletti V, Ravaglia C, Gurioli C, et al. Invasive diagnostic techniques in idiopathic interstitial pneumonias. Respirology. 2016;21:44–50.
6. Hutchinson JP, Fogarty AW, McKeever TM, et al. In-hospital mortality following surgical lung biopsy for interstitial lung disease in the USA: 2000-2011. Am J Respir Crit Care Med. 2016;193:1161–7.
7. Fibla JJ, Molins L, Blanco A, et al. Video-assisted thoracoscopic lung biopsy in the diagnosis of interstial lung disease: a prospective, multicenter study in 224 patients. Arch Bronconeumol. 2012;48:81–5.
8. Kreider ME, Hansen-Flaschen J, Ahmad NN, Rossman MD, Kaiser LR, Kucharczuk JC, Shrager JB. Complications of video-assisted thoracoscopic lung biopsy in patients with interstitial lung disease. Ann Thorac Surg. 2007;83:1140–4.
9. Sheth JS, Belperio JA, Fishbein MC, et al. Utility of transbronchial vs surgical lung biopsy in the diagnosis of suspected fibrotic interstitial lung disease. Chest. 2017;151:389–99.
10. Utz JP, Ryu JH, Douglas WW, et al. High short-term mortality following lung biopsy for usual interstitial pneumonia. Eur Respir J. 2001;17:175–9.
11. Park JH, Kim DK, Kim DS, et al. Mortality and risk factors for surgical lung biopsy in patients with idiopathic interstitial pneumonia. Eur J Cardiothorac Surg. 2007;31:1115–9.
12. Poletti V, Ravaglia C, Dubini A, et al. How might transbronchial cryobiopsy improve diagnosis and treatment of diffuse parenchymal lung disease patients? Expert Rev Respir Med. 2017;11:913–7.
13. Cazzato S, Zompatori M, Burzi M, et al. Bronchoalveolar lavage and transbronchial lung biopsy in alveolar and/or ground glass opacification. Monaldi Arch Chest Dis. 1999;54:115–9.
14. Leslie KO, Gruden JF, Parish JM, et al. Arch Pathol Lab Med. 2007;131:407–23.
15. Colby TV. The pathologist's approach to bronchoscopic biopsies. Pathologica. 2010;102:432–42.

16. Griff S, Schönfeld N, Ammenwerth W, et al. Diagnostic yield of transbronchial cryobiopsy in non-neoplastic lung disease: a retrospective case series. BMC Pulm Med. 2014;14:171.

17. Poletti V, Ravaglia C, Tomassetti S. Transbronchial cryobiopsy in diffuse parenchymal lung diseases. Curr Opin Pulm Med. 2016;22:289–96.

18. Joyner LR, Scheinhorn DJ. Transbronchial forceps lung biopsy through the fiberoptic bronchoscope. Diagnosis of diffuse pulmonary disease. Chest. 1975;67:532–5.

19. Poletti V, Chilosi M, Olivieri D. Diagnostic invasive procedure in diffuse infiltrative lung disease. Respiration. 2004;71:107–19.

20. Tomassetti S, Cavazza A, Colby TV, et al. Transbronchial biopsy is useful in predicting UIP pattern. Respir Res. 2012;13:96.

21. Tomassetti S, Ravaglia C, Poletti V. Diffuse parenchymal lung disease. Eur Respir Rev. 2017;26:170004.

22. Hetzel J, Maldonado F, Ravaglia C, et al. Transbronchial cryobiopsies for the diagnosis of diffuse parenchymal lung diseases: expert statement from the cryobiopsy working group on safety and utility and a call for standardization of the procedure. Respiration. 2018;95:188–200.

23. Casoni GL, Tomassetti S, Cavazza A, et al. Transbronchial lung cryobiopsy in the diagnosis of fibrotic interstitial lung diseases. PLoS One. 2014;9:e86716.

24. Latsi PI, Du Bois RM, Nicholson AG, et al. Fibrotic idiopathic interstitial pneumonia: the prognostic value of longitudinal functional trends. Am J Respir Crit Care Med. 2003;168:531–7.

25. Qiu M, Chen Y, Ye Q. Risk factors for acute exacerbation of idiopathic pulmonary fibrosis: a systematic review and meta-analysis. Clin Respir J. 2017;12:1084–92.

26. Fujimoto K, Taniguchi H, Johkoh T, et al. Acute exacerbation of idiopathic pulmonary fibrosis: high resolution CT scores predict mortality. Eur Radiol. 2012;22:83–92.

27. Ravaglia C, Bonifazi M, Wells AU, et al. Safety and diagnostic yield of transbronchial lung cryobiopsy in diffuse parenchymal lung diseases: a comparative study versus video-assisted thoracoscopic lung biopsy and a systematic review of the literature. Respiration. 2016;91:215–27.

28. Iftikhar IH, Alghothani L, Sardi A, et al. Transbronchial lung cryobiopsy and video-assisted thoracoscopic lung biopsy in the diagnosis of diffuse parenchymal lung disease: a meta-analysis of diagnostic test accuracy. Ann Am Thorac Soc. 2017;14:1197–211.

29. Bango-Alvarez A, Ariza-Prota M, Torres-Rivas H, et al. Transbronchial cryobiopsy in interstitial lung disease: experience in 106 cases—how to do it. ERJ Open Res. 2017;3:00148-2016.

30. Pajares V, Puzo C, Castillo D, et al. Diagnostic yield of transbronchial cryobiopsy in interstitial lung disease: a randomized trial. Respirology. 2014;19:900–6.

31. Schumann C, Hetzel J, Babiak AJ, et al. Cryoprobe biopsy increases the diagnostic yield in endobronchial tumor lesions. J Thorac Cardiovasc Surg. 2010;140:417–21.

32. Babiak A, Hetzel J, Krishna G, et al. Transbronchial cryobiopsy: a new tool for lung biopsies. Respiration. 2009;78:203–8.

33. Griff S, Ammenwerth W, Schonfeld N, et al. Morphometrical analysis of transbronchial cryobiopsies. Diagn Pathol. 2011;6:53.

34. Poletti V, Hetzel J. Transbronchial cryobiopsy in diffuse parenchymal lung diseases: need of procedural standardization. Respiration. 2015;90:275–8.

35. Hagmeyer L, Theegarten D, Wohlschläger J, et al. The role of transbronchial cryobiopsy and surgical lung biopsy in the diagnostic algorithm of interstitial lung disease. Clin Respir J. 2015;10:589–95.

36. Ravaglia C, Wells AU, Tomassetti S, Gurioli C, Gurioli C, Dubini A, Cavazza A, Colby TV, Piciucchi S, Puglisi S, Bosi M, Poletti V. Diagnostic yield and risk/benefit analysis of transbronchial lung cryobiopsy in diffuse parenchymal lung diseases: a large cohort of 699 patients. BMC Pulm Med. 2019;19:16.

37. Tomassetti S, Wells AU, Constabel U, et al. Bronchoscopic lung cryobiopsy increase diagnostic confidence in the multidisciplinary diagnosis of idiopathic pulmonary fibrosis. Am J Resp Crit Care Med. 2016;193:745–52.

38. Poletti V, Casoni GL, Gurioli G, et al. Lung cryobiopsies: a paradigm shift in diagnostic bronchoscopy. Respirology. 2014;19:645–54.

39. Flaherty KR, Travis WD, Colby TV, et al. Histopathologic variability in usual and nonspecific interstitial pneumonias. Am J Respir Crit Care Med. 2001;164:1722–7.

40. Flint A, Martinez FJ, Young ML, et al. Influence of sample and number and biopsy site on the histologic diagnosis of diffuse lung disease. Ann Thorac Surg. 1995;60:1605–8.

41. Winterbauer RH, Hammar SP, Hallman KO, et al. Diffuse interstitial pneumonitis. Clinicopathologic correlations in 20 patients treated with prednisone/azathioprine. Am J Med. 1978;65:661–72.

42. Cherniack RM, Colby TV, Flint A, et al. Quantitative assessment of lung pathology in idiopathic pulmonary fibrosis. The BAL Cooperative Group Steering Committee. Am Rev Respir Dis. 1991;144:892–900.

43. Kreuter M, Ehlers-Tenenbaum S, Palmowski K, et al. Impact of comorbidities on mortality in patients with idiopathic pulmonary fibrosis. PLoS One. 2016;11:e0151425.

44. Wuyts WA, Antoniou KM, et al. Combination therapy: the future of management for idiopathic pulmonary fibrosis? Lancet Respir Med. 2014;2:933–42.

Idiopathic Pulmonary Fibrosis

11

Venerino Poletti, Antonella Arcadu,
Sissel Kronborg-White, and Marco Chilosi

11.1 Introduction

Idiopathic pulmonary fibrosis (IPF) is a disorder mainly affecting the lungs [1, 2]. It affects more frequently males, smokers, or former smokers, in their 60s (average age at diagnosis 64–65). The epidemiology of IPF is difficult to determine, and the available data are still imprecise. However it seems to have an incidence, in Caucasians, of 4–8 new cases/100,000 inhabitants per year. It appears less frequent in Africans or Afro-Americans. This disorder has no known cause identified so far (except the cigarette smoke); therefore, all causes known to be involved in ILD need to be excluded (organic and inorganic exposure, drug/radiation). Symptoms are insidious: dry cough and exertional dyspnea. These symptoms usually are present for longer than 6 months. In about 60–70% of patients, physical examination reveals fine, bibasilar inspiratory crackles ("velcro sounds"). Clubbing is found up to 50% of patients. Familial clinical history is important because up to 20% of cases has a familial form. Presence of idiopathic liver cirrhosis, Fanconi anemia, or myelodysplastic syndromes, or of cases of pulmonary fibrosis in parents, in closer ancestors, or relatives, is a strong clue. Routine laboratory evaluation is not helpful for the diagnosis. In around 30% of patients, autoantibodies (antinuclear antibodies and rarely antineutrophil antibodies—mainly pANCA) may be detected, but these findings have no diagnostic role. The matrix metalloproteinases (MMPs) are proteases involved in the remodelling of extracellular matrix components. MMP-7 appears to be one of the most interesting candidates with regard to a single diagnostic biomarker. Circulating levels of MMP-7 are consistently elevated in the blood of patients with IPF compared to healthy controls and to patients affected by other ILDs. Elevated circulating levels of both SP-D and KL-6 are also detectable. The presence of autoantibodies (anti-heat shock protein 70, anti-periplakin, antiparietal cells, antineutrophils antibodies (ANCA)) and CD28+ lymphocytes and the level of CCL-18 in peripheral blood have been shown to represent valid prognostic

V. Poletti (✉)
Department of Diseases of the Thorax,
Ospedale Morgagni-Pierantoni, Forlì, Italy

Department of Respiratory Diseases and Allergy,
Aarhus University Hospital, Aarhus, Denmark

A. Arcadu
Department of Diseases of the Thorax-Pulmonology
Unit, Azienda Usl della Romagna, Ospedale GB
Morgagni, Forlì, Italy

S. Kronborg-White
Department of Respiratory Diseases and Allergy,
Aarhus University Hospital, Aarhus, Denmark

M. Chilosi
Department of Pathology, P. Pederzoli Hospital,
Peschiera del Garda, Italy

Verona University, Verona, Italy

© Springer Nature Switzerland AG 2019
V. Poletti (ed.), *Transbronchial cryobiopsy in diffuse parenchymal lung disease*,
https://doi.org/10.1007/978-3-030-14891-1_11

biomarkers. The *MUC5B* promoter single-nucleotide polymorphism (SNP) has been identified as a strong risk factor for the development of both familial and sporadic IPF [2, 3].

Pulmonary function tests document a restrictive impairment with mainly reduction of DLCO in the early phases. It is now not infrequent (mainly thanks to the contribution of lung biopsies carried out with cryoprobes) to have a diagnosis of IPF in patients with pulmonary function tests in the so-called normal range. Bronchoalveolar lavage (BAL) is an important ancillary test showing usually a slight increase of neutrophils and eosinophils and a normal lymphocyte count. Rarely neutrophils or even eosinophils may be significantly increased. A lymphocytosis (>30%) militates against a diagnosis of IPF.

The pathogenesis of the disorder may be schematized into three steps [4]. The first step recognizes in the alveolar stem cells failure the *primum movens*. Type II pneumocytes are unable to rebuild lung parenchyma after a variety of insults because of intrinsic defects mainly clearly defined in familial cases [1, 2] [mutations involving telomere-related genes (*TERT, TERC, DKC1, TINF2, RTEL1,* and *PARN*), mutations involving genes coding for the surfactant proteins, etc.] or because of exogenous chronic damage (cigarette smoke) or mechanical stress more evident at the periphery of the secondary pulmonary lobules sited at the lung bases. These senescent cells acquire a secretory phenotype with activation of a variety of pathways (Wnt pathway is one of the most important) with attraction of fibroblasts and induction of myofibroblast transformation, activation of the epithelial-mesenchymal transition, and thereafter deposition of collagen. A profibrotic microenvironment is the final results. During this second step are activated or induced genes and gene networks that are normally associated with lung development and carcinogenesis.

When this damage wave reaches the centrilobular region, the bronchiolar stem cells (that are normal and not prone to apoptosis) are incited to proliferate and migrate (third step). These cells acquire a dysplastic phenotype, and for this reason patients with IPF are more prone to develop peripheral lung cancers with a bronchiolar phenotype [5]. Proliferation of bronchiolar cells and the accompanying fibrosis and smooth muscle cell hyperplasia are the component of the so-called honeycomb areas. This scheme considers the possibility to have two types of fibroblastic foci [6]: one alveolar in which the myofibroblasts and the extracellular matrix reach in tenascin are covered by hyperplastic type II pneumocytes exhibiting epithelial-mesenchymal transition markers and one bronchiolar in which the covering epithelial cells have a bronchiolar phenotype. This last one is present in areas of "honeycombing." The histological background of IPF is named Usual Interstitial Pneumonitis (UIP). In hematoxylin-eosin preps the hallmarks of the UIP pattern are patchy fibrosis (areas of normal lung sharply abutting on areas of fibrosis with deposition of collagen) and fibroblastic foci (ellipsoidal structures having pale extracellular matrix in which myofibroblasts are embedded and covered by hyperplastic type II pneumocytes or by hyperplastic-metaplastic bronchiolar cells). These fibrotic lesions are subpleural and with a periacinar distribution. Honeycomb areas are not formally required to have a diagnosis of UIP pattern. However they are detectable in the majority of cases, mainly when a large sample is analyzed. Inflammation is not an important component in UIP pattern in IPF subjects. Deposition of mucus is evident in the areas of honeycomb changes. UIP pattern is not pathognomonic for IPF because it may be the histological background of other disorders: collagen vascular diseases (mainly rheumatoid arthritis), chronic hypersensitivity pneumonitis, etc. Some clues (presence of inflammation and lymphoid nodules, centrilobular scars and inflammation, poorly formed granulomas, pleural inflammation) may suggest a UIP pattern not related to IPF. Most patients with IPF have a previous or current history of smoking cigarettes, and smoking-related changes may coexist with and complicate the histopathology of UIP in IPF. These changes include emphysema, sometimes associated with scarring; airspace enlargement with fibrosis; respiratory bronchiolitis without or with fibrosis; subpleural hyaline alveolar septal scarring, sometimes stellate and centrilobular scars; desquamative interstitial pneumonia (DIP) with fibrosis; and a pattern that can be described as fibrotic nonspecific interstitial pneumonia (NSIP) in a smoker, resembling DIP but without airspace "smoker" macrophages. Sophisticated immunohistochemical analyses or a "molecular UIP" signature identified from RNA sequencing could in the near future detect a specific tissue pattern related only to IPF [6].

CT scan has a pivotal role in the diagnosis of IPF. A confident diagnosis of IPF may be made in the correct clinical context when the CT shows a pattern of definite (presence of honeycombing in the bibasilar subpleural regions) or probable UIP (reticular pattern with peripheral bronchiectasis in the bibasilar subpleural regions). If the clinical context is indeterminate for IPF or the CT pattern is not definite or probable UIP, biopsy should be considered to confirm the presence of a UIP histologic pattern, and a confident diagnosis of IPF may be made based on multidisciplinary evaluation. If diagnostic tissue is not available, a working diagnosis of IPF may be made after careful multidisciplinary evaluation [7].

The clinical behavior may be—and in the majority of cases is—chronic with constant progressive deterioration of lung function or rapidly progressive, or it may have a chronic course with episodes of acute deterioration with new pulmonary infiltrates and rapidly progressive respiratory failure. These episodes may be determined by infections (bacterial or viral) in the majority of cases. When no cause is identified or identifiable, they are labelled as episodes of "acute exacerbation." In this context the histological background is diffuse alveolar damage or more rarely capillaritis or organizing pneumonia and eosinophilic pneumonia, all superimposed to UIP. The possibility, offered by cryobiopsy, to obtain lung tissue in a larger proportion of patients has shown that features of diffuse alveolar damage or organizing pneumonia, in discrete areas, may be detected also in stable patients that have only some small areas of ground glass attenuation in CT scan suggesting therefore that the clinical entity called "acute exacerbation of IPF" might be the tip of an iceberg with a larger group of patients with mini-

mal and localized features of alveolar damage or organizing pneumonia without any overt clinical manifestation. An attracting hypothesis still to be tested is that the last ones could be the group of rapid progressors. Very rarely the first manifestation of IPF is a rapidly progressive respiratory failure being the "acute exacerbation" the first overt clinical episode. Peripheral lung cancer in most cases originating from areas of honeycombing with peculiar phenotypes occurs in 6–8% of patients. Pulmonary hypertension usually develops in the advanced stages. The familial forms appear more enriched for females and nonsmokers, and we found a statistically significant lower age at onset (mean age 57.8 years versus 74.2 years, p 0.001). Furthermore, in our study, acute exacerbations, IPF progression, and lung cancer were more frequent in the familial IPF group as a cause of death [8]. The differential diagnosis is mainly with chronic hypersensitivity pneumonitis or fibrosing idiopathic NSIP.

Recently, two therapies that slow disease progression, nintedanib and pirfenidone, have been approved for the treatment of IPF, yet the clinical unmet need is still high for IPF patients given their failure to stop disease progression and their potential side effect profiles [9]. New clinical trials [9] are exploring the potential therapeutic role of new drugs: FG-3019 (Fibrogen, Birmingham, AL, USA, NCT 01890265) is a humanized monoclonal antibody (MAB) directed against CTGF; STX-100 (Biogen, Weston, MA, USA, NCT01371305) is a humanized MAB against integrin $\alpha v \beta 6$ being investigated in escalating subcutaneous doses; GSK3008348 (GlaxoSmithKline, London, UK, NCT02612051) is being developed as the first inhaled inhibitor of $\alpha v \beta 6$ integrin; GLPG1690 (Galapagos, Mechelen, Belgium, NCT02738801) is a novel, selective autotaxin inhibitor; PRM-151 (Promedior, Lexington, MA, USA, NCT02550873) is a recombinant form of PTX-2; TD139 (Galecto Biotech AB, Copenhagen, Denmark, NCT02257177) has been developed as a specific inhibitor of the galactoside-binding pocket of galectin-3, and it is administered via inhalation; and IWOO1 (Immuneworks, Indianapolis, IN, USA, NCT01199887) is an oral treatment designed to induce immune tolerance to the Collagen V protein in antibody-positive IPF patients. Stem cells are a new attractive field of research for IPF treatment. Patients fitted for lung transplant (preferably double lung transplant) should be referred early to transplant centers. Finally there are no evidence-based data on treatment of acute exacerbation, and in the daily clinical practice, antibiotics and high-dose steroids are almost always used in combination.

11.2   Case Series

Case 1

A 77-year-old man, former smoker (20 PY, quitted 19 years ago), was referred for dry cough lasting for 1 year. He did not experience dyspnea, and he had no extrapulmonary symptoms. He kept hens and rabbits at his country house, but no daily contact with other animals was elicited. He had no occupational exposures and was on treatment for prostate hyperplasia. Physical examination was normal apart from bibasilar inspiratory crackles. Pulmonary function tests (PFT) were in the normal range except for reduction of DLCO (64% of predicted).

Laboratory tests including autoimmunity work-up and precipitins were not relevant.

HRCT showed mild upper lobe centrilobular emphysema, bibasilar reticulation, and sparse peripheral traction bronchiectasis (probable UIP pattern) (Fig. 11.1a, b). Bronchoscopy with BAL and cryobiopsies (in two segments of the right lower lobe) was carried out.

Differential cell count on BAL fluid was normal, and microbiology tests were negative.

Cryobiopsy samples showed patchy fibrosis and fibroblast foci covered by alveolar epithelium; a few intra-alveolar loose fibrotic buds were also identified (Fig. 11.1c–e).

The diagnosis after multidisciplinary discussion was idiopathic pulmonary fibrosis, and the patient received treatment with specific drugs.

Case 2

A 66-year-old nonsmoker female was referred to the hospital because of 1 year history of shortness of breath (worsened in the last 2 months) and dry cough. She was working in a laundry. No specific professional exposure. In her family one brother died for pneumoconiosis (silicosis). She was on treatment with ramipril and simvastatin. On auscultation inspiratory bibasilar crackles were detected. Digital clubbing was also present. Pulmonary function tests were FVC 108% of predicted, Tiffeneau index = 92%; DLCO 58% of predicted; and 6 MWT 310 m with O_2 saturation from 96 to 90%. Routine blood tests were unremarkable. Autoimmunity work-up was negative.

CT scan showed bibasilar subpleural reticulation (undeterminate UIP pattern) (Fig. 11.2a–c).

A bronchoscopy with BAL in the middle lobe and cryobiopsies from two segments of the lower right lobe were carried out. Bleeding was controlled using two Fogarty balloons.

Total cell count in BAL fluid was in the normal range (110×10^6 cells/L). BAL fluid cytogram: macrophages 79%; lymphocytes 15%; neutrophils 5%; and eosinophils 1%.

Transbronchial cryobiopsy samples documented patchy fibrosis, fibroblastic foci, and honeycomb changes (Fig. 11.2d–f). The definite diagnosis was idiopathic pulmonary fibrosis, and specific treatment was started.

11.3   Discussion

The identification of UIP pattern in samples obtained by transbronchial cryobiopsy is feasible in a significant number of patients with probable or even indeterminate UIP in CT scan. The best strategy to optimize the diagnostic yield capturing the spatial and "temporal" heterogeneity of this morphological pattern is to retrieve samples from at least two different segments [10].

This diagnostic approach may be used in a larger proportion of patients compared to surgical lung biopsy (patients with more advanced disease but also older subjects and patients with comorbidities). The possibility to have lung tissue samples large enough for identification of complex morphological patterns opens new horizons. It might be possible to subclassify IPF patients (assessing the clinical significance of focal superimposed acute lung damage patterns

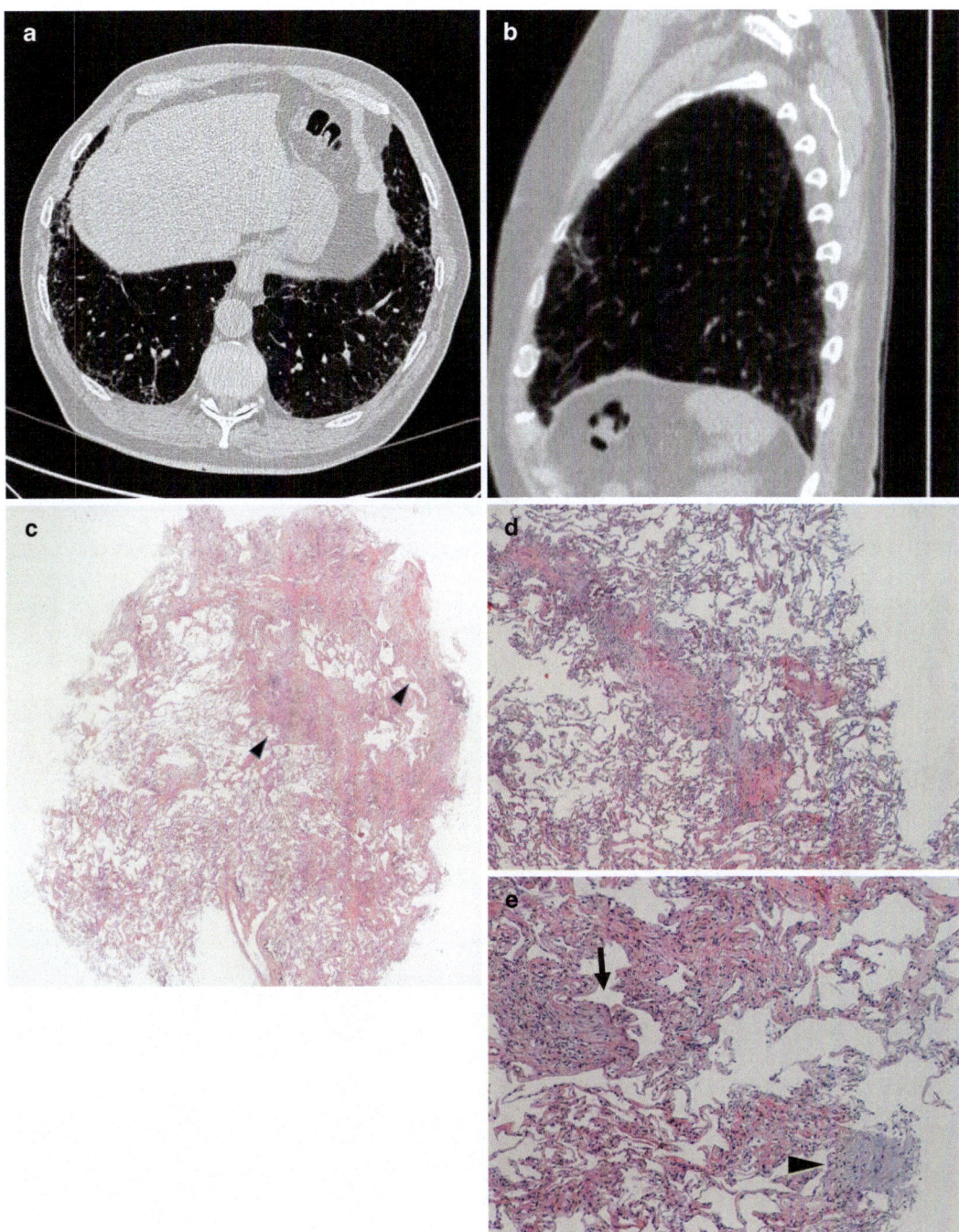

Fig. 11.1 (**a**) CT showing subpleural bibasilar reticulation with some peripheral "traction bronchiectasis". (**b**) CT, sagittal projection showing mild reticulation in the subpleural regions mainly in the lower lobe and mild upper lobe emphysema. (**c**) Transbronchial cryobiopsy. Sample from the lateral segment of the right lower lobe. At low power: fibrotic areas with a periacinar distribution are evident (arrowheads). These areas are sharply demarcated from areas of normal lung (patchy fibrosis) (hematoxylin-eosin). (**d**) Normal lung abutting sharply on a fibrotic area consisting of collagen and foci of "pale fibrosis" (hematoxylin-eosin; low power). (**e**) Transbronchial cryobiopsy. At higher power one fibroblastic focus covered by alveolar, flat epithelium is evident (arrow). One focus of intra-alveolar organizing pneumonia is also present (arrowhead) (hematoxylin-eosin)

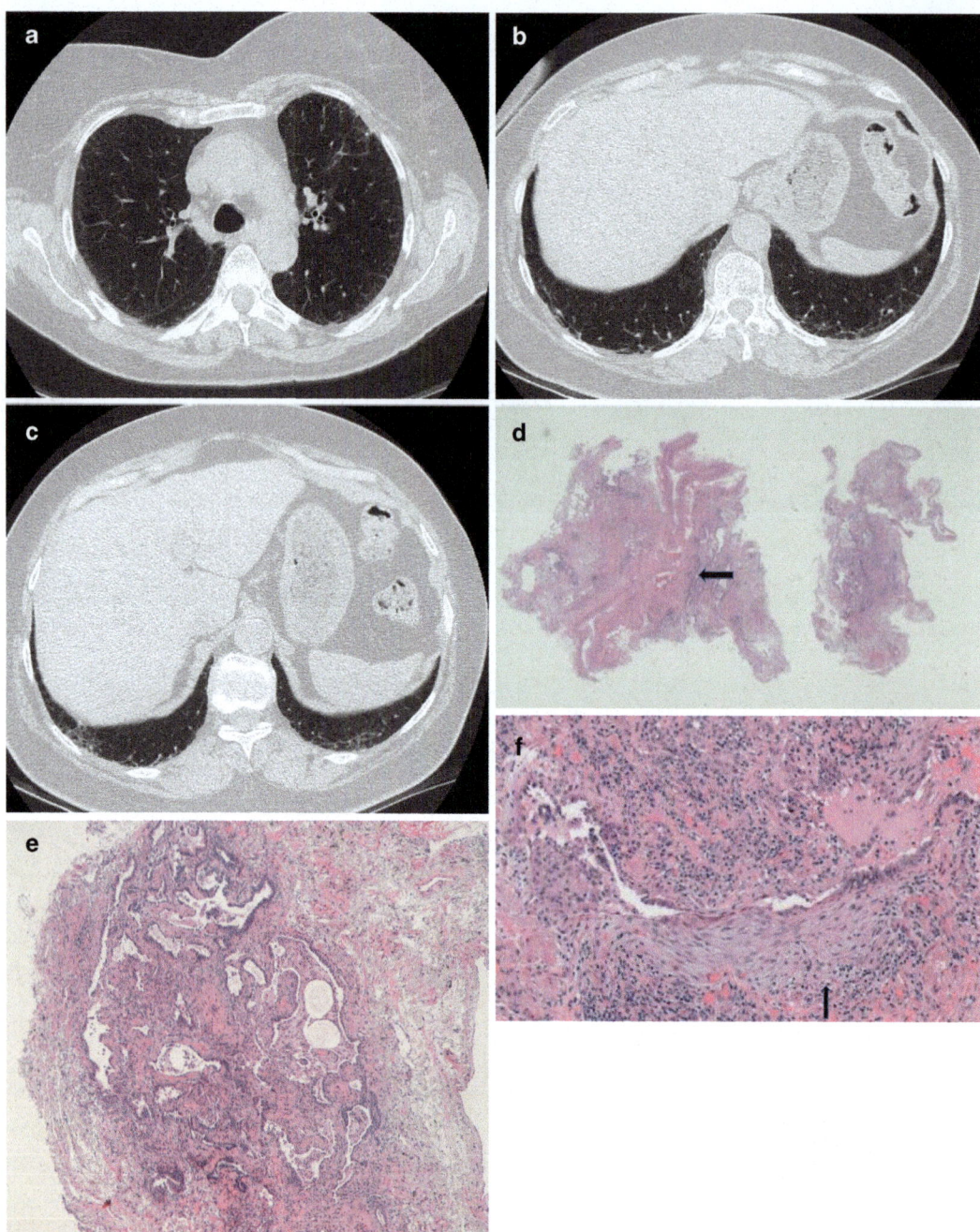

Fig. 11.2 (**a**) CT in the upper lobes: mild subpleural, mainly dorsal reticulation in both lungs. (**b**) CT scan in the lower lobes showing subpleural reticulation in both lungs reticulation. (**c**) CT Reticulation appears more evident in the basilar regions. (**d**) Transbronchial cryobiopsy samples showing significant architectural alterations and fibrosis. Only one small portion consists of normal parenchyma. In one sample a large artery is evident (arrow) (hematoxylin-eosin, low power). (**e**) Visceral pleura on the right border. Just beneath the pleura, dilated bronchiolar dysmorphic structures are identifiable. The epithelium shows focal squamous metaplasia (so-called honeycomb changes) (hematoxylin-eosin, mid power). (**f**) At higher magnification a typical fibroblastic focus (the ellipsoid structure is covered by bronchiolar epithelium) is evident (arrow) (hematoxylin-eosin, high power)

such as organizing pneumonia) and to investigate the morphological background using more sophisticated tools (immunohistochemistry, molecular biology) [11] or even to turn into the possibility to culture cells.

References

1. Barratt SL, Creamer A, Hayton C, Chaudhuri N. Idiopathic pulmonary fibrosis (IPF): an overview. J Clin Med. 2018;7.
2. Martinez FJ, Collard HR, Pardo A, Raghu G, Richeldi L, Selman M, Swigris JJ, Taniguchi H, Wells AU. Idiopathic pulmonary fibrosis. Nat Rev Dis Primers. 2017;3:17074.
3. Chiba H, Otsuka M, Takahashi H. Significance of molecular biomarkers in idiopathic pulmonary fibrosis: a mini review. Respir Investig. 2018;56:384–91.
4. Chilosi M, Carloni A, Rossi A, Poletti V. Premature lung aging and cellular senescence in the pathogenesis of idiopathic pulmonary fibrosis and COPD/emphysema. Transl Res. 2013;162:156–73.
5. Caliò A, Lever V, Rossi A, et al. Increased frequency of bronchiolar histotypes in lung carcinomas associated with idiopathic pulmonary fibrosis. Histopathology. 2017;71:725–35.
6. Raghu G, Flaherty KR, Lederer DJ, Lynch DA, Colby TV, et al. Use of molecular classifier to identify usual interstitial pneumonia in conventional transbronchial lung biopsy samples: a prospective validation study. Lancet Respir Med. 2019. In press.
7. Lynch DA, Sverzellati N, Travis WD, et al. Diagnostic criteria for idiopathic pulmonary fibrosis: a Fleischner Society White Paper. Lancet Respir Med. 2018;6:138–53.
8. Ravaglia C, Tomassetti S, Gurioli C, et al. Features and outcome of familial idiopathic pulmonary fibrosis. Sarcoidosis Vasc Diffuse Lung Dis. 2014;31:28–36.
9. Spagnolo P, Tzouvelekis A, Bonella F. The management of patients with idiopathic pulmonary fibrosis. Front Med (Lausanne). 2018;5:148.
10. Ravaglia C, Wells AU, Tomassetti S, et al. Transbronchial lung cryobiopsy in diffuse parenchymal lung disease: comparison between biopsy from 1 segment and biopsy from 2 segments—diagnostic yield and complications. Respiration. 2017;93:285–92.
11. Choi Y, Liu TT, Pankratz DG, Colby TV, et al. Identification of usual interstitial pneumonia pattern using RNA-Seq and machine learning: challenges and solutions. BMC Genomics. 2018;19(Suppl 2):101.

Chronic Hypersensitivity Pneumonitis

12

Claudia Ravaglia and Venerino Poletti

12.1 Introduction

Hypersensitivity pneumonitism (HP) is a diffuse interstitial lung disease that results from exaggerated immune response to the inhalation of various organic or inorganic particles [1–3]. There is no universally agreed upon definition of HP. However, there is consensus on the following key features of the disease: (1) HP is a pulmonary disease which may or may not be accompanied by systemic manifestations (e.g., fever and weight loss); (2) it is caused by the inhalation of an antigen to which the individual is sensitized and hyperresponsive; and (3) it is defined by exposure to a given antigen, sensitization to this antigen, and the presence of clinical symptoms. Indeed, many exposed individuals develop an antigen-specific immune response limited to the presence of serum IgG antibodies and an increased number of lymphocytes in the lung, but

they never develop the disease. Vice versa, mainly in chronic forms, the inciting antigens may not be recognizable in up to 25% of the cases [4]. HP has been traditionally classified into acute, sub-acute, and chronic forms [3]. Depending on their clinical course, patients with chronic HP are categorized as belonging to one of the two groups: recurrent and insidious [3]. The histopathologic patterns in chronic HP include organizing pneumonia, cellular nonspecific interstitial pneumonia (NSIP), fibrotic NSIP, usual interstitial pneumonia (UIP), and pleuroparenchymal fibroelastosis (PPFE) applying the 2013 American Thoracic Society/European Respiratory Society (ATS/ERS) criteria for the classification of idiopathic interstitial pneumonias [5–7]. Other histopathologic changes identifiable in lung samples obtained from patients with a clinical diagnosis of chronic HP are centrilobular fibrosis, bridging fibrosis, bronchiolitis, granulomas, and scattered giant cells. Recently Yousem SA and Churg A, et al. described a morphological entity named cicatricial organizing pneumonia in which the granulation tissue organized too much dense fibrous tissue but still retained the usual pattern of organizing pneumonia [8, 9]. We have seen such a morphological change in cryobiopsy samples obtained from patients with a diagnosis of chronic HP. Emphysema can occur in patients with CHP independently of smoking history and exposure to specific types of antigens. Emphysematous changes seem to progress at a

C. Ravaglia (✉)
Department of Diseases of the Thorax, Pulmonology Unit, G.B. Morgagni L. Pierantoni Hospital, Forlì, Italy

V. Poletti
Department of Diseases of the Thorax, Ospedale Morgagni-Pierantoni, Forlì, Italy

Department of Respiratory Diseases and Allergy, Aarhus University Hospital, Aarhus, Denmark

© Springer Nature Switzerland AG 2019
V. Poletti (ed.), *Transbronchial cryobiopsy in diffuse parenchymal lung disease*,
https://doi.org/10.1007/978-3-030-14891-1_12

slower pace compared to reticulations/fibrosis [10]. High-resolution CT scan features are reticular opacities, peribronchovascular interstitial thickening, ill-defined centrilobular ground-glass nodules, lobular areas of decreased attenuation and vascularity, mild to moderate extent of ground-glass opacities away from fibrosis, and relative basal sparing [11, 12]. Honeycomb changes may be present [13]. Bronchoalveolar lavage may document a lymphocytosis, but the mere presence of neutrophils does not exclude the diagnosis [1]. Making an accurate diagnosis of chronic HP can be particularly challenging [1–4] but essential as it informs prognosis and requires distinct treatment management [1]. Diagnosis of chronic ILDs ideally is carried out in the setting of a face-to-face multidisciplinary discussion (MDD) [14–17]; however, inter-multidisciplinary team agreement for the diagnosis of chronic HP is usually low [18], and this might be in relation to the absence of evidence-based guidelines to diagnose this disease. Furthermore, features of HP and CTD-ILD (connective tissue disease-related ILD) can overlap with conflicting claims about features that favor one diagnosis or the other [14, 17]; therefore, accurate pathologic contribution to the MDD can be problematic. Distinguishing fibrotic HP from idiopathic pulmonary fibrosis (IPF) might be important, as specific therapy is available for IPF, whereas optimal treatment for fibrotic HP is still poorly defined [1, 14]. However recent data showed that pathogenetic links between chronic fibrotic HP and IPF could be more consistent than previously thought [19].

12.2   Case

A 62-year-old white man has presented to the Thoracic Department of the Morgagni Hospital, Forlì (Italy), with a recent history of persistent dry cough during the last 3 months. The patient reported substantial clinical wellness up to 3 months ago with no signs or symptoms suggestive for collagen vascular disease and no signs or symptoms of gastroesophageal reflux. His general history was negative for other respiratory diseases; he was diagnosed as having benign prostatic hypertrophy and underwent septoplasty and tonsillectomy at a young age. He was a smoker up to 10 years ago (25 pack-year), and he had always worked as a banker, with no other specific exposures. He denied any allergy, and in his family, his mother died for lung cancer, and his father died for lung and larynx cancer. At the point of our presentation, his only medication was alfuzosin.

On examination, pulmonary auscultation revealed vesicular murmur reduction, with some squeaks and no Velcro sounds. The cardiac auscultation and abdominal examination showed no changes; he had no palpable lymphadenopathy or peripheral edema, and the remaining physical examination was normal, and no clubbing was observed. Lung function tests showed Tiffeneau Index 87%, forced vital capacity (FVC) 78% predicted, and diffusing capacity of the lungs for carbon monoxide (DLCO) 38% predicted. The saturation level of oxygen in hemoglobin (SpO_2) was 97% at rest, but in a 6-minute walking test (6-MWT), the patients walked 180 m and underwent oxygen desaturation to 81%. Routine blood tests revealed normal blood count; electrolytes and creatinine were normal; C-reactive protein was normal; plasma lactate dehydrogenase was 274 U/L (normal range 135–225); and coagulation tests, hepatic transaminase, and bilirubin levels were normal. Transthoracic echocardiography showed normal cardiac structures without evidence of pulmonary hypertension. A high-resolution computed tomography (HRCT) showed some bilateral ground-glass opacities with superimposed fine reticulation, areas of decreased attenuation, and vascularity with air trapping on expiratory scans in a lobular distribution (as indirect signs of bronchiolar obstruction); there were also evident traction bronchiectasis and emphysema with rare cysts without a clear apical-basal gradient (Fig. 12.1). Clinical setting and radiological features were reviewed by clinicians and radiologists, but a final multidisciplinary diagnosis was not possible; the possible differential diagnoses included (a) smoking-related lung disease, (b) chronic hypersensitivity pneumonitis, (c) idiopathic pulmonary fibrosis,

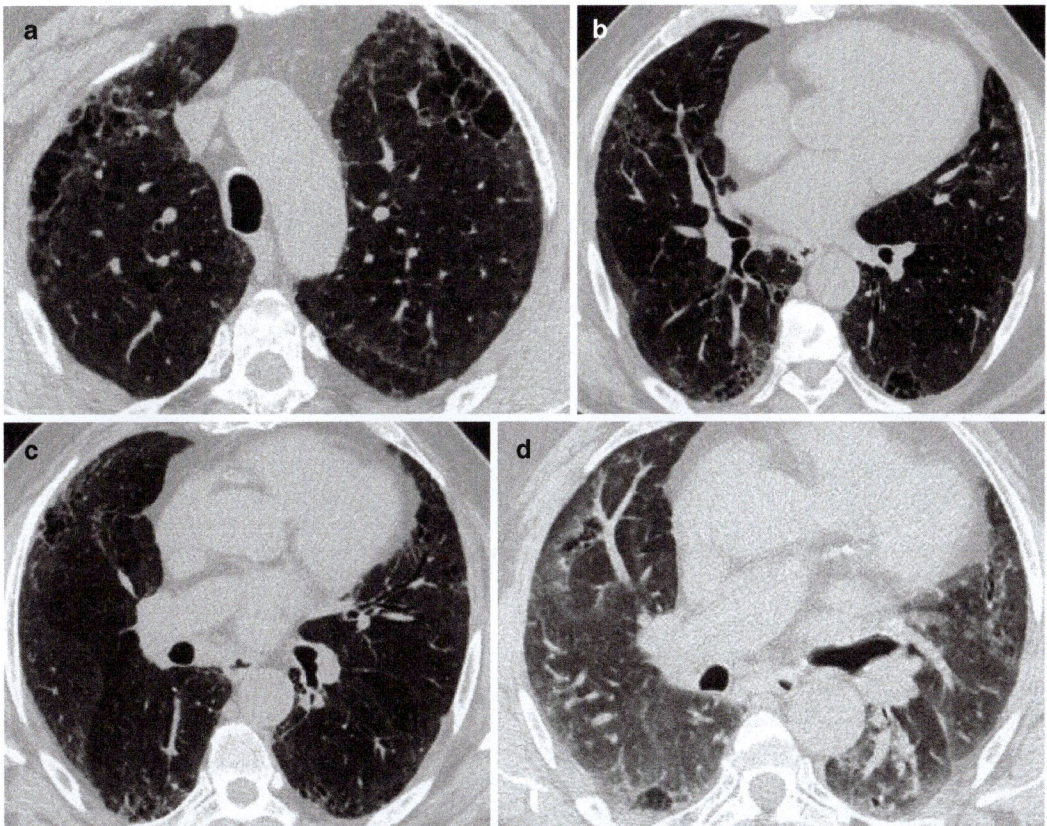

Fig. 12.1 High-resolution computed tomography (HRCT) showing evident traction bronchiectasis and emphysema with rare cysts in the upper lobes (**a**) and lower lobes (**b**), without a clear apical-basal gradient. (**c**) shows bilateral ground-glass opacities with superimposed fine reticulation, areas of decreased attenuation, and vascularity; air trapping on expiratory CT in a lobular distribution (**d**)

and (**d**) other diffuse parenchymal lung diseases. An additional evaluation (including lung biopsy) was therefore considered necessary. Levels of specific antibodies (IgG) against relevant antigens were studied in serum and serum-precipitating antibodies to *Aspergillus fumigatus*, and pigeons and parakeet antigens were positive; autoimmunity screen was negative. Patient underwent a diagnostic fiber-optic bronchoscopy: a 120 mL BAL sample was instilled from the right middle lobe; the total BAL fluid cell count was 109 cells × 10⁶/L. Differential count from BAL fluid showed that 23% of the particles were lymphocytes and 72% were monocyte/macrophages; all lymphocytes were T cells (CD4/CD8 [7, 8]. By method of transbronchial lung cryobiopsy (ERBE, diameter probe 2.4 mm, Tubingen, Germany),

lung tissue samples from the right lower lobe and right upper lobe were gained. The procedure was performed according to the procedure already described [14]: the patient was deeply sedated using propofol and remifentanil and intubated with a rigid tracheoscope; a 2.4 mm cryoprobe was introduced through the operating channel of a fiber-optic bronchoscope; then under fluoroscopic control, transbronchial cryobiopsies were carried out (three samples in the anterior segment of the right lower lobe and one sample in the posterior segment of the right upper lobe). Bleeding was hampered by inflated Fogarty balloon, and no pneumothorax was observed in the days after biopsy.

The fragmented biopsy measured an overall area of 85.2 mm². Microscopic examination of

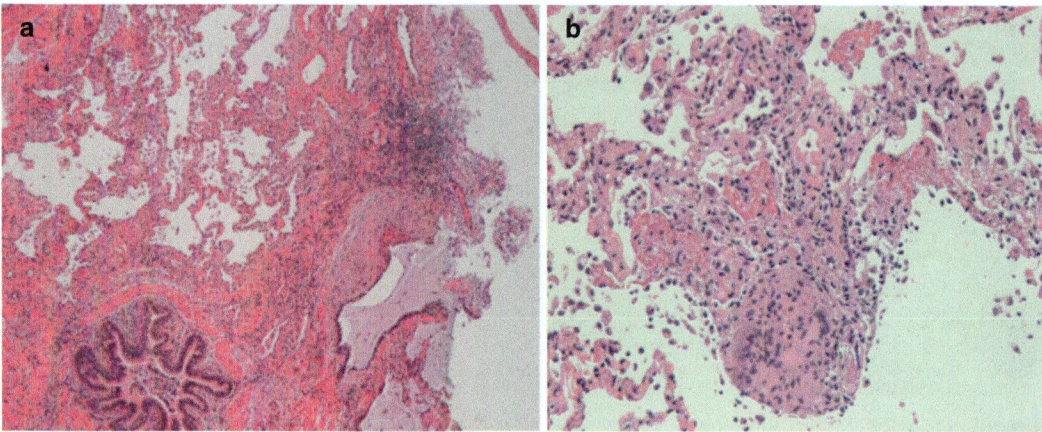

Fig. 12.2 (**a**) Transbronchial lung cryobiopsy (TLCB) performed in the right upper lobe showing bronchiolocentric interstitial fibrosis with honeycomb changes and fibroblastic foci. Note the increased cellularity, represented by an increased blue quality (hematoxylin-eosin). (**b**) Right lower lobe TLCB showing areas of organizing pneumonia and poorly formed granulomas with isolated giant cells containing various cytoplasmic inclusions and rare honeycomb changes (hematoxylin and eosin, mid power)

the samples at low power demonstrated areas of architectural distortion with honeycomb change; scattered throughout were subepithelial interstitial foci comprising linearly oriented myofibroblasts within a pale staining matrix characteristic of fibroblastic foci. The combination of features raised the possibility of a UIP pattern; however, in areas with less well-established fibrosis, a cellular interstitial pneumonia composed of mostly lymphocytes was evident; within the interstitium were poorly formed granulomas, characterized by isolated giant cells containing various cytoplasmic inclusions including cholesterol-like clefts. The lower lobe biopsy lacked fibroblastic foci and instead demonstrated a more airway-centered interstitial fibrosis and poorly formed granulomas associated with honeycomb changes. Based on these findings, the combination of the UIP pattern with a more bronchiolocentric interstitial pneumonia and a characteristic pattern of non-necrotizing granulomatous inflammation was diagnostic of chronic hypersensitivity pneumonitis, and a final multidisciplinary diagnosis of chronic hypersensitivity pneumonitis was confirmed (Figs. 12.2 and 12.3).

Our patient received prednisone at the dose of 12.5 mg/die, and azathioprine was added to the steroid therapy as a steroid-sparing agent (started at 50 mg/day and increased to 150 mg/day). At the first follow-up at our department after

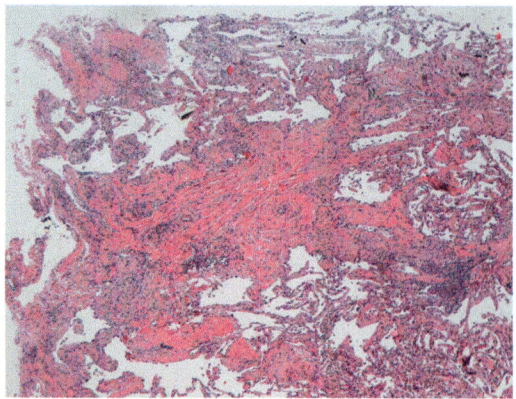

Fig. 12.3 A centrilobular fibrotic lesion is evident with almost complete distortion of the airway structure (hematoxylin and eosin, mid power)

6 months, the patient reported relief in symptoms, and the extent of limitation of lung function remained stable (FVC 82% predicted vs 78%, DLCO 40% predicted vs 38%).

12.3 Discussion

Hypersensitivity pneumonitis is conventionally classified as acute, subacute, and chronic. The nomenclature is only a general basis for the clinical distinction, as there can be significant overlap between these categories. Fibrosis is often already established in patients who present with the chronic form as the onset of respiratory symptoms is often insidious and lung biopsy is often essential to diagnosis. Prognostic indicators could be a low DLCO, low mean FVC, low lymphocyte levels in BAL fluid, and a UIP-like pattern on histology [20, 21]. The chronic presentation of HP can be a result of two distinct events: as a continuum of undiagnosed acute/subacute episodes (recurrent chronic HP) and as the progressive development secondary to low-level, ongoing antigenic exposure, lacking a history of acute episodes (insidious chronic HP). Our patient presented has gone through a history of lung disease with chronic onset, including symptoms like dry cough; the patient was questioned in detail for occupational exposure, domestic exposure, ownership of animals, drug use, and other antigen exposures, but no specific exposure was found. Although reduced respiratory functions are not specific for HP, they suggested that the disease had a serious course. The HRCT was valuable in the diagnostic process: the radiological pattern (ground-glass opacities, mild reticular opacities, and bronchiectasis), the extent, and the distribution of disease showed significant correlations with clinical and functional parameters. Despite not being a specific test for HP cases, BAL analysis may prove useful for differential diagnosis: the BAL fluid more frequently exhibits an increase in total cell count and CD8 T lymphocyte count; however, in our case BAL was not significantly informative. On the other hand, transbronchial lung cryobiopsy (TLCB), as demonstrated in our patient, can play a key role in establishing the diagnosis of hypersensitivity pneumonitis, especially in the absence of an incriminating exposure history.

Multiple biopsies are usually taken to reduce sampling error as we know that diagnosis of interstitial lung diseases can be influenced by the heterogeneity of the disease and by the distribution of the parenchymal pathology. The distribution of disease is also important, as chronic hypersensitivity pneumonitis may have a predilection for the mid to upper lungs, although lower lobe-predominant disease also occurs. Sampling bias may be a factor in separating chronic HP from idiopathic interstitial pneumonias (IIPs), as illustrated in our patient. Trahan et al. reported a

cohort of 15 patients with a multidisciplinary diagnosis of chronic HP who underwent surgical biopsy of 1–3 lobes: some of the patients had discordant findings, showing classic features of HP in 1 specimen and UIP or nonspecific changes in others, and biopsies from 2 showed only UIP and 1 showed NSIP; the conclusion of the paper was that sampling more than 1 lobe may be useful in distinguishing chronic HP from other IIPs [22]. However, the optimal number of biopsies has not been established for cryobiopsy, and different strategies adopted to sample lung tissue are still missing in literature [23]. What we know is that diagnostic yield is significantly influenced by a number of samples and sampling strategy, improving dramatically when >2 samples are performed (instead of only one) and when biopsy is obtained in two different sites (instead of only one site), either from the same lobe or from different lobes [24]. This can be particularly important for chronic HP, in which pathological variability is more challenging and differential diagnosis could be more difficult. In our cohort of 699 patients with suspected diffuse parenchymal lung diseases undergoing TLCB, we observed discordant samples between different sites in almost 30% of cases, with a significant increase in diagnostic yield between one site and two sites (unpublished data). The histologic classification in this 30% of the patients could have differed between HP and NSIP or UIP and HP if biopsy had been obtained in only one site; therefore, it is very important to obtain tissue from two different sites, either from the same lobe or from different lobes when HRCT scan does not show a clear gradient profusion of the pattern or when different patterns are present in different lobes. Significant sampling errors may result from strategies that obtain only one biopsy specimen for ILD. These findings confirm and quantify the frequency of interlobar and intralobar histologic variability in fibrotic ILD and confirm the adequacy of cryobiopsy in identifying this histologic heterogeneity, particularly regarding chronic HP. At last, but still clinically very relevant, cryobiopsy has significantly lower side effects compared to surgical lung biopsy [25, 26].

In conclusion, transbronchial cryobiopsy is a new method that allows to obtain larger samples of the lung tissue without crush artifacts and good diagnostic yield in diffuse parenchymal lung diseases [25], specifically in chronic HP.

References

1. Spagnolo P, Rossi G, Cavazza A, et al. Hypersensitivity pneumonitis: a comprehensive review. J Investig Allergol Clin Immunol. 2015;25:237–50.
2. Lacasse Y, Selman M, Costabel U, et al. Clinical diagnosis of hypersensitivity pneumonitis. Am J Respir Crit Care Med. 2003;168:952–8.
3. Lacasse Y, Girard M, Cormier Y. Recent advances in hypersensitivity pneumonitis. Chest. 2012;142:208–17.
4. Coleman A, Colby TV. Histologic diagnosis of extrinsic allergic alveolitis. Am J Surg Pathol. 1988;12:514–8.
5. Churg A, Sin DD, Everett D, et al. Pathologic patterns and survival in chronic hypersensitivity pneumonitis. Am J Surg Pathol. 2009;33:1765–70.
6. Khiroya R, Macaluso C, Montero MA, et al. Pleuroparenchymal fibroelastosis: a review of histopathologic features and the relationship between histology parameters and survival. Am J Surg Pathol. 2017;41:1683–9.
7. Tanizawa K, Handa T, Kubo T, et al. Clinical significance of radiological pleuroparenchymal fibroelastosis pattern in interstitial lung disease patients registered for lung transplantation: a retrospective cohort study. Respir Res. 2018;30:162.
8. Yousem SA. Cicatricial variant of cryptogenic organizing pneumonia. Hum Pathol. 2017;64:76–82.
9. Churg A, Wright JT, Bilawich AM. Cicatricial organizing pneumonia mimicking a fibrosing interstitial pneumonia. Histopathology. 2018;72:846–54.
10. Soumagne T, Chardon ML, Dournes G, et al. Emphysema in active farmer's lung disease. PLoS One. 2017;12:e0178263.
11. Silva CI, Churg A, Muller NL. Hypersensitivity pneumonitis: spectrum of high-resolution CT and pathologic findings. Am J Roentgenol. 2007;188:334–44.
12. Dias OM, Baldi BG, Pennati F, Aliverti A, Chate RC, Sawamura MVY, Ribeiro de Carvalho CR, Pereira de Albuquerque AL. Computed tomography in hypersensitivity pneumonitis: main findings, differential diagnosis and pitfalls. Expert Rev Respir Med. 2018;12:5–13.
13. Silva CI, Muller NL, Lynch DA, et al. Chronic hypersensitivity pneumonitis: differentiation from idiopathic pulmonary fibrosis and nonspecific interstitial pneumonia by using thin-section CT. Radiology. 2008;246:288–97.
14. Johannson KA, Elicker BM, Vittinghof E, et al. A diagnostic model for chronic hypersensitivity pneumonitis. Thorax. 2016;71:951–4.
15. Morisset J, Johannson KA, Jones KD, Wolters PJ, Collard HR, Walsh SLF, Ley B; HP Delphi Collaborators. Identification of Diagnostic Criteria for Chronic Hypersensitivity Pneumonitis: An International Modified Delphi Survey. Am J Respir Crit Care Med 2018; 197(8):1036–1044.
16. Soumagne T, Dalphin JC. Current and emerging techniques for the diagnosis of hypersensitivity pneumonitis. Expert Rev Respir Med. 2018;12:493–507.
17. Travis WD, Costabel U, Hansell DM, et al.; ATS/ERS Committee on Idiopathic Interstitial Pneumonias. An official American Thoracic Society/European Respiratory Society statement: update of the international multidisciplinary classification of the idiopathic interstitial pneumonias. Am J Respir Crit Care Med. 2013;188:733–48.
18. Walsh SLF, Wells AU, Desai SR, et al. Multicentre evaluation of multidisciplinary team meeting agreement on diagnosis in diffuse parenchymal lung disease: a case-cohort study. Lancet Respir Med. 2016;4:557–65.
19. Ley B, Newton CA, Arnould I, et al. The MUC5B promoter polymorphism and telomere length in patients with chronic hypersensitivity pneumonitis: an observational cohort-control study. Lancet Respir Med. 2017;5:639–47.
20. Gaxiola M, Buendía-Roldán I, Mejía M, et al. Morphologic diversity of chronic pigeon breeder's disease: clinical features and survival. Respir Med. 2011;105:608–14.
21. Wang P, Jones KD, Urisman A, et al. Pathologic findings and prognosis in a large prospective cohort of chronic hypersensitivity pneumonitis. Chest. 2017;152:502–9.
22. Trahan S, Hanak V, Ryu JH, Myers JL. Role of surgical lung biopsy in separating chronic hypersensitivity pneumonia from usual interstitial pneumonia/idiopathic pulmonary fibrosis: analysis of 31 biopsies from 15 patients. Chest. 2008;134:126–32.
23. Hetzel J, Maldonado F, Ravaglia C, et al. Transbronchial cryobiopsies for the diagnosis of diffuse parenchymal lung diseases: expert statement from the cryobiopsy working group on safety and utility and a call for standardization on the procedure. Respiration. 2018;95:188–200.
24. Ravaglia C, Wells AU, Tomassetti S, et al. Transbronchial lung cryobiopsy in diffuse parenchymal lung disease: comparison between biopsy from 1 segment and biopsy from 2 segments—diagnostic yield and complications. Respiration. 2017;93:285–92.
25. Ravaglia C, Wells AU, Tomassetti S, Gurioli C, Gurioli C, Dubini A, Cavazza A, Colby TV, Piciucchi S, Puglisi S, Bosi M, Poletti V. Diagnostic yield and risk/benefit analysis of transbronchial lung cryobiopsy in diffuse parenchymal lung diseases: a large cohort of 699 patients. BMC Pulm Med. 2019;19:16.
26. Fisher JH, Shapera S, Teresa TO, Marras TK, Gershon A, Dell S. Procedure volume and mortality after surgical lung biopsy in interstitial lung disease. Eur Resp J. 2019;53(2):1801164.

Collagen Vascular Diseases

13

Martina Bonifazi, Francesca Barbisan, and Stefani Gasparini

13.1 Introduction

The spectrum of connective tissue diseases (CTDs) includes a heterogeneous group of disorders characterized by circulating autoantibodies and organ-specific autoimmune injuries, leading to variable systemic manifestations. The respiratory system is a common target in this context, and lung involvement may occur as diffuse parenchymal disease, airway dysfunction, pleural lesions, and vascular damages [1]. Diffuse parenchymal lung diseases (DPLDs), the most common manifestations, are hugely heterogenic, as the degree of lung impairment ranges from silent pathological abnormalities to severe progressive diseases associated with significant morbidity and mortality. Thus, a baseline assessment of morphological patterns and ongoing pathogenic activity, as well as a stratification of risk of future complications, has relevant implications in terms of prognostic estimates and therapeutic management. The most common patterns observed in CTDs include nonspecific interstitial pneumonia (NSIP), usual interstitial pneumonia (UIP), organizing pneumonia (OP), NSIP/OP overlap, lymphocytic interstitial pneumonia (LIP), acute interstitial pneumonia (AIP)/diffuse alveolar damage (DAD), and rarely desquamative interstitial pneumonia (DIP). The rheumatic diseases most commonly affected are, in order of descending frequency, systemic sclerosis (SSc)/scleroderma, autoimmune idiopathic myositis (AIM), rheumatoid arthritis (RA), systemic lupus erythematosus (SLE), Sjögren syndrome, and undifferentiated rheumatoid disorders [1]. Onset of respiratory symptoms and subsequent DPLD recognition may occur in patients with an already known rheumatic syndrome or might present as first/concurrent manifestation of CTDs [2]. Moreover, in some cases, there are clinical, serological, or morphological features suggestive of an autoimmune disorder that do not meet criteria for a specific rheumatic disease. Such a condition, currently denominated as interstitial pneumonia with autoimmune features (IPAF) [3], represents a diagnostic challenge for clinicians, and tissue acquisition in this context gains, even more, a relevant role, as the identification of morphological pattern is crucial to estimate patient prognosis and guide management.

Here, we describe three cases of DPLDs associated with CTDs, underlying key points of diagnostic work-up and the valuable role of transbronchial lung cryobiopsy (TLCB) in this context.

M. Bonifazi (✉) · S. Gasparini
Department of Biomedical Sciences and Public Health, Università Politecnica delle Marche, Ancona, Italy

Pulmonary Diseases Unit, Azienda Ospedali Riuniti, Ancona, Italy
e-mail: m.bonifazi@univpm.it; s.gasparini@univpm.it

F. Barbisan
Pathologic Anatomy Unit, Azienda Ospedali Riuniti, Ancona, Italy
e-mail: f.barbisan@ospedaliriuniti.marche.it

© Springer Nature Switzerland AG 2019
V. Poletti (ed.), *Transbronchial cryobiopsy in diffuse parenchymal lung disease*,
https://doi.org/10.1007/978-3-030-14891-1_13

13.2   Case Series

Case 1

A 53-year-old female was admitted to our hospital because of persistent fever, not responsive to antibiotic drugs, dry cough, and subacute dyspnea. She was a former smoker (5 pack/years), and her past medical history was notable for breast cancer, diagnosed 2 years earlier and treated with mastectomy (with subsequent breast implant) and hormonal therapy, still ongoing at the time of hospitalization. Physical examination revealed bibasal fine crackles on auscultation and mechanics hands. Oxygen saturation (SO$_2$) on room air at rest was 95%, but it decreased to 91% during a 6-minute walking test (6MWT).

Pulmonary function tests (PFTs) at baseline showed a restrictive ventilatory impairment, with decreased forced vital capacity (FVC 62% pred), total lung capacity (TLC 66% pred), and markedly reduced diffusion capacity of the lung for carbon monoxide (DLCO 25% pred).

The high-resolution computed tomography (HRCT) scan of the chest revealed ground-glass opacifications and parenchymal consolidations with bibasal distribution and peri-lobular pattern, predominantly in the lower lobes, in absence of lymph adenopathies or pleural effusion (Fig. 13.1).

Laboratory tests showed C-reactive protein 10.7 mg (range 0–5) and erythrocyte sedimentation rate 63 mm/h (range 0–27) with creatine phosphokinase within normal limits. Standard autoimmune investigations revealed only antinuclear antibodies (ANA 1:160 homogeneous, speckled), in absence of autoantibodies against extractable nuclear antigens (ENA) positivity. Because of high pretest probability of antisynthetase syndrome, we explored the complete profile of myositis-specific autoantibodies, finding anti-PL-12 (alanyl) positivity.

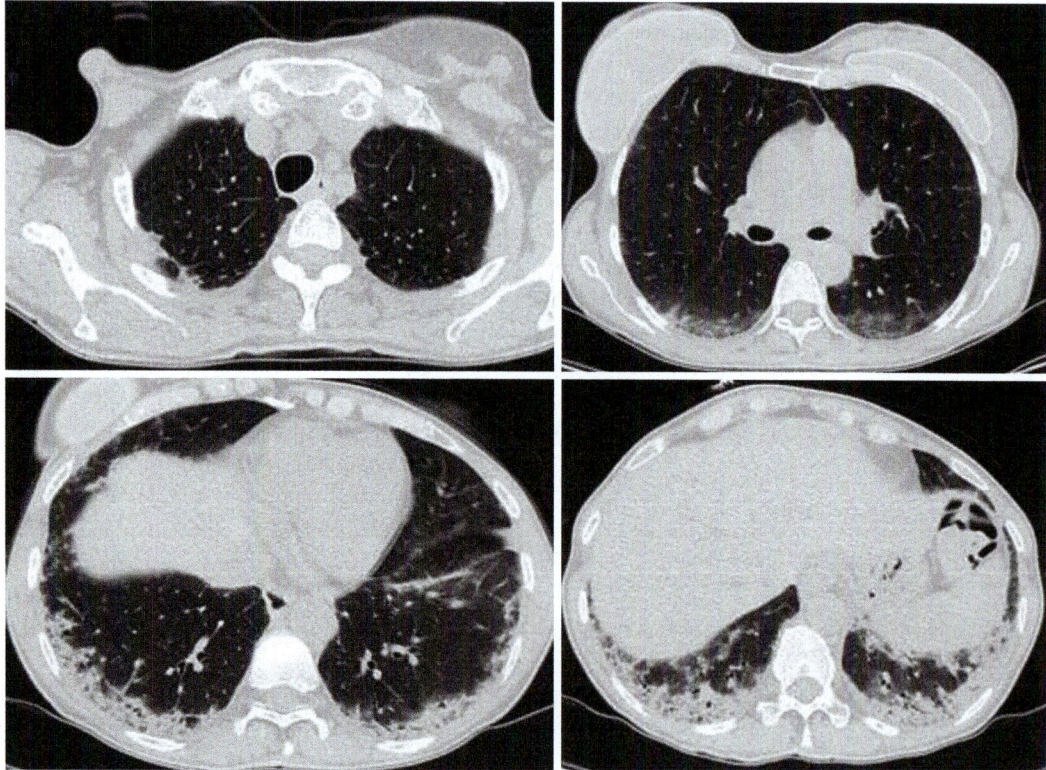

Fig. 13.1 Computed tomography (CT) images at admission, showing ground-glass opacifications and parenchymal consolidations with bibasal distribution and peri-lobular pattern, predominantly in the lower lobes, in absence of lymph adenopathies or pleural effusion

In order to assess the underlying DPLD morphological pattern, a TLCB was performed in the right lower lobe. Histopathologic findings revealed fibrotic non-specific interstitial pneumonia (NSIP) with superimposed organizing pneumonia (OP) pattern (Figs. 13.2, 13.3, and 13.4).

The patient was treated with oral steroids (initially, methylprednisolone 1 mg/kg/die, then progressively tapered) with significant symptomatic, functional, and radiological improvements. Immunosuppressant drugs were contraindicated, due to the recent history of breast cancer. Over

3 years of follow-up, she did not experience any flare or worsening.

13.2.1 Discussion

Anti-synthetase syndrome (ASS) is a rare systemic autoimmune syndrome, characterized by the presence of anti-aminoacyl-tRNA antibodies and the clinical association of fever, Raynaud's phenomenon, myositis, DPLDs, arthritis, and mechanic's hands [4]. It mainly occurs in adult

Fig. 13.2 Transbronchial cryobiopsy of right lower lobe showing alveolated lung parenchyma, with mainly homogeneous fibrosis. Total surface, 15 mm²; alveolated part, 13 mm² (85% of the fragment). Hematoxylin and eosin 20×

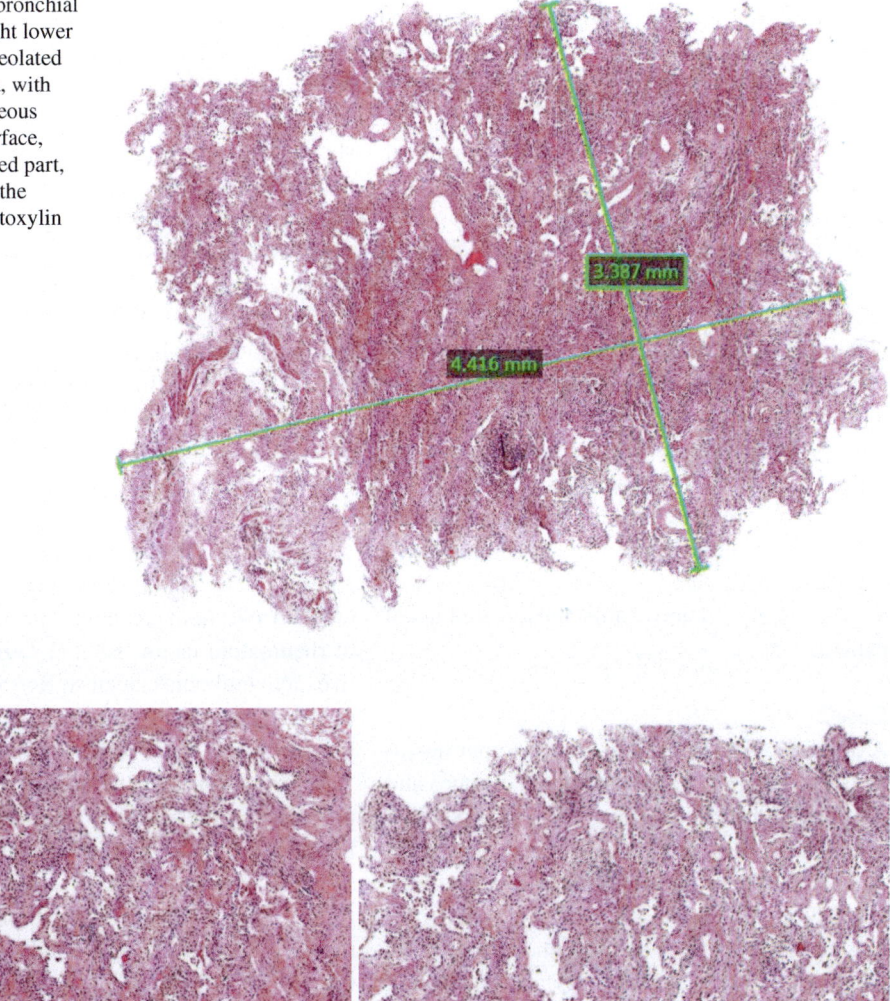

Fig. 13.3 Transbronchial cryobiopsy of right lower lobe, showing diffuse, homogeneous fibrous thickening with mild infiltration of lymphoid cells. Pattern classifiable as fibrotic NSIP. Hematoxylin and eosin 50×

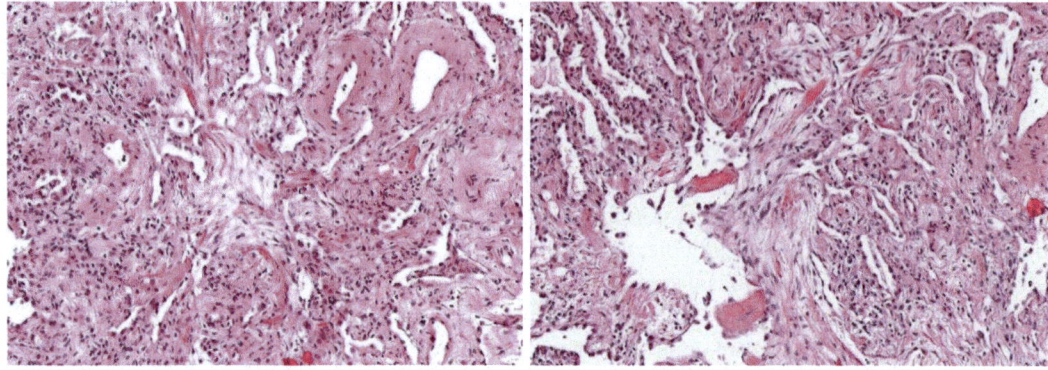

Fig. 13.4 Transbronchial cryobiopsy of right lower lobe, showing endoalveolar plugs of fibro-myxoid tissue in the context of fibrotic NSIP. Pattern suggestive for fibrotic NSIP/OP overlap. Hematoxylin and eosin 100×

females and etiology is not known. Anti-synthetase antibodies are several and include anti-Jo-1, the commonest one, PL-7, PL-12, OJ, EJ, KS, Ha, and Zo, and differences in clinical features according to specific autoantibody have been suggested. Lung involvement in anti-synthetase syndrome is often the major feature, especially in non-anti-Jo1-positive group, and mostly occurs in the absence of myositis (amyopathic ILD) [5]. DPLDs represent a significant cause of morbidity, and the most common patterns are NSIP, OP, NSIP/OP overlap, UIP, and DAD/AIP [1]. Therefore, a prompt identification and an accurate morphologic assessment of this feature, in both myopathic and amyopathic patients, have relevant management implications. The present case clearly shows that TBLC allows to adequately identify this histopathological pattern.

Case 2

A 37-year-old female was admitted to our hospital because of progressive exertional dyspnea and dry cough. She had been diagnosed with Sjögren syndrome 1 year earlier in Pakistan, based on xerophthalmia, xerostomia, and positive salivary gland biopsy findings. Physical examination at presentation revealed bibasal fine crackles on auscultation. Arterial blood gas analysis at rest showed hypoxemia (arterial oxygen partial pressure PaO_2 62 mmHg), carbon dioxide partial pressure within normal limits ($PaCO_2$ 37 mmHg), and SO_2 94%. The 6-minute walking test

(6MWT) was stopped because of significant desaturation (SO_2 80%).

Pulmonary function tests (PFTs) at baseline showed a severe restrictive ventilatory impairment, with markedly decreased forced vital capacity (FVC 34% pred) total lung capacity (TLC 40% pred) and markedly reduced diffusion capacity of the lung for carbon monoxide (DLCO 25% pred).

The high-resolution computed tomography (HRCT) scan of the chest revealed subpleural parenchymal consolidations of upper lobes and ground-glass attenuations with predominantly peribronchovascular distribution in the lower lobes (Fig. 13.5).

Laboratory tests showed polyclonal hyper-gammaglobulinemia, antinuclear antibodies (ANA 1:640 homogeneous, speckled), elevation of rheumatoid factor (RF 121 UI/mL), and positive autoantibodies against Ro/(SS-A) and La/(SS-B). Bronchoalveolar lavage reveals mild lymphocytosis (25%) and neutrophilia (6%).

In order to assess the underlying DPLD morphological pattern and to exclude a lymphoproliferative disease, commonly associated with Sjögren syndrome, a TLCB was performed in the right lower lobe. Histopathologic findings revealed both cellular and fibrotic NSIP (Figs. 13.6 and 13.7).

Due to the severity of symptomatic and functional impairment, the patient was treated with pulse cyclophosphamide and i.v. steroids for 6 months, followed by low-dose steroids and

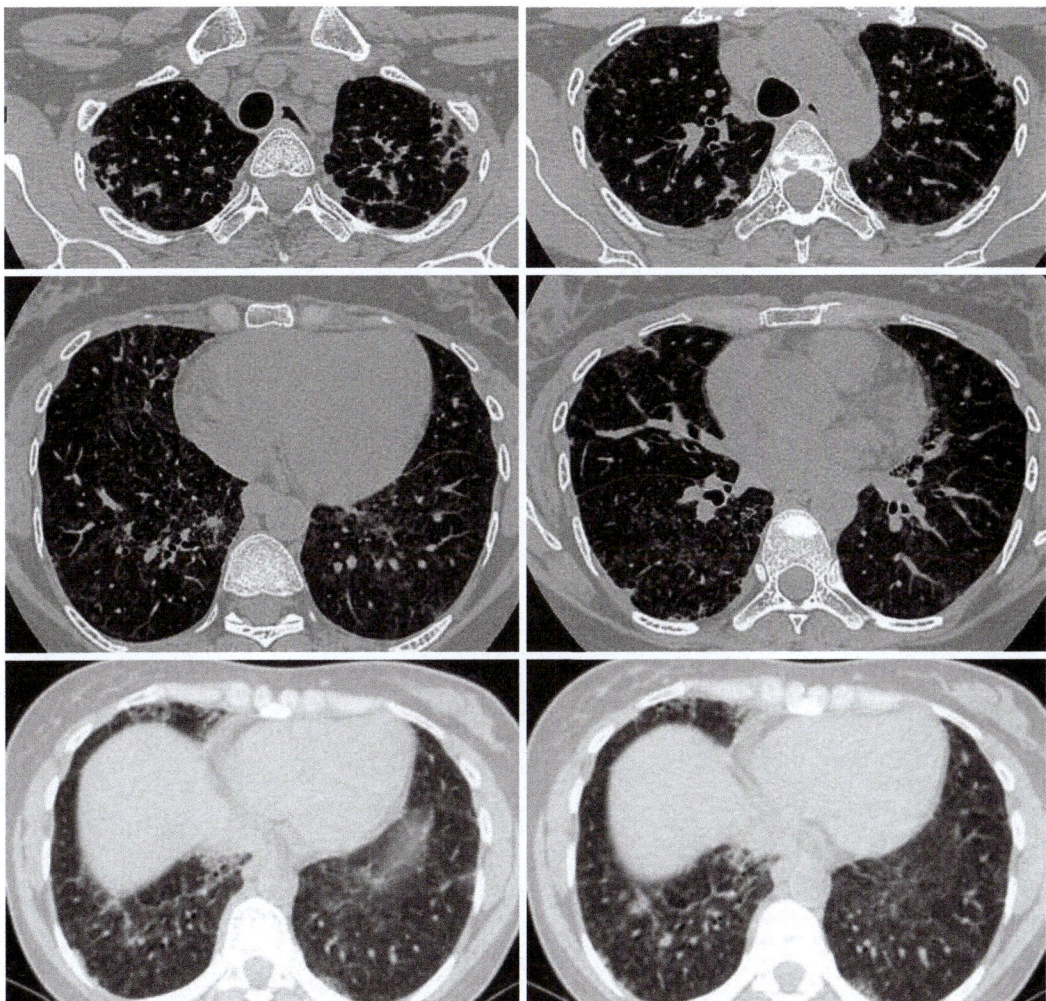

Fig. 13.5 Computed tomography (CT) images at admission, showing ground-glass opacifications and parenchymal consolidations with bibasal distribution and peri-lobular pattern, predominantly in the lower lobes, in absence of lymph adenopathies or pleural effusion

azathioprine. At 1-year follow-up, her PFTs and CT features were stable.

13.2.2 Discussion

Sjögren syndrome is a chronic, multisystem, autoimmune disorder primitively affecting exocrine glands, which can occur in isolation (primary Sjögren) or in combination with other rheumatologic conditions, such as rheumatoid arthritis, systemic lupus erythematosus, or systemic sclerosis (secondary Sjögren). The respiratory tract involvement may manifest as obstructive small airway disease, xerotrachea, pulmonary hypertension, pleuritis, pulmonary amyloidosis, and various DPLDs [6, 7]. These include lymphoid interstitial pneumonia LIP, NSIP, OP, UIP, AIP, amyloidosis, and lymphoproliferative disorders [1]. The diagnosis may be difficult to establish with certainty, especially when autoimmune serology is absent, and, TBLC may be a useful and safe tool for a proper histologic assessment, even in patients in advanced stages, and to exclude lymphoproliferative malignancies.

Fig. 13.6 Transbronchial cryobiopsy of right lower lobe showing alveolated lung parenchyma, with mainly homogeneous fibrosis. Total surface, 12 mm^2; alveolated part, 10.8 mm^2 (90% of the fragment). Hematoxylin and eosin 20×

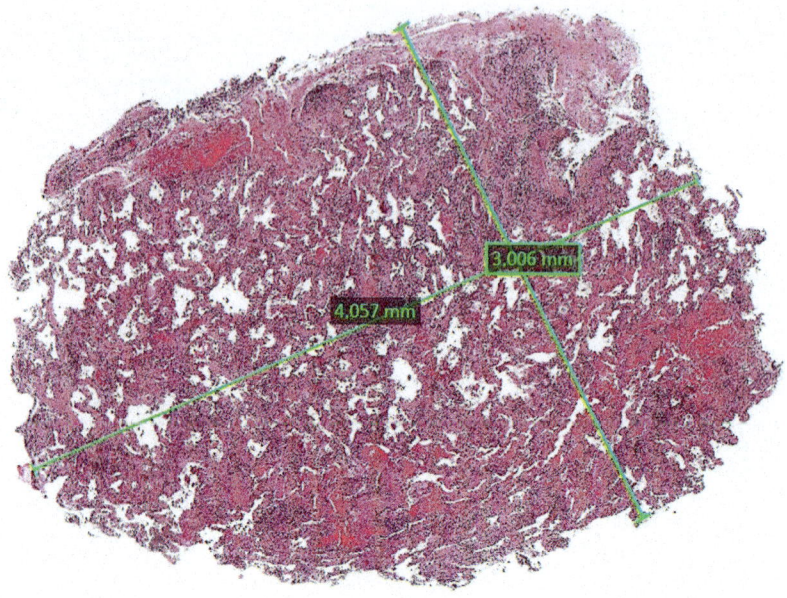

Fig. 13.7 Transbronchial cryobiopsy of right lower lobe, showing the interstitium is evenly widened mostly by inflammatory cells and a little amount of fibrosis. Cellular and fibrotic NSIP. Hematoxylin and eosin 50×

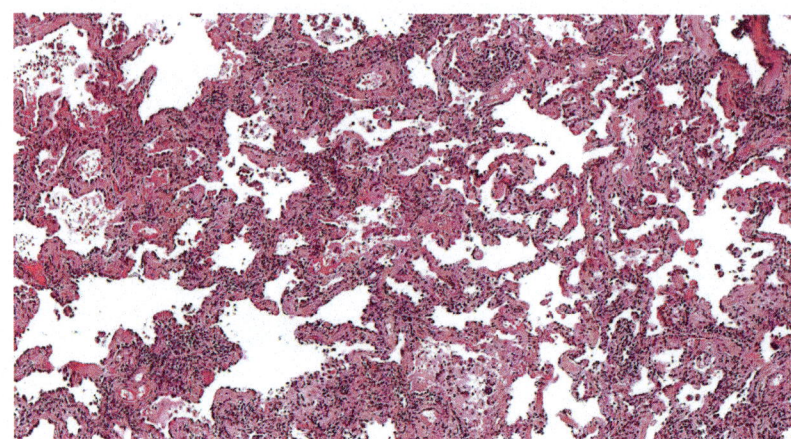

Case 3

A 47-year-old male was admitted to our unit because of progressive dyspnea and persistent dry cough. He was a lifelong no smoker, he had no occupational nor known environmental exposures, his familial history was unremarkable, and his previous medical history was notable only for a recent onset of hand morning stiffness. Physical examination at presentation revealed bibasal fine crackles on auscultation. Arterial blood gas analysis at rest showed mild hypoxemia (arterial oxygen partial pressure PaO$_2$ 73 mmHg), carbon dioxide partial pressure within normal limits (PaCO$_2$ 37 mmHg), and SO$_2$ 96%. The 6-minute walking test (6MWT) revealed a significant desaturation on exertion (SO$_2$ 91%).

Pulmonary function tests (PFTs) at baseline showed a restrictive ventilatory impairment, with decreased forced vital capacity (FVC 79% pred) and slightly reduced diffusion capacity of the lung for carbon monoxide (DLCO 62% pred).

The high-resolution computed tomography (HRCT) scan of the chest revealed fine reticulations with traction bronchiectasis with subpleural distribution predominantly in the lower lobes (Fig. 13.8). The areas of apparent ground-glass

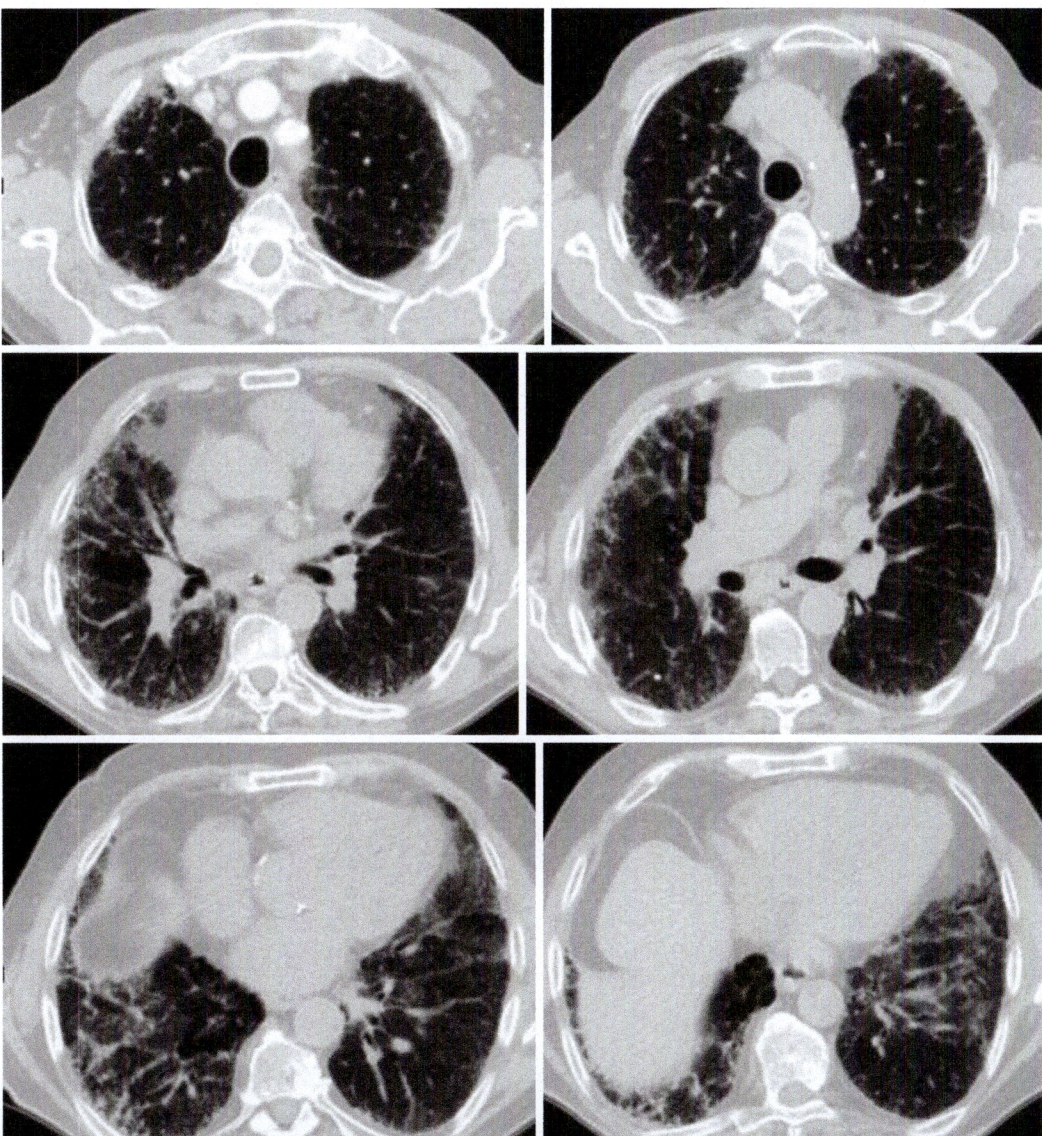

Fig. 13.8 Computed tomography (CT) images at admission, showing fine reticulations with traction bronchiectasis with subpleural distribution predominantly in the lower lobes. The areas of apparent ground-glass abnormalities in the lower lobes are admixed with traction bronchiectasis, and, thus, these should be considered as part of the fibrotic process

abnormalities in the lower lobes are admixed with traction bronchiectasis, and, thus, these should be considered as part of the fibrotic process [8].

Laboratory tests showed C-reactive protein 7.2 mg (range 0–5) and erythrocyte sedimentation rate 85 mm/h (range 0–27), mild elevation of rheumatoid factor (RF 47 UI/mL), and high title positive anti-cyclic citrullinated peptide antibodies (anti-CCP 301 UI/mL).

In order to assess the underlying DPLD morphological pattern, a TLCB was performed in the right lower lobe. Histopathologic findings revealed dense fibrosis causing architecture remodeling with heterogeneous, patchy lung involvement and fibroblast foci at the edge of dense scars; the presence of a moderate chronic cellular infiltrate with a lymphoid aggregate and some aspects of subacute damage were overall suggestive of UIP pattern in the context of an autoimmune disorder (Figs. 13.9, 13.10, 13.11, and 13.12).

During hospital stay, the patient manifested bilateral joint swelling (metacarpophalangeal joints and knees), leading to a final multidisci-

plinary diagnosis of DPLD in rheumatoid arthritis (RA).

13.2.3 Discussion

Interstitial lung diseases in RA, occurring in up to 10% of patients, most commonly manifests as

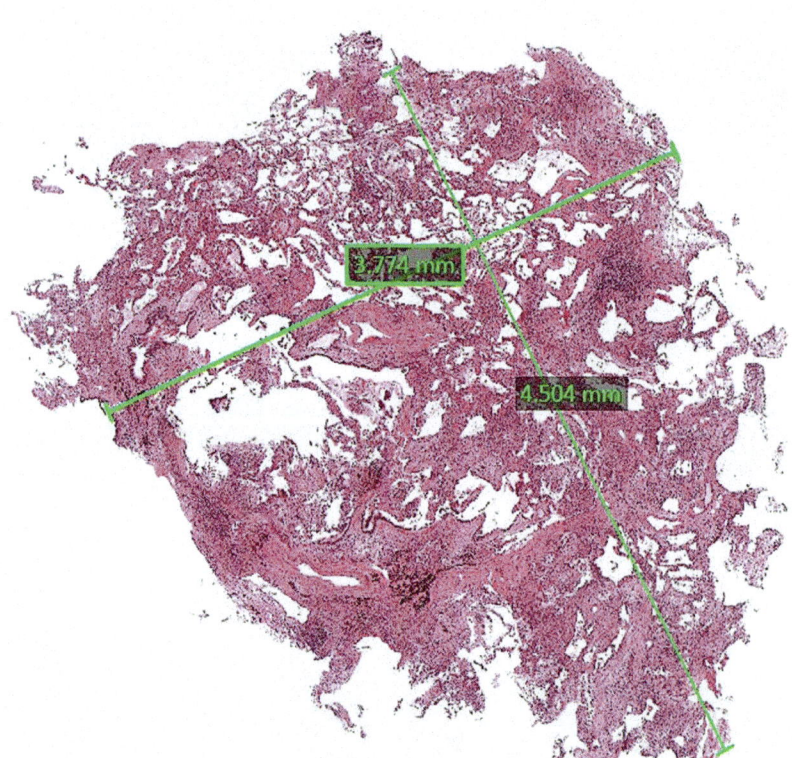

Fig. 13.9 Transbronchial cryobiopsy of right lower lobe showing alveolated lung parenchyma, with heterogeneous, patchy fibrosis and moderate inflammation. Total surface, 16.6 mm^2; alveolated part, 14.5 mm^2 (around 90% of the fragment). Hematoxylin and eosin 20×

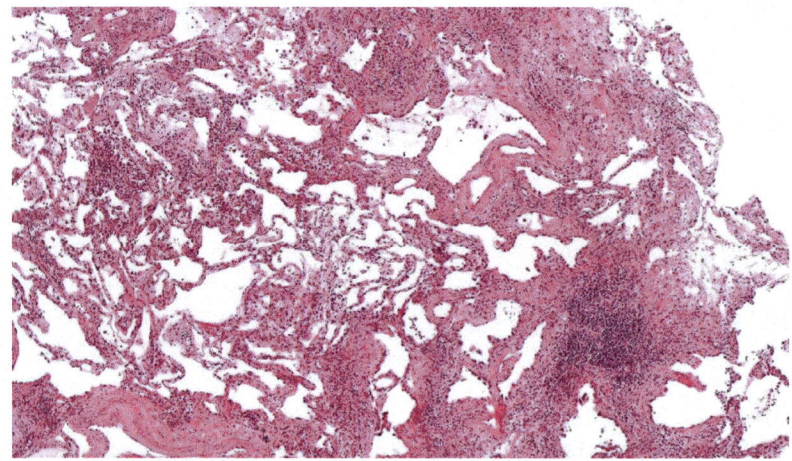

Fig. 13.10 Transbronchial cryobiopsy of right lower lobe showing alveolated lung parenchyma, with heterogeneous, patchy fibrosis and moderate inflammation. Hematoxylin and eosin 20×

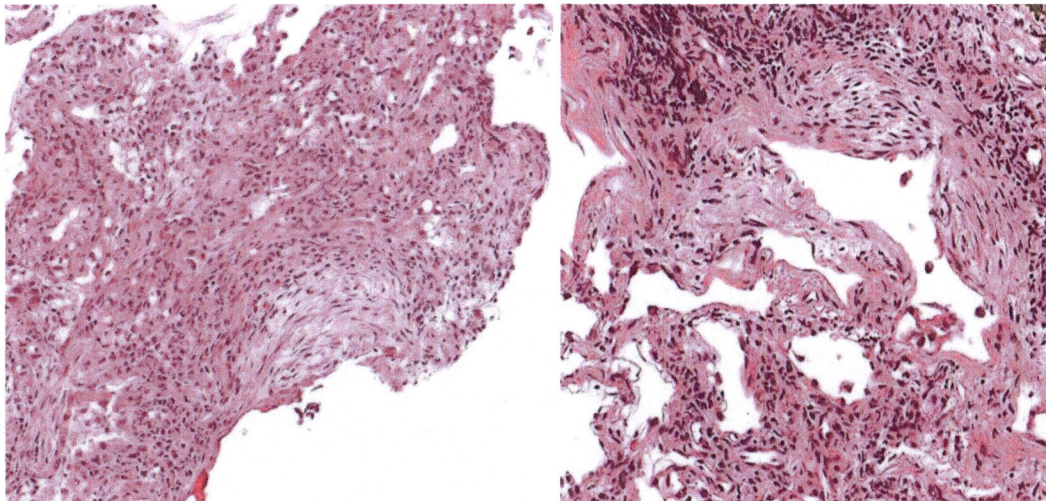

Fig. 13.11 Transbronchial cryobiopsy of right lower lobe, showing fibroblast foci

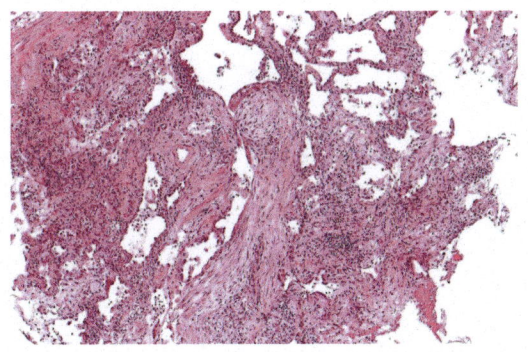

Fig. 13.12 Transbronchial cryobiopsy of right lower lobe, showing subacute damage and diffuse inflammation. Hematoxylin and eosin 50×

UIP pattern, which is associated with significant morbidity and higher mortality risk. In current practice, the discrimination between UIP and non-UIP pattern is mainly based on radiological presentation at HRCT, while histological assessment is rarely obtained [9]. However, the absence of a typical UIP pattern at HRCT is not often adequate for excluding an underlying histological UIP pattern, as clearly shown for other DPLDs. In the present case, indeed, tissue acquisition allowed to reveal a UIP pattern, although

the radiological picture was not suggestive for definite UIP. Moreover, TBLC led to distinguish between a UIP pattern in the context of idiopathic pulmonary fibrosis (UIP/IPF) and a UIP pattern in the context of autoimmune disorders, as it allowed to identify ancillary "secondary" findings, such as lymphoid follicles and moderate inflammation.

References

1. Doyle TJ, Dellaripa PF. Lung manifestations in the rheumatic diseases. Chest. 2017;152(6):1283–95.
2. Kinder BW, Shariat C, Collard HR, et al. Undifferentiated connective tissue disease-associated interstitial lung disease: changes in lung function. Lung. 2010;188(2):143–9.
3. Fischer A, Antoniou KM, Brown KK, et al. An official European Respiratory Society/American Thoracic Society research statement: interstitial pneumonia with autoimmune features. Eur Respir J. 2015;46(4):976–87.
4. Gofrit SG, Yonath H, Lidar M, et al. The clinical phenotype of patients positive for antibodies to myositis and myositis-related disorders. Clin Rheumatol. 2018;37(5):1257–63.
5. Chatterjee S, Prayson R, Farver C. Antisynthetase syndrome: not just an inflammatory myopathy. Cleve Clin J Med. 2013;80(10):655–66.

6. Wight EC, Baqir M, Ryu JH. Constrictive bronchiolitis in patients with primary Sjögren syndrome. J clin Rheumatol. 2019;25(2):74–7.

7. Roca F, Dominique S, Schmidt J, et al. Interstitial lung disease in primary Sjögren's syndrome. Autoimmun Rev. 2017;16(1):48–54.

8. Lynch DA, Sverzellati N, Travis WD. Diagnostic criteria for idiopathic pulmonary fibrosis: a Fleischner Society White Paper. Lancet Respir Med. 2018;6(2):138–53.

9. Paulin F, Doyle TJ, Fletcher EA, et al. Rheumatoid arthritis-associated interstitial lung disease and idiopathic pulmonary fibrosis: shared mechanistic and phenotypic traits suggest overlapping disease mechanisms. Rev Investig Clin. 2015;67(5):280–6.

Lymphangioleiomyomatosis

14

Giulio Rossi, Mirca Valli, Alessandra Dubini, and Paolo Spagnolo

14.1 Introduction

Pulmonary lymphangioleiomyomatosis (LAM) is a rare disease that almost exclusively occurs in women of childbearing age, most often appearing as a diffuse cystic lung disease due to proliferations of distinctive smooth-muscle cell-like cells along lymphatic channels progressively involving the pulmonary parenchyma and the pleura [1–3].

LAM occurs sporadically in patients with no evidence of genetic disease (sporadic form) and in about one third of women with tuberous sclerosis complex (TSC), an autosomal dominant neurocutaneous syndrome characterized by

G. Rossi (✉)
Operative Unit of Pathologic Anatomy,
Hospital St. Maria delle Croci, Azienda USL
della Romagna, Ravenna, Italy
e-mail: giulio.rossi@auslromagna.it

M. Valli
Operative Unit of Pathologic Anatomy,
Hospital "Degli Infermi", Azienda USL
della Romagna, Rimini, Italy
e-mail: mirca.valli@auslromagna.it

A. Dubini
Department of Pathology, Operative Unit
of Pathologic Anatomy, Azienda USL della Romagna,
Ospedale GB Morgagni-L Pierantoni, Forlì, Italy
e-mail: Alessandra.dubini@auslromagna.it

P. Spagnolo
Section of Respiratory Diseases, Department
of Cardiac, Thoracic and Vascular Sciences,
University of Padova, Padova, Italy
e-mail: paolo.spagnolo@unipd.it

mutations of *TSC-1* (located on chromosome 9q34 and encoding for the protein hamartin) and *TSC-2* (located on chromosome 16p13 and encoding for the protein tuberin) genes [4–10]. TSC occurs in 1 of 5800 live births and leads to hamartoma-like tumor growths in different organs, cerebral calcification, seizures, and mental retardation [5, 6]. Sporadic LAM is a relatively uncommon disease with an estimated prevalence of 2.6 per one million women, while a couple of sporadic LAM were documented in a karyotypically normal men without TS [11–13]. The disease tends to present between menarche and menopause, with the mean age at presentation of 34 years [1–3, 14].

The clinical features result from the progressive cystic destruction of the lung parenchyma secondary to widespread growth of LAM cells along lymphatics. Cystic abnormalities and airflow obstruction seem to be related to the constrictive effect on airways of LAM growths, but even the imbalance between matrix metalloproteinases and their inhibitors secreted by LAM cells leading to extracellular matrix degradation is involved in the mechanism of cystic modifications [15–21].

The main pulmonary symptoms consist of progressive dyspnea, recurrent pneumothorax, and chylous pleural effusions [1, 2, 22]. Cough, hemoptysis, and chyloptysis are also reported. Dyspnea is almost always present, while about 60% of patients show concurrent pneumothorax.

© Springer Nature Switzerland AG 2019
V. Poletti (ed.), *Transbronchial cryobiopsy in diffuse parenchymal lung disease*,
https://doi.org/10.1007/978-3-030-14891-1_14

[1, 2, 5, 22] Abdominal symptoms (nausea, abdominal distension, hematuria, flank pain, abdominal hemorrhage) are related to extrapulmonary manifestations such as abdominal lymphangioleiomyomas (retroperitoneum, abdomen, pelvis), lymphadenopathy, chylous abdominal depositions, and angiomyolipoma (kidney and liver) [23–30]. Around 10% of patients will develop chylous ascites due to lymphatic obstruction.

In early phase of LAM, chest X-ray may be normal even in symptomatic patient [31]. However, increased pulmonary volumes, pneumothorax or chylous pleural effusion, and cystic changes are the main radiological features [3].

The distribution of these lesions is generally bilateral and diffuse with some basilar predominance. LAM cysts have a very thin and regular wall and appear equally distributed. In contrast with centrilobular emphysema, LAM cysts show a well-defined wall lacking the centrilobular artery. Centrilobular emphysema predominates in the upper lobes and is smoking-related [1–3, 5]. Cysts of Langerhans cell histiocytosis is another smoking-related interstitial lung disease frequently showing cystic changes. However, cysts are often associated with micronodules and display a thick, irregular wall, also sparing the costophrenic angle [5]. LAM cysts generally have a round shape, do not spare the costophrenic angles, decrease in size on expiration, and tend to progressively increase in number and size. HRCT is also used to evaluate the severity of lung disease. Tiny nodules observed at high-resolution computed tomography consist of small benign proliferation of alveolar type 2 pneumocytes (so-called multifocal nodular type 2 pneumocyte hyperplasia) [3, 5]. Ill-defined ground glass opacities (observed in 25% of the cases) and interlobular septal thickening can be due to alveolar hemorrhage or edema, resulting from the obstruction of pulmonary lymphatic vessels and small veins. In the suspicion of LAM, an abdominal CT scan can provide useful additional findings, namely, renal angiomyolipomas and lymphangioleiomyomas [1–3, 5, 30–36].

High-resolution computed tomography scan should be performed in all young, non-smoking women with unclear recurrent pneumothorax with/without chylous effusion and/or functional obstruction, since imaging findings are quite specific in the hands of expert radiologists [3, 31]. The diagnosis of LAM is consistently performed on a clinical ground with typical clinical symptoms and HRCT pattern without tissue biopsy in presence of other confirmatory findings, such as chylothorax, angiomyolipoma, lymphangioleiomyoma/lymphangiomyoma, tuberous sclerosis complex, and elevated serum vascular endothelial growth factor—VEGF-D $\geq$ 800 pg/mL [31].

In the hands of expert pulmonary radiologists, the sensitivity and specificity of HRCT in identifying LAM among several cystic diseases are 87.5% and 97.5%, respectively [3, 31].

Nevertheless, difficult cases showing characteristic cysts at HRCT in absence of additional confirmatory features require lung tissue examination to achieve a definitive diagnosis. Surgical lung biopsy (SLB) is still considered the gold standard biopsy in interstitial lung diseases (ILD), including those with cystic pattern, but less invasive transbronchial lung biopsy (TBLB) may be considered equally effective and safer than SLB in the diagnosis of LAM [31].

Lung biopsy is performed in suspected LAM patients to exclude other cystic lung diseases [32]. The rarity of the disease and the therapeutic and prognostic implications of the diagnosis make tissue sampling recommended in all clinically uncertain cases. Cytology has a little or no role in LAM diagnosis, but the finding of alveolar hemorrhage with hemosiderin-laden macrophages at bronchoalveolar lavage (BAL) fluid analysis may be helpful [31].

LAM is one of diffuse lung diseases that can be successfully diagnosed on TBLB, which is often attempted before submitting the patient to thoracic surgery [32]. Given the random distribution of the lesions, the diagnostic yield of TBLB increases with the number of biopsies. In TBLBs with clinical and CT findings suspicious for LAM and in all biopsies from patients with cystic disease, the use of immunohistochemical stains is strongly recommended to highlight tiny and focally distributed lesions apparently not visible on hematoxylin-eosin-stained slides [33–35].

Differential diagnosis mainly includes Langerhans cell histiocytosis, emphysema, lymphoid interstitial pneumonia, and non-specific interstitial pneumonia (NSIP) related to connective tissue diseases (e.g., Sjogren's disease), Birt-Hogg-Dubé syndrome, amyloidosis, hypersensitivity pneumonia, and lymphangiomatosis.

In the recent years, several authors and the last 2015 World Health Organization (WHO) classification of lung tumors have suggested to consider LAM as a low-grade tumor arising from peculiar cells spreading through lymphatic channels and possibly metastasizing to lymph nodes [36].

Indeed, LAM cells harbor inactivating mutations in tumor suppressor gene *TSC1* or *TSC2* and activate mammalian target of rapamycin complex 1(mTORC1) leading to cell growth [4]. The 2015 WHO classification has created a group of perivascular epithelioid cell (PEC)-derived tumors including PEComa (formerly clear cell tumor/sugar tumor) and LAM. This view is sustained by the frequent occurrence of extrapulmonary manifestation of LAM, comprising pelvic lymph node infiltration, uterine LAM, and renal angiomyolipoma [36].

In addition, patients with sporadic LAM requiring lung transplantation have developed recurrent LAM in transplanted lungs harboring identical genetic alterations to those originally identified in naïve lungs [37–39]. Furthermore, identical *TSC2* mutations were detected in LAM cells and angiomyolipomas from the same patients, and LAM cells were isolated from blood and other fluids in patients with sporadic LAM [4, 39].

Although data derive from few and limited case series, the diagnostic yield of TBLB is about 60%, and procedure-related complication rate is about 14% (pneumothorax, hemorrhage, thoracic chest pain, pneumonia) [31]. Nevertheless, the most recent American Thoracic Society (ATS)/Japanese Respiratory Society clinical practice guidelines underline the necessity to submit nondiagnostic TBLB samples to expert pathologists for a second opinion, since a significant quote of cases become entirely diagnostic [31].

Limitations of TBLB are related to the small case series published in literature that preclude a confident estimation of the diagnostic yield in LAM, although the diagnostic bar could mainly depend on the percentage of involved lung. Second, data from previous works give no indication in the correct selection of patients undergoing TBLB.

However, once lung tissue examination is required to have a confident diagnosis of LAM, TBLB should be attempted in light of the significant diagnostic yield (up to 50%) and to prevent unnecessary more invasive surgical lung biopsy. The complication rate of TBLB in LAM is acceptable, ranging from 2 to 14%.

Transbronchial fine needle aspiration of enlarged mediastinal lymph nodes could represent an alternative and less invasive approach, as well as the search for LAM cells in chylous effusions using cell block preparation [31].

No studies focused on the efficacy and safety of transbronchial cryobiopsies in LAM have been so far published. Fruchter et al. [40] reported 1 case of LAM among their 75 patients with interstitial lung diseases undergoing histologic examination by transbronchial cryobiopsy. Apparently, the cystic pattern of ILD does not appear a contraindication to transbronchial cryobiopsy.

Survival at 10 years is of 80%, and main treatments include medroxyprogesterone, mTOR inhibitors, and lung transplantation [41–43].

14.1.1 Histology

- Cysts bilaterally distributed through all the lung fields with involvement of costophrenic angles
- Proliferation of smooth-muscle-like cells with cytoplasmic clear vacuolization (LAM cells) along the lymphatic routes lining the cystic formation, even leading to small nodules
- Chronic alveolar hemorrhage around vessels
- Variable immunohistochemical expression of smooth-muscle markers (smooth-muscle actin, desmin), hormonal receptors, melanocytic markers (HMB45, MART-1), and cathepsin-K

Cystic change and LAM cell growth may be very subtle and quite different in each individual case. The distribution of cysts and LAM cells mainly involves lymphatic routes, such as peribronchiolar areas, vessels, pleura, and lymphatic spaces. LAM cells are typically organized in small clusters at the edges of the cysts and along pulmonary lymphatics. Compared to normal smooth-muscle cells, LAM cells have less eosinophilic cytoplasm and a characteristic clear change/vacuolization. LAM cells may vary from small spindle-shaped to round or oval, to large epithelioid cell growing into the cystic spaces or forming small thickening of the cyst wall.

Since LAM cells involve the vessel walls leading to vascular disruption, a careful observation of chronic alveolar hemorrhage with hemosiderin-laden macrophages may indirectly indicate LAM. Serial sections of each formalin-fixed, paraffin-embedded block and the use of immunostains are mandatory in these cases. Indeed, LAM smooth-muscle-like cells generally express melanocytic markers (HMB45, MART-1), hormonal receptors, smooth-muscle actin, and cathepsin-K [44–48].

Multifocal micronodular pneumocyte hyperplasia is another lesion in LAM appearing as tiny nodular proliferations of type 2 pneumocytes with polygonal or cuboidal appearance.

14.1.2 Differential Diagnosis

Basically, all lesions leading to pulmonary cystic modifications may enter in differential diagnosis. Identification of LAM cells around cysts using specific immunostains (e.g., HMB45, cathepsin-K) is unique of LAM. Of note, pathologists should be aware that HMB45 expression may be variable, weak, and restricted to few cells. Since histology of LAM is quite peculiar, the disease may be recognizable even in tiny biopsy.

LAM must be distinguished from other more common cystic pulmonary lesions, as emphysema and pulmonary Langerhans cell histiocytosis. These diseases are characterized by distinctive clinical and HRCT findings, such as association with smoke and upper lobe distribution. LCH is characterized by cystic changes and tiny and cavitate nodules depending on its evolution.

The wall of cysts consists of fascicle of spindle cells resembling smooth-muscle elements. Metastatic low-grade stromal sarcoma may present with several cysts lined by hormonal and CD10 positive bland spindled tumor cells, but clinical history together with imaging studies and lack of expression for melanocytic markers rule out LAM. Even lung endometriosis with/without catamenial pneumothorax and hemoptysis or smooth-muscle lesions (benign metastasizing leiomyoma) enter in the differential diagnosis with LAM.

14.2 Case Presentation

- **Clinical Background**
  - 46-year-old woman
  - Former smoker
  - Unremarkable past medical history
- **Onset of Symptoms**
  - Progressive dyspnea
  - Recurrent pneumothorax
- **Laboratory Findings**
  - Routine laboratory tests: unremarkable
  - Autoimmune serum tests: negative
- **Pulmonary Function Test**
  - FVC 82%; FEV1 61%; FEV1/FVC 58%; RV 88%; DLCO 65%
- **Imaging** (Figs. 14.1, 14.2, and 14.3)
  - CT scan shows numerous and bilateral thin-walled cysts of variable size, diffusely distributed through all pulmonary fields without a preferential location and involving costophrenic angles.
- **Cryobiopsy** (Figs. 14.4, 14.5, 14.6, 14.7, and 14.8)
  - The specimen obtained from the transbronchial cryobiopsy technique consists of three fragments of pulmonary parenchyma ranging from 5 to 8 mm of maximum diameter. Histologically, the lung tissue shows the presence of few cystic spaces characterized by a thin layer of spindled cells with smooth-muscle cell appearance and slightly hyperplastic pneumocytes (Figs. 14.4 and 14.5). Some calcifications are present around spindle cell proliferations. At immunohistochemistry,

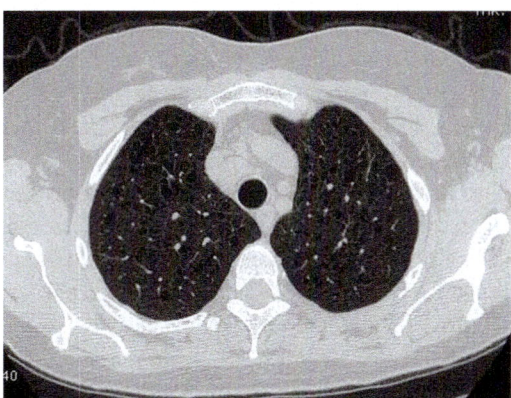

Fig. 14.1 CT scan showing several thin-walled rounded cysts involving bilaterally and diffusely the lung fields without costophrenic angles preservation (upper lobes)

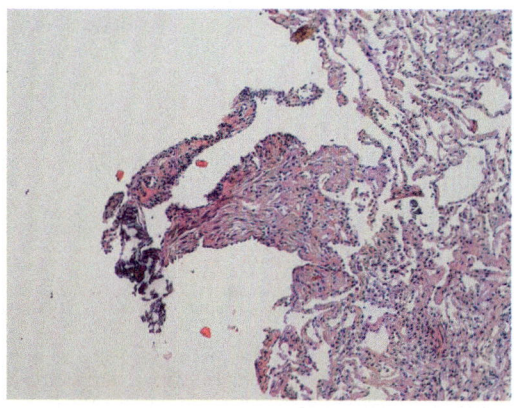

Fig. 14.4 Transbronchial cryobiopsy showing normal lung and subtle aggregates of LAM cells showing smooth-muscle-like appearance and cytoplasmic vacuolization leading to clear changes. Some calcifications are also noted

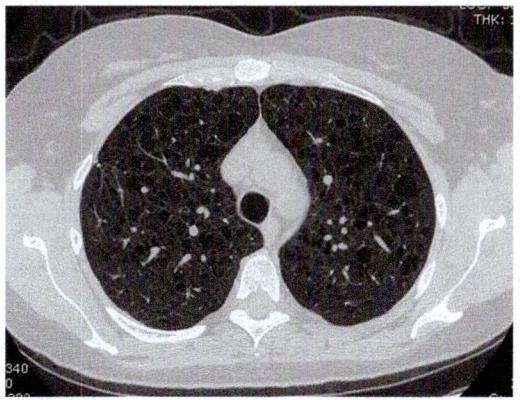

Fig. 14.2 CT scan showing several thin-walled rounded cysts involving bilaterally and diffusely the lung fields without costophrenic angles preservation (upper lobes and middle lobe)

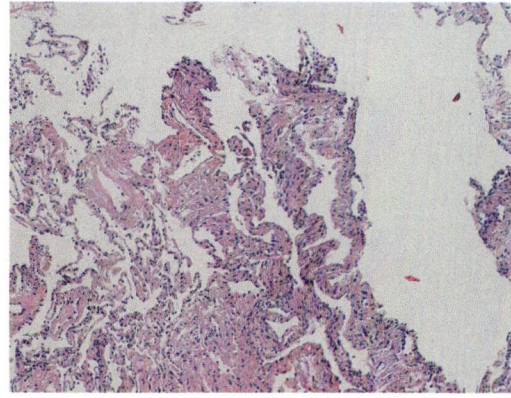

Fig. 14.5 Transbronchial cryobiopsy showing normal lung and subtle aggregates of LAM cells showing smooth-muscle-like appearance and cytoplasmic vacuolization leading to clear changes

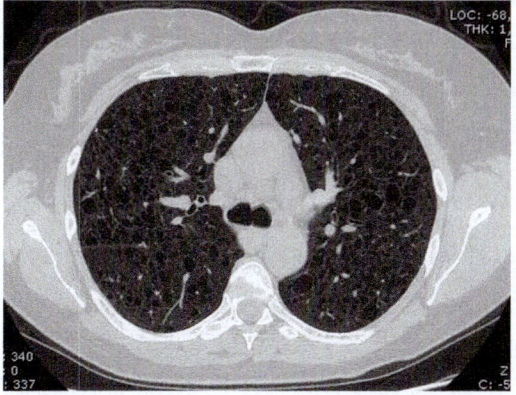

Fig. 14.3 CT scan showing several thin-walled rounded cysts involving bilaterally and diffusely the lung fields without costophrenic angle preservation (lower lobes)

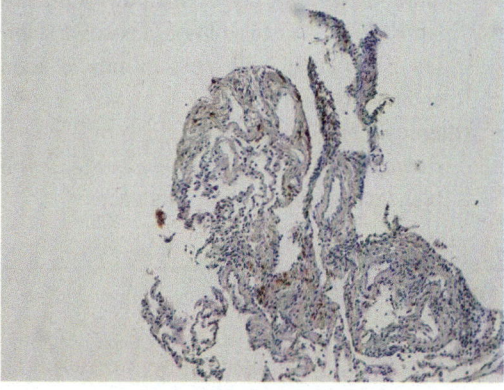

Fig. 14.6 Focal immunohistochemical expression for HMB45 in the cytoplasm of LAM cells

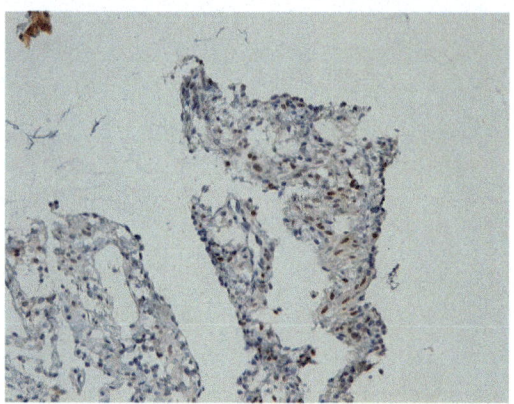

Fig. 14.7 LAM cells showing nuclear staining with estrogen receptor

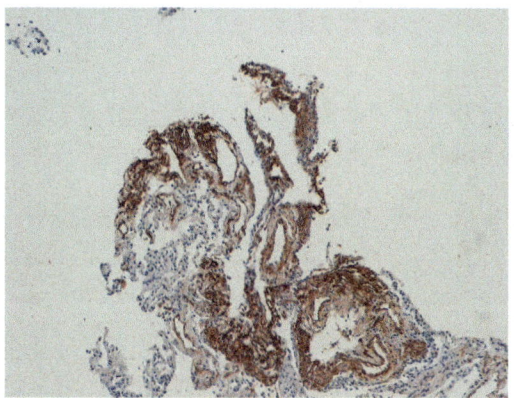

Fig. 14.8 Consistent immunohistochemical expression for cathepsin-K in LAM cells

these cells show a patchy, weak, and focal expression for HMB45 (Fig. 14.6), nuclear positivity with estrogen receptors (Fig. 14.7), and consistent and diffuse staining for cathepsin-K (Fig. 14.8). In addition, a positive staining is observed with smooth-muscle actin and focally with MART-1.

- **Diagnosis**
  - *Pulmonary lymphangioleiomyomatosis* with high level of diagnostic confidence.

14.3 Discussion

Transbronchial cryobiopsy may be used in patients with suspected LAM. Anecdotic reports also suggest that lung complications related to

the procedure have a limited clinical impact. Lung tissue samples so obtained are well preserved, and immunohistochemical analyses or even molecular investigations may be done easily. Recently an increased PD-L1 expression in lung tissue from LAM patients has been proven suggesting new opportunities for therapeutic targeting [49]. The need of lung tissue that is now limited to cases that do not meet all the criteria required for a clinic-radiologic- and laboratory-based diagnosis will probably gain importance.

References

1. McCormack FX. Lymphangioleiomyomatosis: a clinical update. Chest. 2008;133:507–16.
2. Taylor JR, Ryu J, Colby TV, Raffin TA. Lymphangioleiomyomatosis. Clinical course in 32 patients. N Engl J Med. 1990;323:1254–60.
3. Abbott GF, Rosado de Christenson ML, Frazier AA, Franks TJ, Pugatch RD, Galvin JR. From the archives of the AFIP: lymphangioleiomyomatosis: radiologic-pathologic correlation. Radiographics. 2005;25:803–28.
4. Juvet SC, McCormack FX, Kwiatkowski DJ, Downey GP. Molecular pathogenesis of lymphangioleiomyomatosis: lessons learned from orphans. Am J Respir Cell Mol Biol. 2007;36:398–408.
5. Morbini P, Guddo F, Contini P, Luisetti M, Schiavina M, Zompatori M. Rare diffuse diseases of the lung. Pulmonary alveolar proteinosis, lymphangioleiomyomatosis, amyloidosis. Pathologica. 2010;102:547–56.
6. Krymskaya VP, McCormack FX. Lymphangioleiomyomatosis: a monogenic model of malignancy. Annu Rev Med. 2017;68:69–83.
7. Carsillo T, Astrinidis A, Henske EP. Mutations in the tuberous sclerosis complex gene TSC2 are a cause of sporadic pulmonary lymphangioleiomyomatosis. Proc Natl Acad Sci U S A. 2000;97:6085–90.
8. Smolarek TA, Wessner LL, McCormack FX, Mylet JC, Menon AG, Henske EP. Evidence that lymphangiomyomatosis is caused by TSC2 mutations: chromosome 16p13 loss of heterozygosity in angiomyolipomas and lymph nodes from women with lymphangiomyomatosis. Am J Hum Genet. 1998;62:810–5.
9. Dibble CC, Elis W, Menon S, et al. TBC1D7 is a third subunit of the TSC1-TSC2 complex upstream of mTORC1. Mol Cell. 2012;47:535–46.
10. Goncharova EA, Goncharov DA, Eszterhas A, et al. Tuberin regulates p70 S6 kinase activation and ribosomal protein S6 phosphorylation. A role for the TSC2 tumor suppressor gene in pulmonary lymphangioleiomyomatosis (LAM). J Biol Chem. 2002;277:30958–67.

11. Schiavina M, Di Scioscio V, Contini P, Cavazza A, Fabiani A, Barberis M, et al. Pulmonary lymphangioleiomyomatosis in a karyotypically normal man without tuberous sclerosis complex. Am J Respir Crit Care Med. 2007;176:96–8.
12. Aubry MC, Myers JL, Ryu JH, et al. Pulmonary lymphangioleiomyomatosis in a man. Am J Respir Crit Care Med. 2000;162:749–52.
13. Miyake M, Tateishi U, Maeda T, et al. Pulmonary lymphangioleiomyomatosis in a male patient with tuberous sclerosis complex. Radiat Med. 2005;23:525–7.
14. Kitaichi M, Nishimura K, Itoh H, Izumi T. Pulmonary lymphangioleiomyomatosis: a report of 46 patients including a clinicopathologic study of prognostic factors. Am J Respir Crit Care Med. 1995;151:527–33.
15. Finlay G. The LAM cell: what is it, where does it come from, and why does it grow? Am J Physiol Lung Cell Mol Physiol. 2004;286:L690–3.
16. Crooks DM, Pacheco-Rodriguez G, DeCastro RM, et al. Molecular and genetic analysis of disseminated neoplastic cells in lymphangioleiomyomatosis. Proc Natl Acad Sci U S A. 2004;101:17462–7.
17. Chang WY, Cane JL, Blakey JD, Kumaran M, Pointon KS, Johnson SR. Clinical utility of diagnostic guidelines and putative biomarkers in lymphangioleiomyomatosis. Respir Res. 2012;13:34.
18. Matsui K, Takeda K, Yu ZX, Travis WD, Moss J, Ferrans VJ. Role for activation of matrix metalloproteinases in the pathogenesis of pulmonary lymphangioleiomyomatosis. Arch Pathol Lab Med. 2000;124:267–75.
19. Hayashi T, Fleming MV, Stetler-Stevenson WG, et al. Immunohistochemical study of matrix metalloproteinases (MMPs) and their tissue inhibitors (TIMPs) in pulmonary lymphangioleiomyomatosis (LAM). Hum Pathol. 1997;28:1071–8.
20. Glassberg MK, Elliot SJ, Fritz J, et al. Activation of the estrogen receptor contributes to the progression of pulmonary lymphangioleiomyomatosis via matrix metalloproteinase-induced cell invasiveness. J Clin Endocrinol Metab. 2008;93:1625–33.
21. Odajima N, Betsuyaku T, Nasuhara Y, Inoue H, Seyama K, Nishimura M. Matrix metalloproteinases in blood from patients with LAM. Respir Med. 2009;103:124–9.
22. Urban T, Lazor R, Lacronique J, et al. Pulmonary lymphangioleiomyomatosis. A study of 69 patients. Groupe d'Etudes et de Recherche sur les Maladies "Orphelines" Pulmonaires (GERM"O"P). Medicine (Baltimore). 1999;78:321–37.
23. Cudzilo CJ, Szczesniak RD, Brody AS, et al. Lymphangioleiomyomatosis screening in women with tuberous sclerosis. Chest. 2013;144:578–85.
24. Astrinidis A, Khare L, Carsillo T, et al. Mutational analysis of the tuberous sclerosis gene TSC2 in patients with pulmonary lymphangioleiomyomatosis. J Med Genet. 2000;37:55–7.
25. Gupta R, Kitaichi M, Inoue Y, Kotloff R, McCormack FX. Lymphatic manifestations of lymphangioleiomyomatosis. Lymphology. 2014;47:106–17.
26. Hayashi T, Kumasaka T, Mitani K, et al. Prevalence of uterine and adnexal involvement in pulmonary lymphangioleiomyomatosis: a clinicopathologic study of 10 patients. Am J Surg Pathol. 2011;35:1776–85.
27. Matsui K, Tatsuguchi A, Valencia J, et al. Extrapulmonary lymphangioleiomyomatosis (LAM): clinicopathologic features in 22 cases. Hum Pathol. 2000;31:1242–8.
28. Torres VE, Björnsson J, King BF, et al. Extrapulmonary lymphangioleiomyomatosis and lymphangiomatous cysts in tuberous sclerosis complex. Mayo Clin Proc. 1995;70:641–8.
29. Kerr LA, Blute ML, Ryu JH, Swensen SJ, Malek RS. Renal angiomyolipoma in association with pulmonary lymphangioleiomyomatosis: forme fruste of tuberous sclerosis? Urology. 1993;41:440–4.
30. De Pauw RA, Boelaert JR, Haenebalcke CW, Matthys EG, Schurgers MS, De Vriese AS. Renal angiomyolipoma in association with pulmonary lymphangioleiomyomatosis. Am J Kidney Dis. 2003;41:877–83.
31. Gupta N, Finlay GA, Kotloff RM, Strange C, Wilson KC, Young LR, Taveira-DaSilva AM, Johnson SR, Cottin V, Sahn SA, Ryu JH, Seyama K, Inoue Y, Downey GP, Han MK, Colby TV, Wikenheiser-Brokamp KA, Meyer CA, Smith K, Moss J, McCormack FX, ATS Assembly on Clinical Problems. Lymphangioleiomyomatosis diagnosis and management: high-resolution chest computed tomography, transbronchial lung biopsy, and pleural disease management. An official American Thoracic Society/Japanese Respiratory Society clinical practice guideline. Am J Respir Crit Care Med. 2017;196(10):1337–48.
32. Leslie KO, Gruden JF, Parish JM, Scholand MB. Transbronchial biopsy interpretation in the patient with diffuse parenchymal lung disease. Arch Pathol Lab Med. 2007;131:407–23.
33. Koba T, Arai T, Kitaichi M, Kasai T, Hirose M, Tachibana K, Sugimoto C, Akira M, Hayashi S, Inoue Y. Efficacy and safety of transbronchial lung biopsy for the diagnosis of lymphangioleiomyomatosis: a report of 24 consecutive patients. Respirology. 2018;23(3):331–8.
34. Meraj R, Wikenheiser-Brokamp KA, Young LR, Byrnes S, McCormack FX. Utility of transbronchial biopsy in the diagnosis of lymphangioleiomyomatosis. Front Med. 2012;6(4):395–405.
35. Harari S, Torre O, Cassandro R, Taveira-DaSilva AM, Moss J. Bronchoscopic diagnosis of Langerhans cell histiocytosis and lymphangioleiomyomatosis. Respir Med. 2012;106(9):1286–92.
36. Travis WD, Brambilla E, Nicholson AG, et al. The 2015 World Health Organization classification of lung tumors: impact of genetic, clinical and radiologic advances since the 2004 classification. J Thorac Oncol. 2015;10(9):1243–60.
37. Karbowniczek M, Astrinidis A, Balsara BR, et al. Recurrent lymphangiomyomatosis after transplantation: genetic analyses reveal a metastatic mechanism. Am J Respir Crit Care Med. 2003;167:976–82.

38. Bittmann I, Rolf B, Amann G, Löhrs U. Recurrence of lymphangioleiomyomatosis after single lung transplantation: new insights into pathogenesis. Hum Pathol. 2003;34:95–8.

39. Steagall WK, Zhang L, Cai X, Pacheco-Rodriguez G, Moss J. Genetic heterogeneity of circulating cells from patients with lymphangioleiomyomatosis with and without lung transplantation. Am J Respir Crit Care Med. 2015;191:854–6.

40. Fruchter O, Fridel L, El Raouf BA, Abdel-Rahman N, Rosengarten D, Kramer MR. Histological diagnosis of interstitial lung diseases by cryo-transbronchial biopsy. Respirology. 2014;19(5):683–8.

41. Rossi GA, Balbi B, Oddera S, Lantero S, Ravazzoni C. Response to treatment with an analog of the luteinizing-hormone-releasing hormone in a patient with pulmonary lymphangioleiomyomatosis. Am Rev Respir Dis. 1991;143:174–6.

42. Taveira-DaSilva AM, Stylianou MP, Hedin CJ, Hathaway O, Moss J. Decline in lung function in patients with lymphangioleiomyomatosis treated with or without progesterone. Chest. 2004;126:1867–74.

43. McCormack FX, Gupta N, Finlay GR, Young LR, Taveira-DaSilva AM, Glasgow CG, Steagall WK, Johnson SR, Sahn SA, Ryu JH, Strange C, Seyama K, Sullivan EJ, Kotloff RM, Downey GP, Chapman JT, Han MK, D'Armiento JM, Inoue Y, Henske EP, Bissler JJ, Colby TV, Kinder BW, Wikenheiser-Brokamp KA, Brown KK, Cordier JF, Meyer C, Cottin V, Brozek JL, Smith K, Wilson KC, Moss J, ATS/JRS Committee on Lymphangioleiomyomatosis. Official American Thoracic Society/Japanese Respiratory Society clinical practice guidelines: lymphangioleiomyomatosis diagnosis and management. Am J Respir Crit Care Med. 2016;194(6):748–61.

44. Nijmeh J, El-Chemaly S, Henske EP. Emerging biomarkers of lymphangioleiomyomatosis. Expert Rev Respir Med. 2018;12(2):95–102.

45. Tanaka H, Imada A, Morikawa T, et al. Diagnosis of pulmonary lymphangioleiomyomatosis by HMB45 in surgically treated spontaneous pneumothorax. Eur Respir J. 1995;8:1879–82.

46. Fetsch PA, Fetsch JF, Marincola FM, Travis W, Batts KP, Abati A. Comparison of melanoma antigen recognized by T cells (MART-1) to HMB-45: additional evidence to support a common lineage for angiomyolipoma, lymphangiomyomatosis, and clear cell sugar tumor. Mod Pathol. 1998;11:699–703.

47. Chilosi M, Pea M, Martignoni G, Brunelli M, Gobbo S, Poletti V, et al. Cathepsin-k expression in pulmonary lymphangioleiomyomatosis. Mod Pathol. 2009;22:161–6.

48. Martignoni G, Pea M, Reghellin D, et al. Molecular pathology of lymphangioleiomyomatosis and other perivascular epithelioid cell tumors. Arch Pathol Lab Med. 2010;134:33–40.

49. Maisel K, Merrilees M, Atochina-Vassermaqn EN, et al. Immune checkpoint ligand PD-L1 is upregulated in pulmonary lymphangioleiomyomatosis. Am J Respir Cell Mol Biol. 2018;59(6):723–32.

Pleuroparenchymal Fibroelastosis

15

Maria Cecilia Mengoli, Thomas Colby,
Alessandra Dubini, Giulio Rossi,
and Alberto Cavazza

15.1 Introduction

Pleuroparenchymal fibroelastosis (PPFE) is a rare and possibly underrecognized interstitial pneumonia, as defined by the updated 2013 ATS/ERS Classification [1].

There are two groups of patients, those with a known cause and those without known association, the latter being termed idiopathic PPFE [2].

The first group includes cases of PPFE associated with lung transplantation (late posttransplant complication in 2–7.5% of lung transplant recipients), hematopoietic stem cell transplantation (late complication in 0 and 2% of patients), previous chemotherapy (alkylating agents) and/or radiotherapy, occupational dust exposure (asbestos, aluminum), recurrent pulmonary infections (*Aspergillus* sp., *Mycobacterium avium-intracellulare*), autoimmune diseases (ankylosing spondylitis, ulcerative colitis, psoriasis, lupus, rheumatoid arthritis), and familial cases with a possible underlying genetic predisposition (e.g., a short telomere syndrome characterized by telomere-related gene mutations of TERT, TERC, RTEL1, and PARN): the latter are prevalent among female patients [2–6].

When all these causes may be excluded or no specific clinical settings are identified, the disorder is labeled as idiopathic [4].

Curiously PPFE is morphologically similar to a spontaneous syndrome of aged donkeys with a high prevalence (35%) that analogously involves the upper lung zones. PPFE as an effect of aging in humans has also been speculated upon [7].

PPFE is also classified into pure PPFE and PPFE combined with other interstitial pneumonias, such as usual interstitial pneumonia (UIP) and non-specific interstitial pneumonia (NSIP), often involving the lower lung zones [8].

There is a wide age range at diagnosis (13–87 years, mean 53 years) and a bimodal distribution of presentation with an early peak in the third and a later peak in the sixth decade; a striking predominance of female cases in the earlier peak is observed.

A frequent association with a low body mass index (BMI) and with a "platythorax" (reduction

M. C. Mengoli (✉) · A. Cavazza
Anatomia Patologica, Azienda Unità Sanitaria
Locale-IRCCS di Reggio Emilia,
Reggio Emilia, Italy
e-mail: alberto.cavazza@ausl.re.it

T. Colby
Department of Laboratory Medicine and Pathology,
Mayo Clinic Scottsdale, Scottsdale, AZ, USA
e-mail: Colby.Thomas@mayo.edu

A. Dubini
Department of Pathology, Operative Unit
of Pathologic Anatomy, Azienda USL della Romagna,
Ospedale GB Morgagni-L Pierantoni, Forlì, Italy
e-mail: alessandra.dubini@auslromagna.it

G. Rossi
Operative Unit of Pathologic Anatomy, Hospital
St. Maria delle Croci, Azienda USL della Romagna,
Ravenna, Italy

© Springer Nature Switzerland AG 2019
V. Poletti (ed.), *Transbronchial cryobiopsy in diffuse parenchymal lung disease*,
https://doi.org/10.1007/978-3-030-14891-1_15

in the anterior-posterior diameter of the chest wall) has also been demonstrated [2–4].

Recently a possible association between idiopathic PPFE and hypothyroidism ("lung-thyroid syndrome") and cutaneous manifestations of PPFE that clinically simulate telangiectasia macularis eruptiva perstans, but lacking mast cell infiltrate, have been reported [9, 10].

The most common presenting symptoms are dyspnea, cough, hemoptysis, weight loss, low-grade fever, recurrent infection, pleuritic chest pain, and spontaneous pneumothorax [2–4].

Pulmonary function tests typically show a restrictive pattern or a mixed restrictive-obstructive pattern with an increased residual volume/total lung capacity (RV/TLC) ratio, which is a peculiar functional impairment that differs from that seen in IPF [11].

Serum laboratory data show elevation of KL-6 with the disease progression, and also surfactant protein D may be elevated. About a half of patients with PPFE demonstrates increased titers of a variety of serum autoantibodies such as rheumatoid factor, double-stranded DNA, and antinuclear antibody, suggesting a possible role of autoimmune mechanism in the pathogenesis of the disease [3, 4].

Chest radiograph at the early stage of PPFE shows bilateral, apical, irregular thickening of the pleura. Later the elevation of bilateral hila is detected. The lateral view often demonstrates an abnormally narrowed anterior-posterior thoracic dimension [2, 3].

Radiologic criteria for the diagnosis of PPFE are proposed by Reddy as follows: a definite diagnosis of PPFE at HRCT requires upper lobe pleural thickening and subpleural fibrosis (traction bronchiectasis, architectural distortion, upper lobe volume loss, superior hilar retraction), with involvement of the lower lobes being less marked or absent. The presence of a clear demarcation between the affected and the normal lung is a characteristic feature. Pneumothorax, platythorax, parenchymal consolidations, subpleural cysts, and ground glass areas might be present, mainly in the upper zones. A consistent diagnosis of PPFE is considered when there is pleural thickening and subpleural fibrosis that are not concentrated in the upper lobe or there is presence of coexistent disease elsewhere [3].

At the advanced stage, fibrotic shadows extend to lower lung fields, and the diaphragm is elevated with the loss of bilateral lung volume. Multiple bullae and large cysts often appear in the upper lung fields [3].

The radiological differential diagnosis includes familial pulmonary fibrosis, connective tissue disease (particularly ankylosing spondylitis), fibrotic sarcoidosis, and chronic hypersensitivity pneumonitis (HP) [3, 11].

Once PPFE becomes symptomatic, patients may remain stable for a long period of time or progress rapidly (60% of cases) to hypoxemic and hypercapnic respiratory failure [1–4].

Urinary desmosines (degradation product of mature elastin) have been proposed as a novel, noninvasive diagnostic biomarker, since urinary levels are significantly higher in patients with PPFE than those in patients with IPF or healthy controls [12].

At present, there are no established therapeutic options for PPFE, except for transplantation. Patients have been treated empirically with corticosteroids, N-acetylcysteine, prophylactic antibiotics, and immunosuppressant (cyclophosphamide, azathioprine) although none have demonstrated clear evidence of efficacy except for supportive care (oxygen therapy). A potential efficacy of pirfenidone in preventing lung function decline has been suggested in single cases of PPFE combined with UIP/IPF, leading to the consideration that a subset of PPFE may potentially benefit from antifibrotic drugs, especially in the setting of PPFE combined with UIP/IPF [13].

15.1.1 Histology

- Upper lobes and peripheral predominant distribution.
- Collagenous fibrosis of the visceral pleura with haphazardly arranged elastic fibers.
- Subpleural intra-alveolar elastotic fibrosis.
- Alveolar septal elastosis.
- Increase in subpleural network of elastin fibers best appreciated at histochemistry with elastic tissue stains.
- Abrupt transition between the areas of fibro-elastosis and the surrounding unaffected

parenchyma with occasional fibroblastic foci at the leading edge of fibrosis (i.e., interface of PPFE and adjacent lung).

- Mild and patchy chronic inflammation within areas of fibrosis.
- Vascular fibrointimal thickening with partial stenosis in arteries and/or vascular microthrombi.
- Absence of classic honeycombing.
- Possible coexistence of other histologic features and/or patterns: granulomas, UIP/IPF, HP, NSIP.
- Diffuse alveolar damage, alveolar hemorrhage, and obliterative bronchiolitis are possible concomitant findings in lung or hematopoietic stem cell transplant recipients.

15.1.2 Differential Diagnosis

The main histologic differential diagnosis is between PPFE and UIP, either in its idiopathic form (IPF) or secondary to other known causes such as chronic HP, connective tissue disease-related interstitial lung disease (CTD-related ILD), drug reaction, asbestosis, or chronic fibrosing sarcoidosis. In the pure forms, PPFE and UIP are readily distinguishable. As the name implies, PPFE is a morphologically descriptive term denoting intense elastotic fibrosis of the visceral pleura and adjacent lung parenchyma. Elastosis is a distinctive form of chronic scarring in the lung that differs from the common scarring associated with extensive remodeling of the lung parenchyma and honeycomb changes which are appreciable in UIP pattern. Usually, PPFE lungs contain twice as much elastin fibers compared to UIP/IPF appreciable both on hematoxylin and eosin and using elastic stains in the upper lobes. The distinction between PPFE and UIP/IPF relies above all in the different predominant involvement of the lung parenchyma as follows: PPFE is an upper lobe-dominant elastotic fibrosis, whereas IPF is a lower lobe-dominant collagenous fibrosis. Both PPFE and UIP/IPF are characterized by a similar abrupt transition between fibrotic areas and spared juxtaposed lung, but PPFE lacks honeycombing and shows a smaller number of fibroblastic foci. In addition PPFE is prevalent among non-smok-

ers (62–85%), while the majority of patients with UIP/IPF are smokers [2–4].

Since UIP/IPF and PPFE can coexist in the same patient, the histologic interpretation becomes more difficult. These cases represent a disease entity distinct from UIP/IPF. Compared with patients with IPF, patients with PPFE and UIP/IPF had (1) higher complication rate of pneumothorax or pneumomediastinum, (2) lower BMI, (3) flattened chest, and (4) distinct pulmonary function with restrictive pattern, alveolar hypoventilation, and increased RV/TLC ratio and $PaCO_2$. The prognosis is worse, and the survival time is shorter in patients with PPFE and UIP/IPF than in patients with IPF [8]. The histologic problem centers on whether a PPFE-like change or UIP-like regions are significant or not, and the issue is best addressed with clinical and radiologic correlation.

The secondary UIP pattern seen in chronic HP should be differentiated from PPFE for its bronchiolocentric/centrilobular involvement with frequent sparing of the pleural surfaces and presence of scattered interstitial granulomas and/or giant cells. In addition a diagnosis of PPFE should only be made in absence of a relevant history of exposure to inhaling antigens.

The fibrotic stage of Langerhans cell histiocytosis may present with upper lobe fibrosis, and the distinction with PPFE depends on the identification of CD1a-positive Langerhans cells within fibrotic areas, on the stellate bronchiolocentric scars, and/or on the coexistent smoking-related damage typical of Langerhans cell histiocytosis.

The differential diagnosis out of PPFE also includes the residua of infections (previous history of tuberculosis and tuberculosis pneumothorax treatment, aspergillosis), as well as asbestos exposure, advanced chronic fibrotic sarcoidosis, or connective tissue disease.

The histological pattern of asbestos-related fibrosis tends to display more prominent parietal pleural thickening and more advanced remodeling and architectural distortion than PPFE.

Nonetheless, a confident diagnosis of PPFE should only be made in absence of a relevant occupational exposure history to asbestos as well as the lack of asbestos bodies, sarcoid-like granulomas, microorganisms at special stains, dense lymphoplasmacytic infiltrates, and/or numerous follicles with germinal centers suggestive of a CTD-related ILD.

The incidental lesion that morphologically and radiologically closely mimics PPFE is apical cap.

Apical cap is a localized lesion of lung apices in the form of subpleural pyramidal fibroelastotic scar, often resected for a radiologically suspected carcinoma. Characteristically, apical caps occur in older asymptomatic males, mostly smokers and are stable in time, while PPFE also affects younger, non-smoker patients, who present with symptoms and poor clinical outcome. Radiologically, apical caps do not involve the pleura circumferentially like PPFE. Histologically, apical caps consist of dense collagenous fibrosis and are often associated with pleural plaques, extensive alveolar collapse, and smoking-related damage of the adjacent parenchyma, which are not typically present in PPFE [2–4].

Finally, an upper lobe pulmonary fibrosis, radiologically consistent with PPFE but limited to unilateral lung, has been observed as an iatrogenic reaction in patients with a history of thoracotomy for resecting lung or esophageal cancers. In these cases the lesions are limited to the operated side [14].

15.1.3 Role of Cryobiopsy in the Diagnosis of PPFE

The pathologic diagnostic criteria of PPFE on cryobiopsy are the same as those on surgical lung biopsies: "Definite PPFE" is assigned when there are upper zone pleural fibrosis with subjacent intra-alveolar fibrosis accompanied by alveolar septal elastosis and sparing of the parenchyma distant from the pleura, at most mild patchy lymphoplasmacytic infiltrates and at most small numbers of fibroblastic foci; "Consistent with PPFE" is considered when intra-alveolar fibroelastosis is present, but it is not (1) associated with significant pleural fibrosis, (2) not predominantly beneath the pleura, or (3) not in an upper lobe biopsy; and "Inconsistent with PPFE" is the definition for cases lacking the requisite features above described [3].

Due to the transbronchial method of sampling, the pleura is included in cryobiopsies in about a third of cases; as a consequence the multidisciplinary discussion team including pulmonologists, radiologists, and pathologists with careful revision of imaging findings and knowledge of the clinical background of the patient (drug reaction, infection, inhalation exposures, lung/bone marrow transplantation, etc.) is always necessary to reach the proper diagnosis of PPFE [2–4]. However, the morphologic evidence of a prominent interstitial and/or intra-alveolar fibroelastosis in a cryobiopsy of symptomatic patient with a predominant upper lobe disease at imaging could be highly suggestive of PPFE.

15.2 Case Presentation

- **Clinical Background**
  - 55-year-old female
  - Non-smoker
  - Family history: no family history of ILD
  - Past medical history: Hashimoto thyroiditis on therapy with L-thyroxine; negative for prior chemotherapy or transplant
- **Onset of Symptoms**
  - Exertional dyspnea for a year and half
  - Cough, fever, weight loss, and fatigue for 6 months
- **Laboratory Findings**
  - Laboratory findings: unremarkable
  - Autoimmune status: negative
  - Quantiferon: negative
- **Pulmonary Function Test**
  - Slight reduction of DLCO
- **Imaging** (Figs. 15.1 and 15.2)
  - High-resolution computed tomography (HRCT) showed pleural and subpleural irregular fibrosis with traction bronchiectasis and tiny subpleural cysts in the apices and middle zones of both lungs.
- **Bronchoscopy with Cryobiopsy** (Figs. 15.3, 15.4, 15.5, and 15.6)
  - Cryobiopsies of the right upper lobe were obtained: two fragments of tissue 7.5 and 6.9 mm in maximum diameter, respectively (Fig. 15.3).

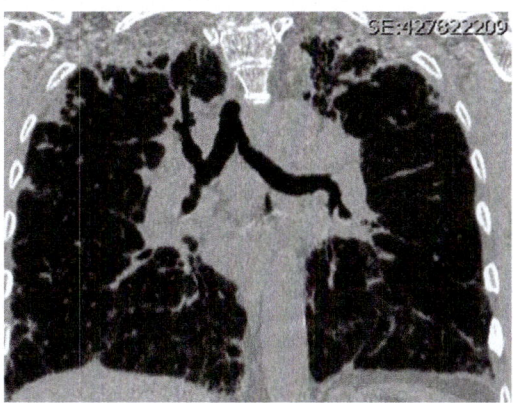

Fig. 15.1 HRCT of upper lung lobes evidenced pleural and subpleural thickening, fibrotic changes in the marginal parenchyma, traction bronchiectasis, architectural distortion, and fine subpleural cyst

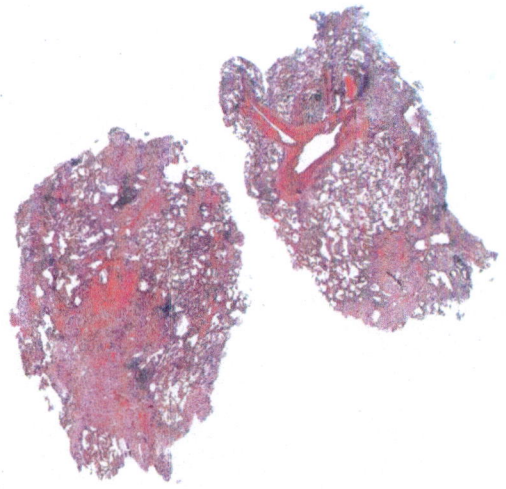

Fig. 15.3 Low-power view of the two cryobiopsies of 7.5 and 6.9 mm of maximum diameter. The sharp demarcation between the affected and the normal lung parenchyma was appreciable also at low-power

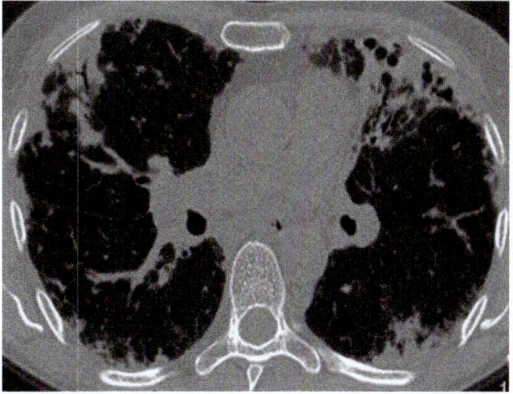

Fig. 15.2 A sharp demarcation between the affected and the normal lung was appreciated as well as an apical-caudal gradient

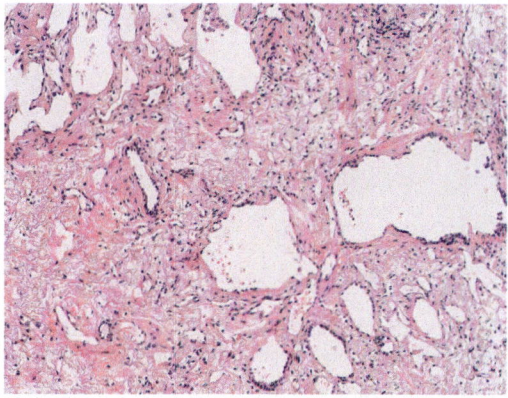

Fig. 15.4 Prominent septal fibroelastosis. Haphazardly arranged elastic fibers were detected at hematoxylin and eosin stains as short, curled, intensely eosinophilic fragments within a loose edematous fibroelastotic interstitium. A mild and patchy lymphoplasmacytic infiltrate coexisted

- The biopsies showed a subpleural and bronchiolocentric fibroelastotic process characterized by interstitial fibroelastosis with focal/mild inflammatory infiltrate (Fig. 15.4). Abrupt transition to the normal parenchyma was present, and scattered fibroblastic foci were also appreciated (Fig. 15.5).
- Histochemistry with Elastic van Gieson staining evidenced the prominent network of elastic fibers (Fig. 15.6).
- **Diagnosis**
  - Idiopathic pleuroparenchymal fibroelastosis.

15.3 Discussion

It has been recently showed that transbronchial cryobiopsy may be a valid method to obtain a histopathologic diagnosis in patients with suspected idiopathic PPFE and even airway-centered FE

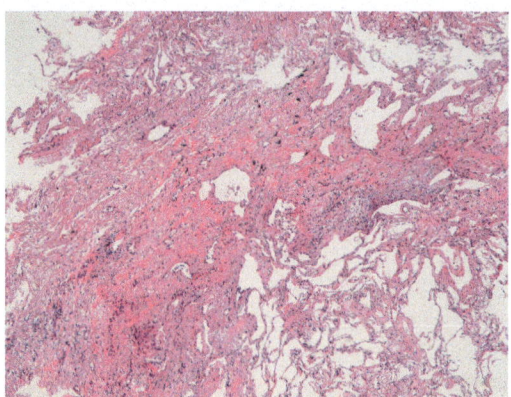

Fig. 15.5 The parenchyma adjacent to the fibroelastotic area was unremarkable, and a small fibroblastic focus was visible

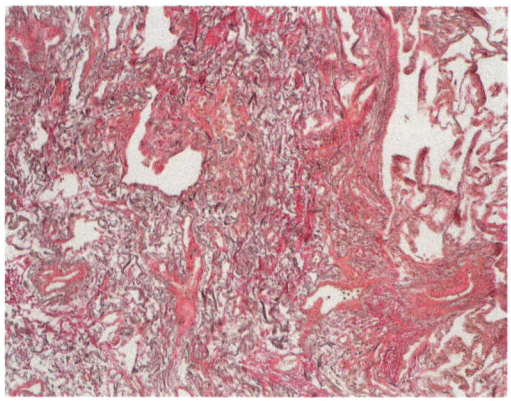

Fig. 15.6 Histochemistry with elastic stain showed short, curled, and randomly oriented elastic fibers within alveolar septa

and that it can be obtained with an acceptable complication rate. In fact, no bleeding (mild, moderate, or severe) was observed, and pneumothorax was documented in three out of eight cases, none of them requiring drainage or lasting more than 3 days. No death, acute lung injury, persistent fever, prolonged air leak, pneumonia/empyema, or other adverse events occurred after the procedure in any of the cases [15]. The critical point, mainly in cases of idiopathic PPFE, is to stay very peripheral with the probe (around 1 cm from the pleura) in order to retrieve tissue containing pleural-subpleural structures. The use of smaller cryoprobes (1.9 instead of 2.4) is

recommended to reach the upper portion of the lungs mainly in smaller subjects or in patients with bronchial malacia.

References

1. Travis WD, Costabel U, Hansell DM, King TE Jr, Lynch DA, Nicholson AG, Ryerson CJ, Ryu JH, Selman M, Wells AU, Behr J, Bouros D, Brown KK, Colby TV, Collard HR, Cordeiro CR, Cottin V, Crestani B, Drent M, Dudden RF, Egan J, Flaherty K, Hogaboam C, Inoue Y, Johkoh T, Kim DS, Kitaichi M, Loyd J, Martinez FJ, Myers J, Protzko S, Raghu G, Richeldi L, Sverzellati N, Swigris J, Valeyre D. An official American Thoracic Society/European Respiratory Society statement: update of the international multidisciplinary classification of the idiopathic interstitial pneumonias. Am J Respir Crit Care Med. 2013;188(6):733–48.
2. Camus P, von der Thüsen J, Hansell DM, Colby TV. Pleuroparenchymal fibroelastosis: one more walk on the wild side of drugs? Eur Respir J. 2014;44(2):289–96.
3. Reddy TL, Tominaga M, Hansell DM, von der Thusen J, Rassl D, Parfrey H, Guy S, Twentyman O, Rice A, Maher TM, Renzoni EA, Wells AU, Nicholson AG. Pleuroparenchymal fibroelastosis: a spectrum of histopathological and imaging phenotypes. Eur Respir J. 2012;40(2):377–85.
4. von der Thüsen JH. Pleuroparenchymal fibroelastosis: its pathological characteristics. Curr Respir Med Rev. 2013;9(4):238–47.
5. Mariani F, Gatti B, Rocca A, Bonifazi F, Cavazza A, Fanti S, Tomassetti S, Piciucchi S, Poletti V, Zompatori M. Pleuroparenchymal fibroelastosis: the prevalence of secondary forms in hematopoietic stem cell and lung transplantation recipients. Diagn Interv Radiol. 2016;22(5):400–6.
6. Newton CA, Batra K, Torrealba J, Kozlitina J, Glazer CS, Aravena C, Meyer K, Raghu G, Collard HR, Garcia CK. Telomere-related lung fibrosis is diagnostically heterogeneous but uniformly progressive. Eur Respir J. 2016;48(6):1710–20.
7. Miele A, Dhaliwal K, Du Toit N, Murchison JT, Dhaliwal C, Brooks H, Smith SH, Hirani N, Schwarz T, Haslett C, Wallace WA, McGorum BC. Chronic pleuropulmonary fibrosis and elastosis of aged donkeys: similarities to human pleuroparenchymal fibroelastosis. Chest. 2014;145(6):1325–32.
8. Oda T, Ogura T, Kitamura H, Hagiwara E, Baba T, Enomoto Y, Iwasawa T, Okudela K, Takemura T, Sakai F, Hasegawa Y. Distinct characteristics of pleuroparenchymal fibroelastosis with usual interstitial pneumonia compared with idiopathic pulmonary fibrosis. Chest. 2014;146(5):1248–55.
9. Awano N, Izumo T, Fukuda K, Tone M, Yamada D, Takemura T, Ikushima S, Kumasaka T. Is

hypothyroidism in idiopathic pleuroparenchymal fibroelastosis a novel lung-thyroid syndrome? Respir Investig. 2018;56(1):48–56.

10. Lowther CM, Morrison AO, Candelario NM, Khalafbeigi S, Cockerell CJ. Novel cutaneous manifestations of pleuroparenchymal fibroelastosis. Am J Dermatopathol. 2016;38(10):e140–3.

11. Enomoto Y, Nakamura Y, Satake Y, Sumikawa H, Johkoh T, Colby TV, Yasui H, Hozumi H, Karayama M, Suzuki Y, Furuhashi K, Fujisawa T, Enomoto N, Inui N, Iwashita T, Kuroishi S, Yokomura K, Koshimizu N, Toyoshima M, Imokawa S, Yamada T, Shirai T, Hayakawa H, Suda T. Clinical diagnosis of idiopathic pleuroparenchymal fibroelastosis: a retrospective multicenter study. Respir Med. 2017;133:1–5.

12. Oyama Y, Enomoto N, Suzuki Y, Kono M, Fujisawa T, Inui N, Nakamura Y, Kuroishi S, Yokomura K, Toyoshima M, Imokawa S, Oishi K, Watanabe S, Kasahara K, Baba T, Ogura T, Ishii H, Watanabe K, Nishioka Y, Suda T. Evaluation of urinary desmosines as a noninvasive diagnostic biomarker in patients with idiopathic pleuroparenchymal fibroelastosis (PPFE). Respir Med. 2017;123:63–70.

13. Sato S, Hanibuchi M, Takahashi M, Fukuda Y, Morizumi S, Toyoda Y, Goto H, Nishioka Y. A patient with idiopathic pleuroparenchymal fibroelastosis showing a sustained pulmonary function due to treatment with pirfenidone. Intern Med. 2016;55(5):497–501.

14. Sekine A, Satoh H, Iwasawa T, Matsui K, Ikeya E, Ikeda S, Yamakawa H, Okuda R, Kitamura H, Shinohara T, Baba T, Komatsu S, Kato T, Hagiwara E, Ogura T. Unilateral upper lung field pulmonary fibrosis radiologically consistent with pleuroparenchymal fibroelastosis after thoracotomy: a new disease entity related to thoracotomy. Respiration. 2017;94(5):431–41.

15. Kronborg-White S, Ravaglia C, Dubini A, et al. Cryobiopsies are diagnostic in pleuroparenchymal and airway-centered fibroelastosis. Respir Res. 2018;19:135.

Acute Lung Injury

16

Venerino Poletti, Giovanni Poletti,
Christian Gurioli, Carlo Gurioli,
and Alessandra Dubini

16.1 Introduction

Rapidly progressive respiratory failure (from days to a few weeks) with diffuse parenchymal lung infiltrates in CT scan is a clinical setting that may be determined by a variety of clinical and pathologic conditions [1]. The term acute lung injury may be used to define this setting. CT scan features are usually characterized by alveolar consolidation and/or ground glass attenuation [2]. Some peculiar aspects may address a specific diagnosis: alveolar consolidation surrounded by ground glass attenuation (the "halo sign") is seen mainly in infections and in organizing pneumo-

V. Poletti (✉)
Department of Diseases of the Thorax,
Ospedale Morgagni-Pierantoni, Forlì, Italy

Department of Respiratory Diseases and Allergy,
Aarhus University Hospital, Aarhus, Denmark

G. Poletti
Hematologic Section, Corelab, Azienda USL
Romagna, Pievesestina, Cesena, Italy

C. Gurioli · C. Gurioli
Department of Diseases of the Thorax,
Ospedale Morgagni-Pierantoni, Forlì, Italy

A. Dubini
Department of Diseases of the Thorax-Pulmonology
Unit, Azienda Usl della Romagna, Ospedale GB
Morgagni, Forlì, Italy

nia; the reversed "halo sign" (atoll sign) is more typically observed in cases with organizing pneumonia; and the perilobular sign may suggest the diagnosis of antisynthetase syndrome manifesting mainly as lung involvement or a diagnosis of Niemann-Pick disease. The pathologic background is highly heterogenous. Usually however this background may be identified without the need of biopsies because bronchoalveolar lavage (BAL) is diagnostic. Atypical type II pneumocytes with evident nucleoli and with finely textured cyanophilic cytoplasm and frequently fine or large cytoplasmic vacuoles appearing singly in flat plaques or in rosettes or pseupapillae are grouped around extracellular amorphic and metachromatic material and are the cytological hallmark of the histopathologic patterns called "diffuse alveolar damage" [3]. Inflammatory cells may consist of neutrophils (in classical diffuse alveolar damage pattern), eosinophils (in acute eosinophilic pneumonia), or even lymphocytes with a "Lutzner-like" appearance (in explosive organizing pneumonia or in a minority of cases of the yet not well-known idiopathic entity labeled by the morphological term "acute fibrinous and organizing pneumonia," in cases of antisynthetase syndrome, in drug-induced lung injury) [4–8]. The coexistence of hemosiderin-laden macrophages and red cells is diagnostic of alveolar hemorrhage/capillaritis (typically observed in ANCA-associated vasculitis or systemic lupus erythematosus). Infectious causes (from bacteria to DNA viruses) may be detected also. Finally microbiological investigation in BAL fluid, including molecular biological tests, is very sensitive and specific for identification of causative agents. Rarely rapidly progressive respiratory failure may be due to lung neoplasms (carcinomatous lymphangitis or neoplastic thrombotic microangiopathy, acute myeloid leukemia, metastatic melanoma) or to fat embolism. In this context however BAL may again contribute significantly to the final diagnostic [9].

Therefore lung biopsy is indicated only when BAL result to be inconclusive [10].

16.2 Case Series

Case 1

A 48-year-old male, non-smoker, truck-driver, was admitted to the hospital for acute dyspnea. Physical examination was not relevant. Gas analysis documented a severe hypoxemia (PaO_2 while breathing room air at rest = 54 mmHg) and hypocapnia. Pulmonary function tests were not performed due to the severe dyspnea. Routine laboratory tests were not relevant except a significant reduction of absolute lymphocyte count (lymphocytes = 385×10^9/L). High-resolution CT scan documented diffuse ground glass attenuation with superimposed interlobular septal thickening and intralobular reticular thickening ("crazy paving" pattern) (Fig. 16.1a). BAL was diagnostic of *Pneumocystis jiroveci* and *Cytomegalovirus* pneumonia (Fig. 16.1b, c). Further investigations documented an HIV infection and a marked CD4+ lymphopenia.

Case 2

A 54 year-old, housewife, non-smoker female was admitted to the hospital for low-grade fever since 1 month and rapidly progressive dyspnea in the last week. Family history was not relevant. Pulmonary function tests documented a restrictive defect with FVC = 58% of predicted and DLCO = 35% of predicted. Gas analysis, while breathing room air at rest, showed a PaO_2 of 59 mmHg and $PaCO_2$ of 31 mmHg. Physical examination showed only inspiratory rales

and a high-pitched, mid-systolic crescendo-decrescendo murmur at the apex of the heart (mitral valve prolapse). CT scan showed alveolar consolidations and ground glass opacities distributed in the upper and lower parts of the lung with a gradient and mainly in the subpleural regions with a perilobular pattern (Fig. 16.2a).

Bronchoalveolar lavage fluid cell count documented an increase of total cells (450,000/mm^3) and an increase of lymphocytes (39%, in the great majority CD3+, with a CD4/CD8 ratio of 0.7) and of neutrophils (19%) with scattered eosinophils and mast cells. Some reactive type II pneumocytes singly or in small cluster were also present. Transbronchial cryobiopsies were taken from the lateral segment of the lower right lobe and the dorsal segment of the upper right lobe (Fig. 16.2b, c).

Autoimmune tests were not relevant except positivity for autoantibodies against PL-7 (threonyl-tRNA synthetase).

A diagnosis of idiopathic organizing pneumonia (with fibrin) and nonspecific interstitial pneumonia with an autoimmune background was rendered. This case has all the characteristics to be classified as idiopathic interstitial pneumonia with autoimmune features (IPAF). This is not a diagnosis but a heterogenous category. The morphologic features (perilobular pattern in CT scan and a mixed pattern in histology-organizing pneumonia with fibrin and nonspecific interstitial pneumonia) predict a good response to steroids and immunosuppressors. In fact the patient improved significantly after treatment with steroids (high doses at the beginning) and mycophenolate.

Case 3

A 37-year-old male, bank employee and smoker (11 packs/year), was admitted to intensive care unit for rapidly progressive respiratory failure. He had two previous episodes of acute dyspnea in the last 2 years diagnosed as community-acquired pneumonia and treated with a short course of antibiotics and steroids. CT scan showed a diffuse "crazy paving" pattern (Fig. 16.3a).

Laboratory tests documented normal functional renal indexes and a significant increase of

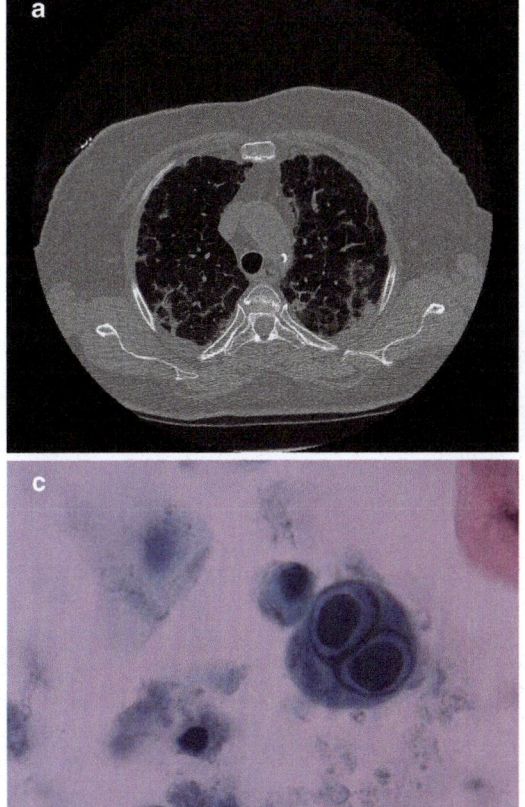

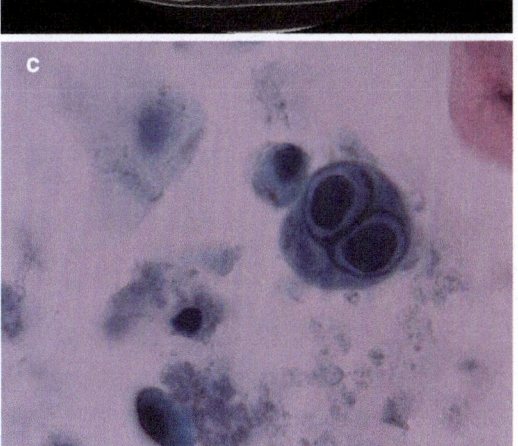

Fig. 16.1 (**a**) HRCT: crazy paving pattern and some alveolar consolidations in the upper lobes. (**b**) A cluster of extracellular foamy material consisting of spherical "cysts" with a thin wall containing one or two dot-like trophozoites. These casts are essentially diagnostic of *Pneumocystis jiroveci* (May Grunwald Giemsa). (**c**) A markedly enlarged cell with large, basophilic intranuclear inclusions surrounded by a clear halo and tiny satellite basophilic inclusions in the cytoplasm. Extracellular foamy exudate is also present. These cytological aspects are typically due to *Cytomegalovirus*. The foamy exudate represents casts of *Pneumocystis* (Papanicolaou)

C-reactive protein and of LDH and a slight increase of neutrophils. Autoimmunity tests, including ANCA autoantibodies, were negative.

Bloody lavage (increase on sequential aliquots of bloody fluid) was macroscopically evident, and the microscopic analysis documented fresh red cells, neutrophils, and siderophages.

Transbronchial cryobiopsy samples showed typical features of neutrophilic capillaritis (Fig. 16.3b). Because of the primary lung involvement, negative autoimmunity tests, negative tests for cocaine abuse, and a clinical history excluding use of drugs known to elicit an alveolar hem-

orrhage, a diagnosis of idiopathic pulmonary capillaritis was done. The patient was treated with steroids and cyclophosphamide.

16.3 Discussion

Lung biopsy is rarely useful in patients with acute lung failure and bilateral lung infiltrates, mainly when they are in noninvasive or mechanical ventilation. In fact in the majority of cases, blood laboratory tests are pivotal for a definite diagnosis. BAL may support the diagnosis in

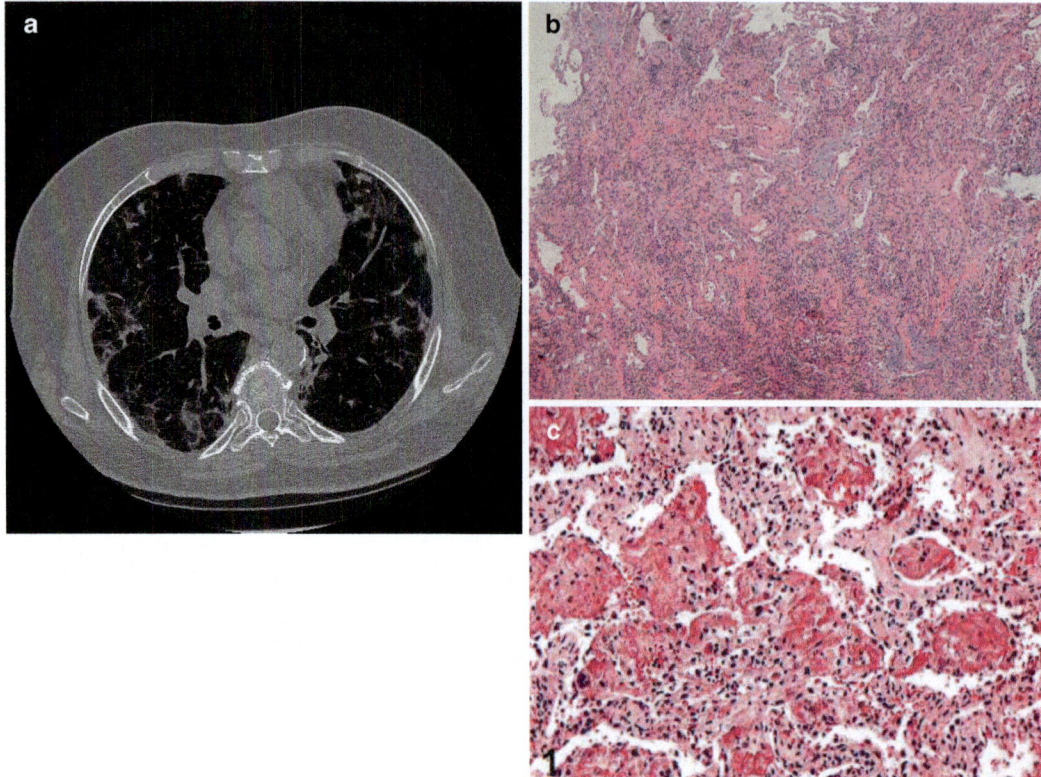

Fig. 16.2 (a) Peripheral alveolar consolidation and ground glass opacities predominantly located at the bounderies of the lobules with a poorly defined arcadelike or polygonal appearance (perilobular pattern) in the upper and lower parts of both lungs. (b) Nonspecific interstitial pneumonia. Preserved alveolar lung architecture with widened alveolar septa for fibrosis and chronic inflamma-tory cells infiltration. Ellipsoidal intra-alveolar buds of granulation tissue—pale in H and E—rich in extracellular matrix are also present (hematoxylin-eosin, low power). (c) In some areas intra-alveolar ball of fibrin with embed-ded inflammatory cells are also present (hematoxylin-eosin, mid power)

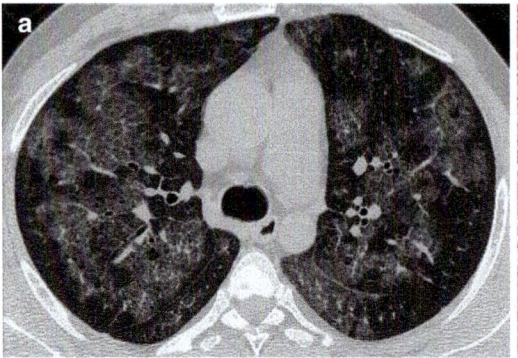
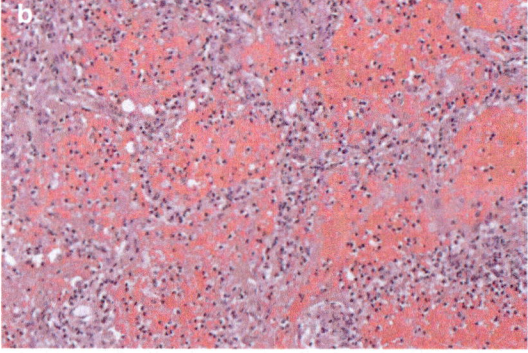

Fig. 16.3 (a) CT scan. Ground glass opacities and super-imposed reticulation with sparing of the subpleural regions. (b) Alveolar walls are infiltrated and partly destroyed by neutrophils that spill into the adjacent alveo-lar spaces. Alveolar spaces contain also numerous red blood cells and fibrin (hematoxylin-eosin, mid power)

cases in which these tests will not be conclusive. Recent papers considering the role of surgical lung biopsy in this context did not explore the role of BAL and mainly they did not investigate the diagnostic value of cytological analysis of BAL fluid [10, 11]. Transbronchial forceps biopsy in combination with BAL was shown to increase the diagnostic confidence with no associated important complications [12]. The potential role of transbronchial cryobiopsy in acute respiratory distress syndrome has been recently addressed [13]. Transbronchial cryobiopsy in ventilated patients is done without the use of fluoroscopic guide, and an increase of pneumothorax rate or even bleeding is expected. This last complication may be reduced using bronchial blockers and stopping immediately the retrieval of the bronchoscope—after having frozen the probe—when resistance is felt. Transbronchial cryobiopsy may provide with large and well-preserved samples to have a diagnosis of organizing pneumonia (with or without fibrin), diffuse alveolar damage, or pulmonary capillaritis or confirm the histopathologic background in subjects with acute-subacute disease that may be categorized as IPAF [14].

References

1. Katzenstein AL. Acute lung injury pa Fourth Edtterns: diffuse alveolar damage and bronchiolitis obliterans-organizing pneumonia. In: Katzenstein AL, editor. Katzenstein and Askin's non-neoplastic lung disease. 4th ed. Philadelphia: Saunders Elsevier; 2006. p. 17–49.
2. Dalpiaz G, Cancellieri A. Alveolar pattern. In: Dalpiaz G, Cancellieri A, editors. Atlas of diffuse lung disease. Cham: Springer; 2017. p. 145–201.
3. Linssen KC, Jacobs JA, Poletti V, van Mook W, Cornelissen EI, Drent M. Reactive type II pneumocytes in bronchoalveolar lavage fluid. Acta Cytol. 2004;48:497–504.
4. Cazzato S, Zompatori M, Baruzzi G, et al. Bronchiolitis obliterans-organizing pneumonia: an Italian experience. Respir Med. 2000;94:702–8.
5. Nishino M, Mathai SK, Schoenfeld D, Digumarthy SR, Kradin RL. Clinicopathologic features associated with relapse in cryptogenic organizing pneumonia. Hum Pathol. 2014;45:342–51.
6. Torrealba JR, Fisher S, Kanne JP, et al. Pathology-radiology correlation of common and uncommon computed tomographic patterns of organizing pneumonia. Hum Pathol. 2018;71:30–40.
7. Ravaglia C, Gurioli C, Casoni G, Romagnoli M, Tomassetti S, Gurioli C, Corso RM, Poletti G, Dubini A, Marinou A, Poletti V. Diagnostic role of rapid on-site cytologic examination (ROSE) of broncho-alveolar lavage in ALI/ARDS. Pathologica. 2012;104:65–9.
8. Poletti V, Poletti G, Murer B, Saragoni L, Chilosi M. Bronchoalveolar lavage in malignancy. Semin Respir Crit Care Med. 2007;28:534–45.
9. Fan E, Brodie D, Slutsky AS. Acute respiratory distress syndrome: advances in diagnosis and treatment. JAMA. 2018;319:698–710.
10. Park J, Lee YJ, Lee J, et al. Histopathologic heterogeneity of acute respiratory distress syndrome revealed by surgical lung biopsy and its clinical implications. Korean J Intern Med. 2018;33:532–40.
11. Pillipponet C, Cassagnes L, Pereira B, et al. Diagnostic yield and therapeutic impact of open lung biopsy in the critically ill patient. PLoS One. 2018;13:e0196795.
12. Bulpa PA, Dive AM, Mertens L, et al. Combined bronchoalveolar lavage and transbronchial lung biopsy: safety and yield in ventilated patients. Eur Respir J. 2003;21:489–94.
13. Dincer HE, Zamora F, Gibson H, Cho RJ. The first report of safety and feasibility of transbronchial cryoprobe lung biopsy in ARDS. Intensive Care Med. 2018;44:971–2.
14. Poletti V, Casoni GL, Cancellieri A, Piciucchi S, Dubini A, Zompatori M. Diffuse alveolar damage. Pathologica. 2010;102:453–63.

Disseminated Neoplasms

17

Venerino Poletti, Angelo Carloni, and Marco Chilosi

17.1 Introduction

Disseminated pulmonary neoplasms mimicking interstitial lung disorders (ILDs) represent a heterogenous group including metastases from neoplasms originating in the lungs or from outside the lungs and disseminated neoplasms appearing also or mainly in the lungs [1–3]. Carcinomatous lymphangitis, neoplastic thrombotic microangiopathy, and metastatic angiosarcoma are the prototypes of the first group; lymphoproliferative lung disorders, lymphangioleiomyomatosis, pulmonary epithelioid hemangioendothelioma, primary pulmonary angiosarcoma, and Kaposi sarcoma are good examples in the second group. Langerhans cell histiocytosis and Erdheim-Chester disease are now considered inflammatory myeloid neoplasms, and they may appear as limited to the lungs [4, 5]. Other rare dissemi-

nated tumors manifesting in the lungs that may mimic ILDs are minute pulmonary meningothelial-like nodules [6], diffuse idiopathic pulmonary neuroendocrine cell hyperplasia with obliterative bronchiolitis (DIPNECH) [7] and the socalled pulmonary benign metastasizing leiomyoma. Inflammatory myofibroblastic tumor may occur as scattered nodules or infiltrates in the lungs. Whether it is a low-grade mesenchymal neoplasm or a nonneoplastic reactive inflammatory lesion is still controversial; however based on the identification of consistent clonal abnormalities (recently EML4-ALK rearrangement was documented in inflammatory myofibroblastic tumors) [8] as well as local recurrence, local invasion, and metastases in some cases, it is included in the group of mesenchymal and miscellaneous tumors by many authors.

The clinical manifestations are quite variegated. The most acute pulmonary symptoms (dyspnea, cough, hemoptysis) are observed in carcinomatous lymphangitis, neoplastic thrombotic microangiopathy, intravascular lymphoma, and metastatic angiosarcoma. Pneumothorax may be the first clinical sign of Langerhans cell histiocytosis. Laboratory tests are not specific although a significant increase of LDH and gas analysis values consisting with pulmonary thromboembolism are typically present in cases of intravascular lymphoma. New onset pulmonary hypertension may reveal a neoplastic thrombotic microangiopathy.

V. Poletti (✉)
Department of Diseases of the Thorax, Ospedale
Morgagni-Pierantoni, Forlì, Italy

Department of Respiratory Diseases and Allergy,
Aarhus University Hospital, Aarhus, Denmark

A. Carloni
Department of Radiology, Ospedale di Terni,
Terni, Italy

M. Chilosi
Verona University, Verona, Italy

Department of Pathology, P. Pederzoli Hospital,
Peschiera del Garda, Italy
e-mail: marco.chilosi@univr.it

© Springer Nature Switzerland AG 2019
V. Poletti (ed.), *Transbronchial cryobiopsy in diffuse parenchymal lung disease*,
https://doi.org/10.1007/978-3-030-14891-1_17

CT scan features are quite characteristic even if not diagnostic. Hematogenous metastases from solid tumors are usually characterized by nodules with a random distribution, sometimes with the "feeding vessel" sign. In carcinomatous lymphangitis, interlobular, more frequently nodular, septal thickening, peribronchovascular cuffing, enlarged hilar and/or mediastinal lymph nodes, and not infrequently small pleural effusion are the imaging hallmarks. The classic imaging features of pulmonary Kaposi sarcoma are peribronchovascular consolidations with flame-shaped hilar radiation. Other CT findings include poorly defined lung nodules, interlobular septal thickening, patchy ground-glass opacities, fissural nodularity with distortion, and small pleural effusion. In neoplastic thrombotic microangiopathy, the so-called pseudo tree in bud pattern is present. Metastatic angiosarcoma may manifest with alveolar nodules surrounded by ground-glass attenuation ("halo sign"). Lung parenchymal capillary infiltration of acute myeloid leukemia (M4 and M5 subtypes) or by melanoma cells determines an acute alveolar hemorrhage with ground-glass opacities. CT scan features of DIPNECH are mosaic oligemia with expiratory air-trapping and some scattered small nodules. Cysts and nodules are typical of Langerhans cells histiocytosis and of metastatic epithelial tumors ("cheerios" in the lung), and cysts are the hallmark of LAM but may be also due to other metastatic low-grade sarcomas. In Erdheim-Chester disease, interlobular septal thickening, pulmonary nodules, airway wall thickening, and ground-glass opacities are found in the large majority of cases. However extrathoracic findings are an important clue for the diagnosis: symmetric osteosclerosis involving the metaphyses and diaphyses of the long bones, the "coated aorta," the "hairy" kidneys, and coronary artery sheathing.

The new therapeutic approaches deriving from a great progress in comprehension of pathogenetic mechanisms at the molecular level require enough material for identification of targetable genetic modifications. Therefore biopsy is gaining the role it had in the past also in the diagnosis of disseminated tumors in the lungs.

17.2   Case Series

Case 1

A 55-year-old-male, a plumber, nonsmoker, was admitted to the hospital for a 3-month history of dry cough, fatigue, shortness of breath, and weight loss. His medical history was relevant because he was treated 10 years ago for chronic myeloid leukemia (chemotherapy, allogeneic bone marrow transplant, and then imatinib). Current treatment: none. Medical examination was unremarkable (no digital clubbing, no Velcro sounds). Saturation of O_2 at rest while breathing room air = 93%. Laboratory tests documented only a slight increase of reactive C protein. Pulmonary function tests: FVC = 60% of predicted; DLCO = 56% of predicted. Gas analysis: PaO_2 = 88 mmHg; $PaCO_2$ = 46.6 mmHg; pH = 7.355. CT scan documented multiple nodules prevalent into the basal portions of both lungs with variable size and with hypodense centers (so-called "cheerios in the lung" pattern) (Fig. 17.1a).

A previous transbronchial lung biopsy with regular forceps and BAL were not diagnostic. Transbronchial cryobiopsies using a 2.4 probe were carried out in the right lower lobe in different segments. A diagnosis of adenocarcinoma with enteric phenotype was done (Fig. 17.1b–e).

Case 2

A 51-year-old-male was admitted to the hospital for rapidly progressive dyspnea. Saturation at rest while breathing room air was 89%.

CT scan showed nodular thickening of interlobular septa. A "vascular" tree in bud pattern was also present (Fig. 17.2a).

Transbronchial cryobiopsies in the lower right lobe documented carcinomatous lymphangitis and neoplastic thrombotic microangiopathy (Fig. 17.2b, c).

Case 3

A 63-year-old female, former smoker (quitted 8 years ago: 20 packs/year). Housewife. Right pneumonia in 2008.

Episodes of acute bronchitis since 2008. Arterial hypertension under treatment (beta-blocker).

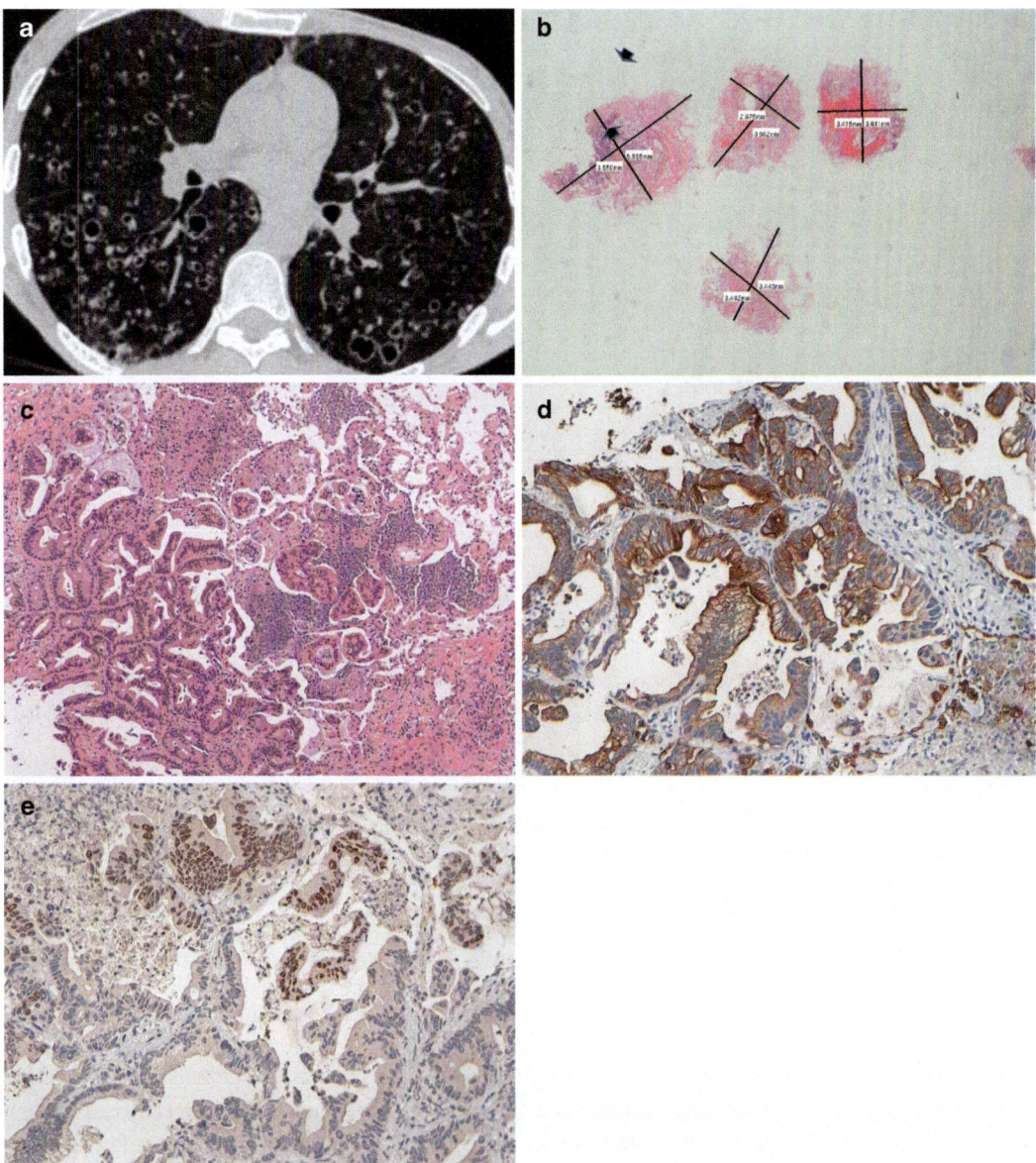

Fig. 17.1 (**a**) CT scan showing nodules of variable size, in the lower lobes, with hypodense centers. (**b**) Four samples obtained by using a cryoprobe. Only one documents part of a cavitated nodule. The wall is made by neoplastic cells (arrows) that appear blue at low power in contrast with the normal lung parenchyma that appear pink (hematoxylin-eosin, low power). (**c**) Cryobiopsy sample. Malignant cells growing with a glandular/papillary pattern and with intervening cellular debris (hematoxylin-eosin, midpower). (**d**) The neoplastic cells are clearly marked by anti-cytokeratin antibodies (CK 7). (**e**) Part of the neoplastic cells show a nuclear positivity for CDX2, a marker of enteric phenotype

Admitted to the hospital for mild dyspnea on effort, arthromyalgias. She claimed also for a Raynaud phenomenon since 2 years. Routine laboratory tests were not relevant. Autoimmunity tests revealed a positivity for Ku and Ro52 antibodies. In serum a small IgG-lambda monoclonal peak was also detected. Spirometry was normal and DLCO was moderately reduced (55% of predicted.

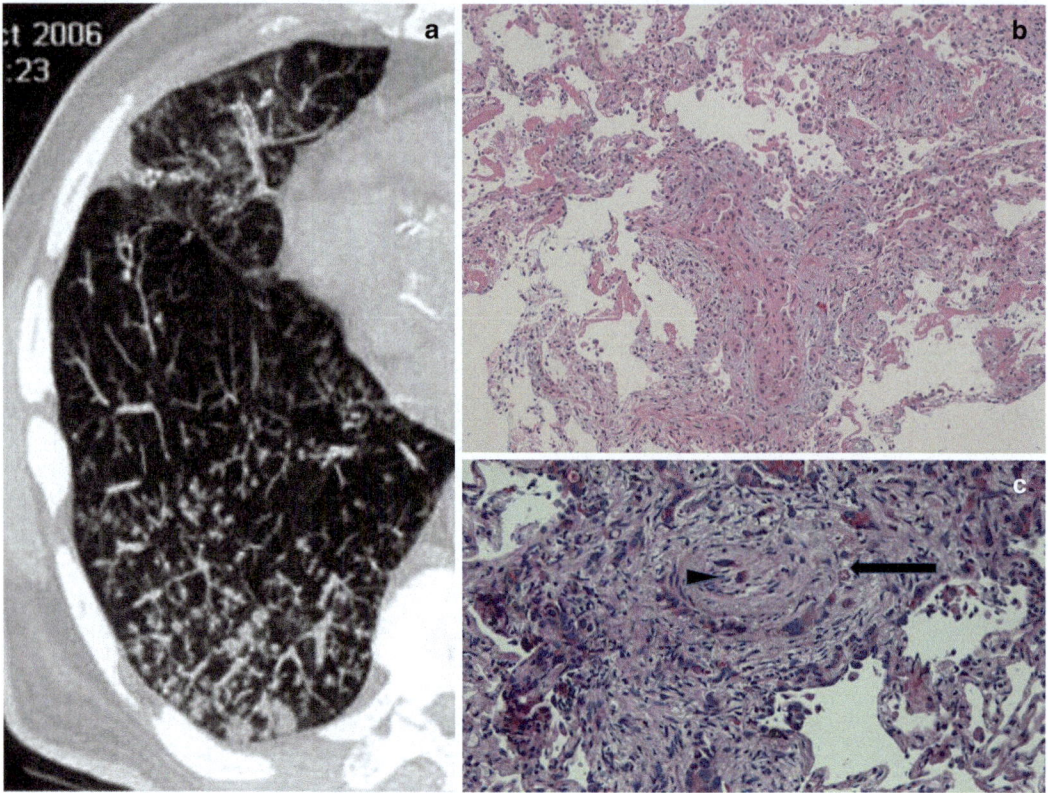

Fig. 17.2 (**a**) Nodular thickening of the interlobular septa more evident in the middle lobe and "vascular" tree in bud pattern in the lower right lobe. Nodules are evident at the end of small pulmonary arteries. (**b**) Transbronchial cryobiopsy. A dilated lymphatic containing neoplastic cells clustered in a glandular structure (carcinomatous lymphangitis). Features of acute diffuse alveolar damage are also present (hyaline membranes, thickening of the alveolar walls for edema and accumulation of extracellular matrix and myofibroblasts) (hematoxylin-eosin, midpower). (**c**) The lumen of a small pulmonary artery is completely occluded (arrow) by an organized thrombus with embedded scattered neoplastic cells containing mucin (arrowhead) (PAS, midpower)

CT scan documented alveolar nodular consolidations, areas of ground-glass attenuation along the bronchovascular bundles, and some cysts (Fig. 17.3a, b). BAL cytogram: macrophages 73%, lymphocytes 23%, neutrophils 1%, eosinophils 1%. Lymphocyte subsetting by flow cytometry documented 15% of CD 19 lymphocytes (mature B cells) with a monoclonal restriction (lambda). Transbronchial lung biopsies were carried out in the left lower lobe after identification of the lesion with a radial echography. Identification of lymphoid infiltration and identification of a monoclonal restriction allowed a diagnosis of MALT lymphoma.

Case 4

A 45-year-old female, smoker (20 packs/year), employed in a shopping mall, was referred to the hospital for detection of an interstitial disease in the chest X-ray film. The chest X-ray was required for not relevant clinical reasons.

Laboratory examinations were unremarkable. Pulmonary function tests showed a slight obstructive impairment (FEV1FVC = 69%) and a slight decrease of DLCO (71% of predicted). Physical examination was negative.

CT scan showed irregular cysts and some nodules in the upper lobes with sparing of the lung bases.

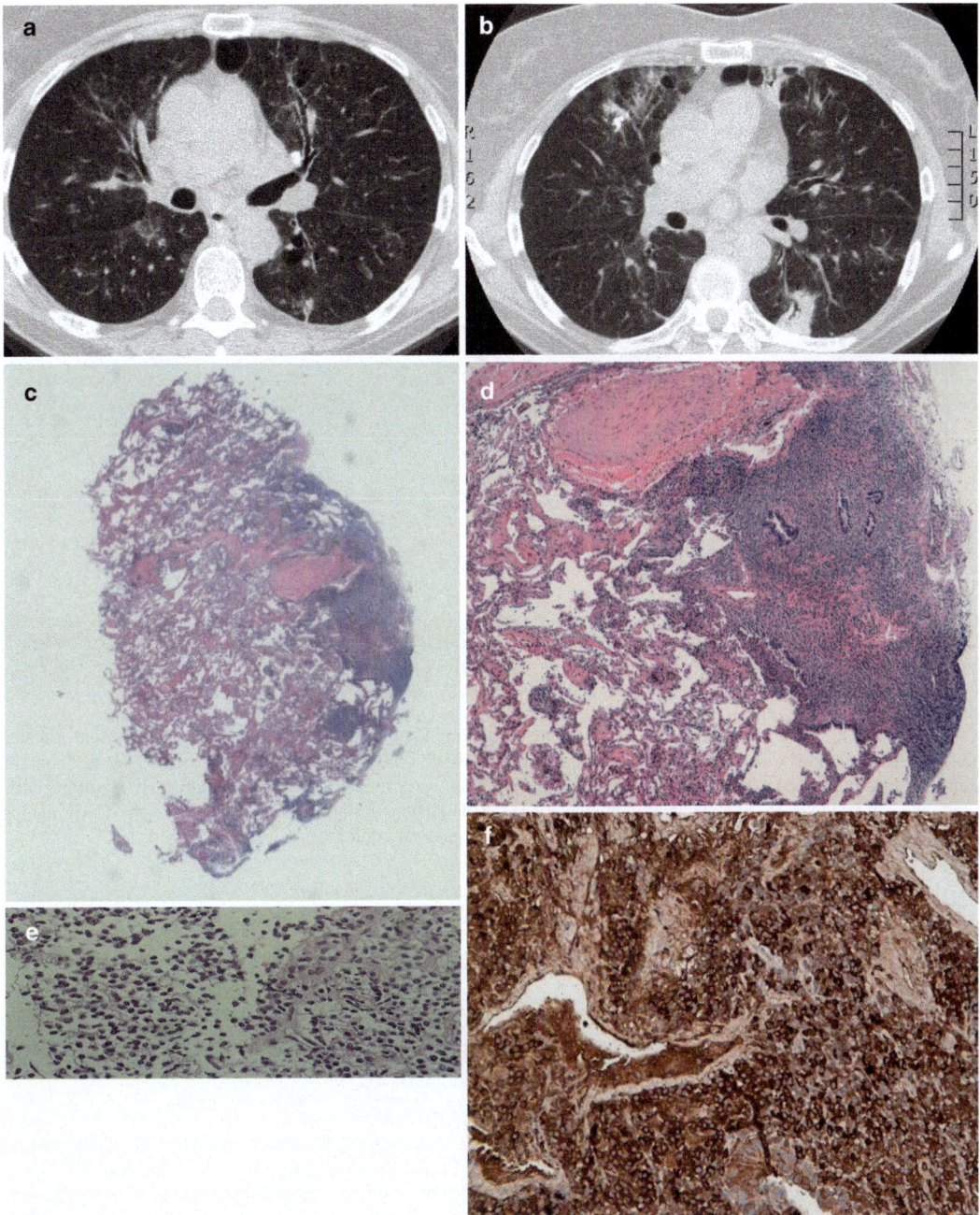

Fig. 17.3 (**a**) CT showing areas of ground-glass attenuation mainly along the bronchovascular bundles and some cysts. (**b**) Alveolar consolidation with air bronchogram is evident in the left lower lobe. (**c**) Transbronchial cryobiopsy sample showing a lymphoid infiltrate with a perilymphatic distribution (mainly sited along a bronchovascular bundle with sparing of the surrounding alveolar spaces) (hematoxylin-eosin, low power). (**d**) At higher power is possible to see that the lymphoid infiltrate tends to obstruct the small airways (hematoxylin-eosin, midpower). (**e**) At higher magnification epithelial-lymphoid complexes are identifiable (small lymphocytes infiltrate the bronchiolar epithelium) (hematoxylin-eosin, high power). (**f**) Lymphoid cells express surface lambda chains (monoclonal restriction)

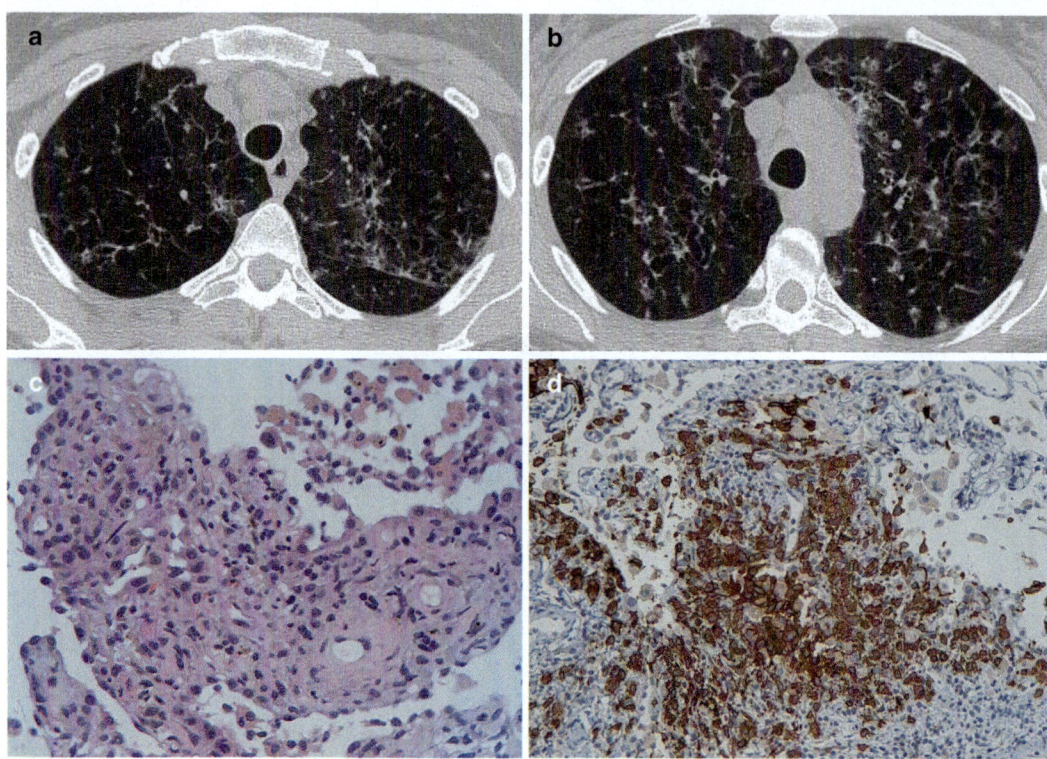

Fig. 17.4 (a) CT scan showing irregular cysts, emphysematous changes, and some centrilobular nodules with central hypodensity. (b) CT scan. Centrilobular "escavated" and solid nodules are more evident in the lower portions of the upper lobes. (c) Transbronchial cryobiopsy. A cluster of cells with grooved nuclei mixed with scattered lymphocytes and eosinophils is evident around a small vessel. The surrounding alveolar spaces contain "smoker" macrophages (hematoxylin-eosin, midpower). (d) Histiocytes are strongly marked by anti-CD1a monoclonal antibodies

BAL showed an increase of total cells (550×10^6/L) with a normal cytogram (Fig. 17.4a, b). The majority of macrophages had a cytoplasm laden by brown granules. Immunohistochemical analysis with CD1a antibodies marked the 2% of the macrophages.

Transbronchial cryobiopsies using a 1.9 cryoprobe were taken from the upper left lobe. The pathologic report was diagnostic for Langerhans cell histiocytosis (Fig. 17.4c, d). Detection of BRAF >V600E mutation by immunohistochemistry was negative. A diagnosis of Langerhans cell histiocytosis primary in the lung was done.

References

1. Murer B, Chilosi M, Hasleton P, Flieder DB. Metastases involving the lungs. In: Hasleton P, Flieder DB, editors. Spencer's pathology of the lung, vol. 2. Cambridge: Cambridge University Press; 2013. p. 1375–407.
2. Allen TC, Cagle PT, Flieder DB. Mesenchymal and miscellaneous neoplasms. In: Hasleton P, Flieder DB, editors. Spencer's pathology of the lung, vol. 2. Cambridge: Cambridge University Press; 2013. p. 1224–315.
3. Poletti V, Ravaglia C, Tomassetti S, et al. Lymphoproliferative lung disorders: clinicopathological aspects. Eur Respir Rev. 2013;22:427–36.

4. Milne P, Bigley V, Bacon CM, et al. Hematopoietic origin of Langerhans cell histiocytosis and Erdheim-Chester disease in adults. Blood. 2017;130:167–75.
5. Ozkaya N, Rosenblum MK, Durham DH, et al. The histopathology of Erdheim Chester disease: a comprehensive review of a molecularly characterized cohort. Mod Pathol. 2018;31:581–97.
6. Weissferdt A, Tang X, Suster S, Wistuba II, Moran C. Pleuroparenchymal meningothelial proliferations: evidence for a common histogenesis. Am J Surg Pathol. 2015;39:1673–8.
7. Mengoli MC, Rossi G, Cavazza A, et al. Diffuse idiopathic pulmonary neuroendocrine cell hyperplasia (DIPNECH) syndrome and carcinoid tumors with or without NECH: a clinicopathologic, radiologic and immunomolecular comparison study. Am J Surg Pathol. 2018;42:646–55.
8. Vargas-Madueno F, Gould E, Valor R, Ngo N, Zhang L, Villalona-Calero MA. EML4-ALK rearrangement and its therapeutic implications in inflammatory myofibroblastic tumors. Oncologist. 2018;23(10):1127–32.

Miscellaneous

18

Venerino Poletti, Antonella Arcadu,
Christian Gurioli, Fabio Sultani,
Linda Tagliaboschi, Carlo Gurioli,
and Giovanni Poletti

18.1 Pulmonary Alveolar Proteinosis

Pulmonary alveolar proteinosis (PAP) syndrome was first described in 1958 by Samuel H. Rosen et al. [1]. Since that time, clinicians' understanding of this rare lung disease has improved dramatically [2]. It is characterized by the accumulation of surfactant in the alveoli and terminal airways eventually resulting, in the majority of cases, in hypoxemic respiratory failure.

There are three separate pathways to the development of surfactant accumulation within alveoli: congenital, secondary, and autoimmune. All three of these pathways result in decreased clearance of surfactant, rather than increased production. Autoimmune PAP is the most common pathophysiologic mechanism accounting for 90% of documented cases. Autoimmune PAP is initi-

ated by immunoglobulin (Ig)-G anti-granulocyte macrophage colony-stimulating factor (anti-GM-CSF) antibodies, which decrease functional alveolar macrophages. Secondary PAP lacks anti-GM-CSF antibodies but has decreased functional macrophages secondary to hematological malignancies (myelodysplastic syndrome, chronic myelogenous leukemia, among others) or primary immunodeficiency diseases (common variable immunodeficiency, DiGeorge syndrome, among others) or GATA2 deficiency, an immunodeficiency and bone marrow failure disorder caused by pathogenic variants of GATA2 (a defect inherited in an autosomal-dominant pattern or due to de novo sporadic germline mutation) [3]. In this disorder morphological alterations include also sarcoid-like granulomas and pulmonary fibrosis. Secondary PAP has also been associated with inhalation of several environmental exposures. These environmental exposures include silica, talc, cement, kaolin, aluminum, titanium, indium, and cellulose. Reports suggest a link between indium inhalation and anti-GM-CSF antibodies, suggesting these toxic inhalations might induce autoantibodies. Hereditary dysfunction in one of many proteins responsible for surfactant regulation causes congenital PAP. This includes mutations in the GM-CSF receptor alpha-subunit or beta-subunit, surfactant protein B, surfactant protein C, ATP-binding cassette 3, NK2 homeobox 1, or the lysinuric protein intolerance disease. Mutations in the telomerase complex may lead to

V. Poletti (✉)
Department of Diseases of the Thorax,
Ospedale Morgagni-Pierantoni, Forlì, Italy

Department of Respiratory Diseases and Allergy,
Aarhus University Hospital, Aarhus, Denmark

A. Arcadu · C. Gurioli · F. Sultani · L. Tagliaboschi
C. Gurioli
Department of Diseases of the Thorax,
Ospedale Morgagni-Pierantoni, Forlì, Italy

G. Poletti
Hematologic Section, Corelab, Azienda USL
Romagna, Pievesestina, Cesena, Italy

© Springer Nature Switzerland AG 2019
V. Poletti (ed.), *Transbronchial cryobiopsy in diffuse parenchymal lung disease*,
https://doi.org/10.1007/978-3-030-14891-1_18

pulmonary fibrosis, cirrhosis, bone marrow failure, or cutaneous diseases. A 35-year-old patient with initial diagnosis of PAP and evolution to lung fibrosis associated with TERT mutation had been recently described [4]. Congenital PAP is the least common form. The predominant high-resolution CT (HRCT) feature of PAP is reported to be a crazy-paving pattern (i.e., smoothly thickened intralobular interstitial lines and interlobular septal lines against a background of widespread ground-glass opacities) often with lobular or geographic sparing. In several articles, investigators have reported that pulmonary fibrosis (traction bronchiectasis, honeycombing changes) developed in patients with PAP and was detected at long-term follow-up [5]. Patients with secondary PAP are more prone to pulmonary fibrosis or to atypical radiological features. The diagnosis is usually made by bronchoalveolar lavage (macroscopically the fluid may appear milky; microscopically extracellular plaques of eosinophilic material and macrophages filled granules with similar characteristics are detected; sometimes a frank lymphocytosis may be associated to these typical features). However in a minority of cases, mainly in patients with hematologic disorders or immunocompromised, or in patients with atypical radiologic features, biopsy is required for a morphological diagnosis. Furthermore the appearance of PAP reaction in a lung biopsy specimen from a compromised host should prompt vigorous search for an infection [6].

18.2 Drug-Induced Lung Disease

Drug-induced lung injury is common and can be induced by a wide variety of drugs used for treatment of many different clinical conditions. More than 600 prescribed medications have been reported to cause drug-induced pulmonary toxicity [7, 8]. Adverse drug reactions have been estimated to occur in approximately 5% of all patients receiving any drug and are responsible for up to 0.03% of all hospital deaths. Although less frequent than liver or cutaneous manifesta-

tions, pulmonary involvement deserves special attention due to the potential for severe disease presentations. Four mechanisms of drug injury to the lungs are recognized: (1) oxidant injury, such as during chronic nitrofurantoin ingestion; (2) direct cytotoxic effects (and these effects may be aggravated by oxidant injuries); (3) deposition of phospholipids within cells, such as those produced by cationic amphophilic drugs such as amiodarone; and (4) immune-mediated injury through drug-induced *systemic lupus erythematosus* (SLE). Although clues indicating that other forms of immune system-mediated mechanisms could be involved, they have not yet been proven. Cofactors may be important for triggering the drug-related injury: radiation and oxygen when chemotherapeutic drugs are involved, infections, analogs of human granulocyte colony-stimulating factor (G-CSF) when bleomycin is involved, and surgery or trauma as reported for amiodarone drug induced lung injury. Because most associations are based on anecdotal reports, a definite linkage between a potential etiologic agent and the lung injury observed in a specific patient is not always achievable, so in some cases a particular agent may be considered a "probable" or "possible" cause of the lung injury encountered. Although CT scan features might be useful to consider a drug as a cause of the lung infiltrates, a higher degree of diagnostic confidence may be reached only after results provided by invasive procedures. Bronchoalveolar lavage cellular profiles indicating a drug-induced lung injury may be characteristic but not pathognomonic: lymphocytosis, eosinophilia, presence of dysplastic type II pneumocytes and extracellular hyaline material, and alveolar hemorrhage have all been reported to be associated with drug-induced lung injury. Histopathologic findings are again not pathognomonic being however quite characteristic in the appropriated clinic-radiologic context. Finally all these tests, when feasible without significant increase of risks, are useful to exclude another cause that could explain the clinical features (infections, neoplasms) [9].

18.3 Granulomatous-Lymphocytic Interstitial Lung Disease (GLILD)

Granulomatous-lymphocytic ILD is the pulmonary component of a systemic disease characterized by adenopathy, splenomegaly, and granulomatous inflammation that may affect not only the lungs but also the liver, bone marrow, and lymph nodes [10]. The prevalence of GLILD in patients with primary antibody deficiencies is unknown; however, it is found in common variable immunodeficiency disease (CVID) and an increasing number of monogenic disorders. Approximately 20% of patients with GLILD present with polyclonal lymphocytic infiltration or nonmalignant hyperplasia of the lymph nodes in addition to non-necrotizing granulomas. GLILD typically occurs in the context of CVID; so far, GLILD has not been recently reported in patients with 22q11.2 deletion syndrome (22q11.2DS) [11]. In these patients immunodeficiency is secondary to thymic dysplasia as a result of the chromosomal microdeletion, and it varies from the more common mild-to-moderate T-cell lymphocytopenia to the rarer severe combined immunodeficiency phenotype. The key histopathological features of GLILD are lymphocytic interstitial pneumonia, follicular bronchiolitis, and non-necrotizing granulomas. Foci of organizing pneumonia and areas of pulmonary interstitial fibrosis may also be present. The predominant cells in the infiltrate are CD4+ T cells, but nodules of CD20+ B cells surrounded by CD4+ T cells are also found, predominantly localized to the interstitium. Surprisingly, regulatory T cells are absent in the lungs in GLILD. Granulomas are non-necrotizing, poorly formed to well-formed, surrounded by lymphocytes, and widely distributed, but with lower lung zone predominance, HRCT is the gold-standard imaging technique for ILDs and, in specific cases and in the context of a multidisciplinary team evaluation, can lead to a diagnosis without need for histologic confirmation. In GLILD patients it may show bronchiec-tasis, bronchial wall thickening, air trapping, parenchymal consolidation, emphysema, reticular and/or nodular changes, and/or fibrosis, with or without ground-glass opacities, predominantly affecting the lower lobes. The differential diagnosis of GLILD includes infections, other defined ILDs (sarcoidosis, chronic hypersensitivity pneumonitis, NSIP, and usual interstitial pneumonia), and malignant lymphoproliferative diseases. Thus, definitive diagnosis relies on a high index of suspicion, a clinical and microbiological correlation, and a histopathologic confirmation in individuals with the right clinical setting.

Case 1

A 49-year-old man with myelodysplastic syndrome AREB I was admitted to the hospital for fever, exertional dyspnea, and night sweats. HRCT: ground-glass and "crazy paving" pattern (Fig. 18.1).

BAL showed a dirty extracellular background and globules of eosinophilic amorphous extracellular material typical for alveolar proteinosis (Fig. 18.2). Transbronchial cryobiopsy samples (Fig. 18.3) documented the presence of pink granular material filling the airspaces in a patchy distribution. Microbiological investigations on BAL fluid and on lung tissue resulted to be negative. GM-CSF autoantibodies were not detected in serum. A final diagnosis of secondary alveolar proteinosis was eventually rendered.

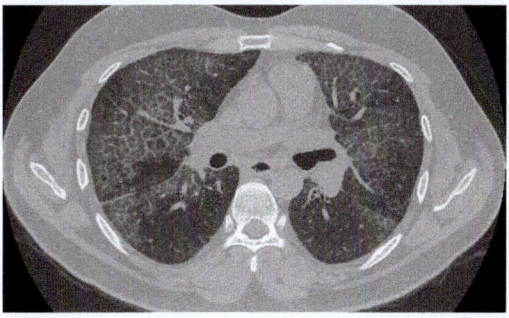

Fig. 18.1 HRCT: ground-glass and "crazy paving" pattern

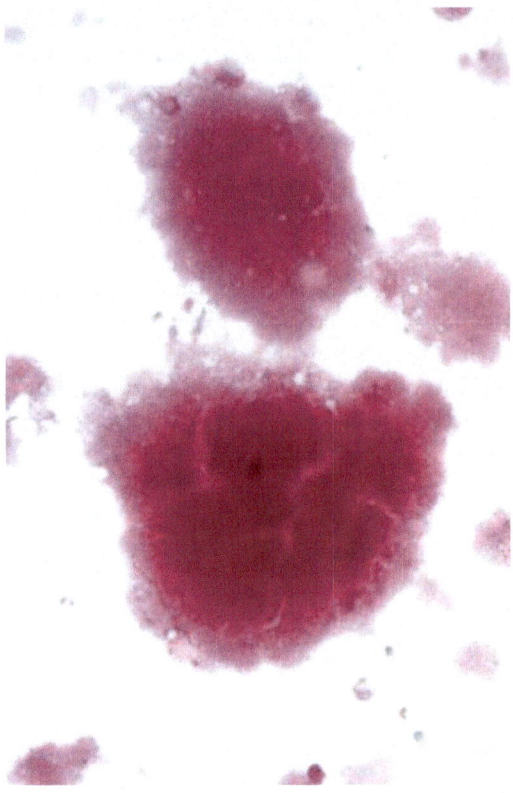

Fig. 18.2 Bronchoalveolar lavage: Eosinophilic amorphous extracellular material typical for alveolar proteinosis (Papanicolaou, high power)

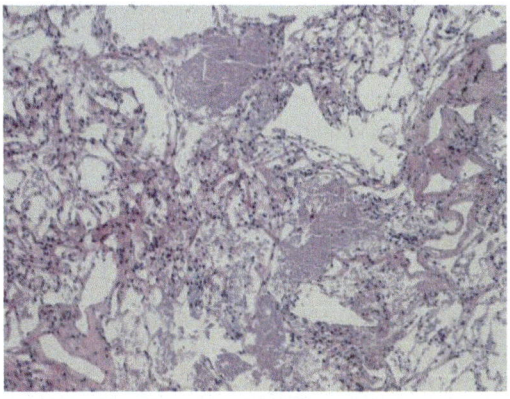

Fig. 18.3 Transbronchial cryobiopsy: Amorphous eosinophilic intra-alveolar material with acicular clefts left by cholesterol crystals dissolved during the process. Scattered interalveolar lymphocytes are evident. (Hematoxylin and eosin, low power)

Case 2

A 54-year-old male, carpenter and current smoker (19 packs/year), seeks medical advice for 1-month history of dry cough and shortness of breath. No professional exposures were clearly documented. Family history was not relevant. No known allergy to drugs. He had a 5-year history of recurrent episodes of atrial fibrillation, treated with propafenone, flecainide, pulmonary vein encircling ablation ($n = 3$), and amiodarone (for 9 months, until 1 year ago). No collagen vascular disease-related symptoms and no fever were documented. Examination: no clubbing, no Velcro sounds, no signs of right heart failure. At rest and on room air saturation of O_2 was 95%. Current medications were warfarin and flecainide. Pulmonary functions tests documented a slight reduction of volumes and a significant impairment of DLCO (44% of predicted). HRCT scan showed alveolar and ground-glass attenuation with a perilobular pattern evident in the lower lobes and emphysematous change (Fig. 18.4a, b). After information provided by bronchoalveolar lavage (lymphocytosis) and cryobiopsy (a mixed pattern with nonspecific interstitial pneumonia and organizing pneumonia) (Figs. 18.5 and 18.6), a diagnosis of flecainide-related lung injury was rendered.

Case 3

An 84-year-old male, a former smoker affected by COPD, was seen by a pulmonologist because of worsening dyspnea in the last 3 months. His clinical history was relevant for radical cystectomy and prostatectomy performed 2 years before because of urothelial tumor of the bladder (Tis, N1, M0) and adenocarcinoma of the prostate (T2a, N0, Mo). Five months before PET-CT had documented areas of increased uptake of radiolabeled [^{18}F]-2-fluoro-2-deoxy-d-glucose in multiple retroperitoneal lymph nodes [retrocaval (SUV = 14.9); left iliac (SUV = 20.6)], and thereafter the patient started treatment with atezolizumab (an anti-PD-L1 humanized antibody). Saturation of oxygen at rest while breathing room air was 90% and blood gas analysis showed hypocapnia. Pulmonary function tests documented a restrictive impairment with significant reduction of DLCO (43% of predicted). Routine laboratory peripheral blood tests were not relevant. High-resolution CT scan features were bilateral peripheral alveolar consolidations and

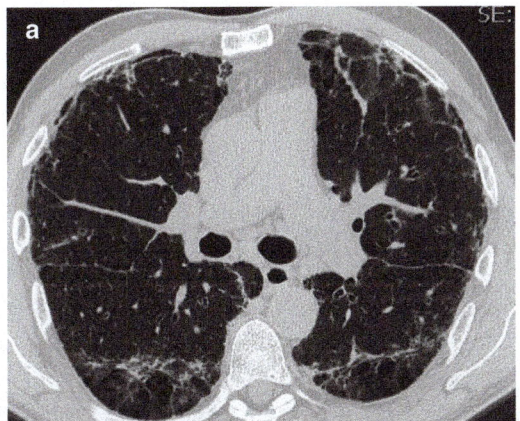

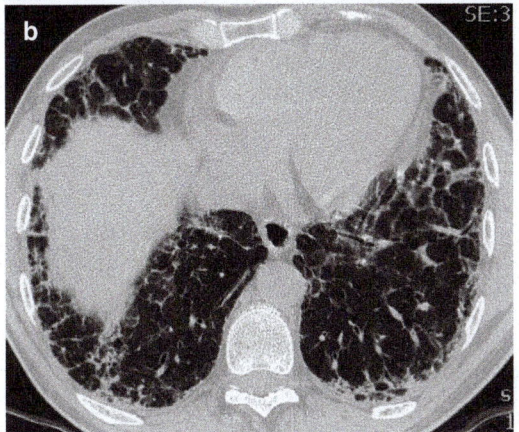

Fig. 18.4 (**a, b**) Alveolar consolidation with a perilobular distribution, sparing of the subpleural region and areas of emphysema

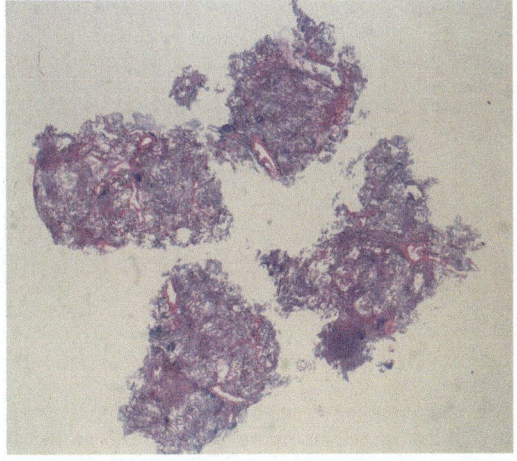

Fig. 18.5 Transbronchial cryobiopsy of four specimens documenting a preserved alveolar architecture with thickening of the alveolar septa due to inflammatory cells and an alveolar filling process (hematoxylin and eosin, low power)

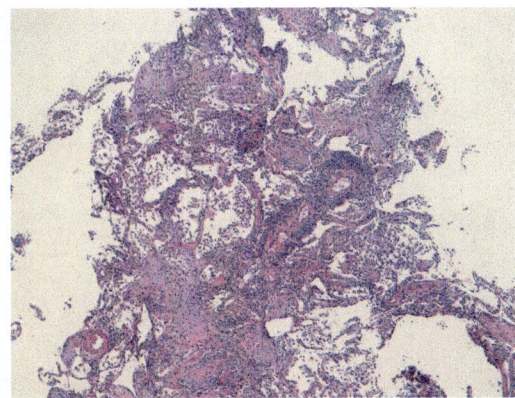

Fig. 18.6 Lymphoid cells in the alveolar septa and cuffing a pulmonary vein and granulation tissue in the alveolar spaces (organizing pneumonia pattern) (hematoxylin and eosin, mid power)

areas of ground glass (Fig. 18.7). Bronchoalveolar lavage documented a lymphocytosis (41%) with a CD4/CD8 ratio of 4. Microbiological investigations on BAL fluid were negative. A cryobiopsy was carried out with four samples obtained from the lateral segment of the lateral right lower lobe (Figs. 18.8, 18.9, and 18.10). A diagnosis of drug (atezolizumab)-related lung injury was eventually done.

Case 4

A 44-year-old female with a previous diagnosis of common variable immunodeficiency syndrome presented with shortness of breath, hypoxemia, a restrictive ventilatory impairment, and reduction of DLCO. High-resolution CT scan showed reticulation and ground glass with reduction of volumes in upper (Fig. 18.11a) and lower lobes (Fig. 18.11) with no clear predominance. BAL showed a slight increase of lymphocytes (32%) with a CD4/CD8 ratio of 3.9. Microbiological investigations on BAL fluid and serum were negative. A transbronchial cryobiopsy was carried out with samples from the lateral segment of the right lower lobe (Figs. 18.12 and 18.13). The diagnosis of granulomatous-lymphocytic interstitial lung disease in a patient with common variable immunodeficiency syndrome was done, and a treatment with rituximab and azathioprine was started.

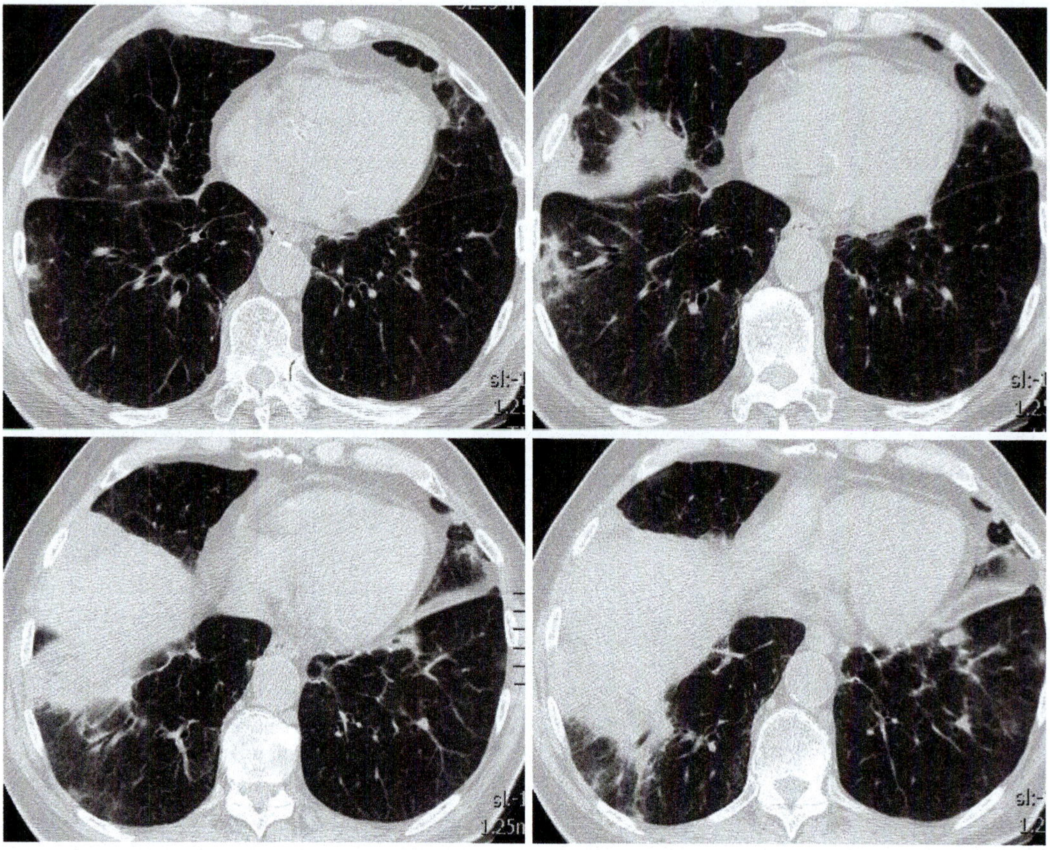

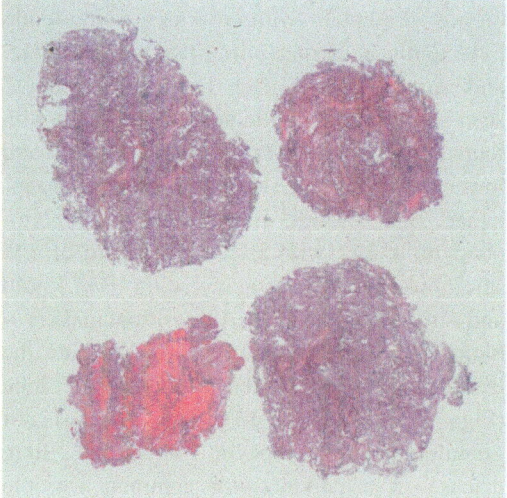

Fig. 18.7 High-resolution CT. Areas of alveolar subpleural consolidation and ground-glass attenuation are evident in both lungs with a predominance in the right lower lobe. The first radiological diagnostic hypothesis was organizing pneumonia

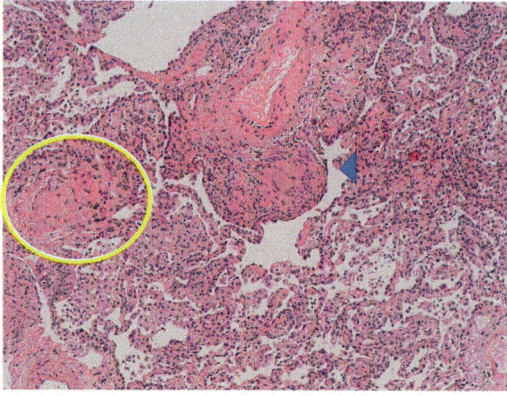

Fig. 18.8 Four fragments obtained from the lateral segment of the right lower lobe. In one (in the right lower corner), artifacts due to bleeding are evident (hematoxylin and eosin, low power)

Fig. 18.9 Areas of organizing pneumonia (circle) and a sarcoid-like granuloma (arrowhead) are evident (hematoxylin and eosin, mid power)

Fig. 18.10 At higher power a lymphocytic perivenular infiltrate is also evident (hematoxylin and eosin, high power)

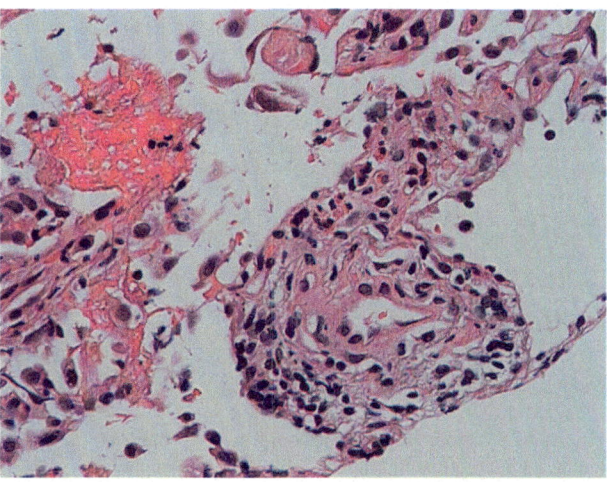

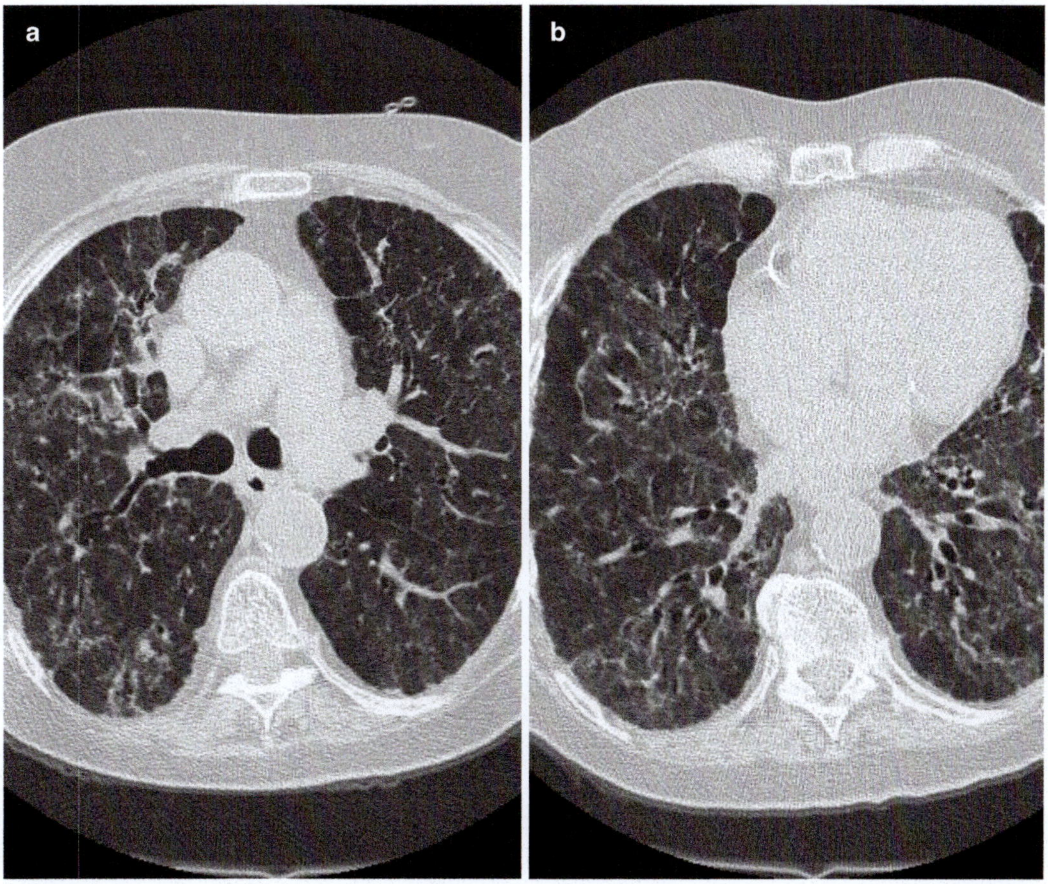

Fig. 18.11 High-resolution CT scan showed reticulation and ground glass with reduction of volumes in upper (**a**) and lower lobes (**b**)

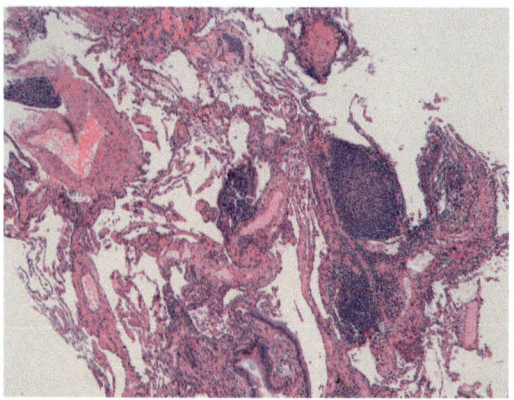

Fig. 18.12 Transbronchial cryobiopsy sample from the lateral segment of the right lower lobe showing lymphoid follicles with germinal centers in the centrilobular region (follicular bronchiolitis) (hematoxylin and eosin, low power)

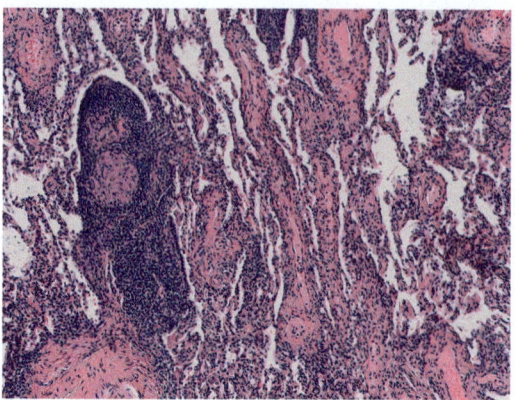

Fig. 18.13 Transbronchial cryobiopsy sample from the posterior segment of the right lower lobe showing lymphocytic interstitial inflammation and acellular fibrosis. Two perivascular non-necrotizing granulomas are rimmed by mature lymphocytes (hematoxylin and eosin, mid power)

References

1. Rosen SH, Castleman B, Liebow AA. Pulmonary alveolar proteinosis. N Engl J Med. 1958;258:1123–42.
2. Kumar A, Abdelmalak B, Inoue Y, Culver DA. Pulmonary alveolar proteinosis: pathophysiology and clinical approach. Lancet Respir Med. 2018;6:554–65.
3. McReynolds LJ, Calvo KR, Holland SM. Germline GATA2 mutation and bone marrow failure. Hematol Oncol Clin North Am. 2018;32:713–28.
4. Marchand-Adam S, Diot B, Magro P, et al. Pulmonary alveolar proteinosis revealing a telomerase disease. Am J Respir Crit Care Med. 2013;188:402–4.
5. Akira M, Inoue Y, Arai T, et al. Pulmonary fibrosis on high-resolution CT of patients with pulmonary alveolar proteinosis. AJR. 2016;207:544–51.
6. Colby TV, Carrington CB. Interstitial lung disease. In: Thurlbeck WM, Churg AM, editors. Pathology of the lung. Stuttgart: Thieme Medical Publishers; 1995. p. 589–737.
7. www.pneumotox.com.
8. Dulohery MM, Maldonado F, Limper AH. Drug induced pulmonary disease. In: Broaddus VC, Mason RJ, Ernst JD, King TE, Lazarus SC, Murray JF, Nadel JA, Slutsky AS, Gotway MB, editors. Murray & Nadel's textbook of respiratory medicine. Philadelphia: Saunders; 2016. p. 1275–94.
9. Romagnoli M, Bigliazzi C, Casoni G, et al. The role of transbronchial lung biopsy for the diagnosis of diffuse drug-induced lung disease: a case series of 44 patients. Sarcoidosis Vasc Diffuse Lung Dis. 2008;25:36–45.
10. Cinetto F, Scarpa R, Rattazzi M, Agostini C. The broad spectrum of lung diseases in primary antibody deficiency. Eur Respir Rev. 2018;27:180019.
11. Sood AK, Funkhouser W, Handly B, Weston B, Wu EY. Granulomatous-lymphocytic interstitial lung disease in 22q11.2 deletion syndrome: a case report and literature review. Curr Allergy Asthma Rep. 2018;18:14.

The manufacturer's authorised representative in the EU is Springer
Nature Customer Service Centre GmbH, Europaplatz 3, 69115 Heidelberg,
Germany. If you have any concerns regarding our products, please
contact ProductSafety@springernature.com

Printed and bound by CPI Group (UK) Ltd, Croydon, CR0 4YY
23/04/2026
02095586-0008